Toothwear: The ABC of the Worn Dentition

Toothwear: The ABC of the Worn Dentition

Edited by

Dr Farid Khan

and

Professor William George Young

WILEY-BLACKWELL

A John Wiley & Sons, Ltd., Publication

This edition first published 2011 by John Wiley & Sons Ltd
© 2011 John Wiley & Sons Ltd

Wiley-Blackwell is an imprint of John Wiley & Sons, formed by the merger of Wiley's global Scientific, Technical and Medical business with Blackwell Publishing.

Registered office: John Wiley & Sons Ltd, The Atrium, Southern Gate, Chichester, West Sussex, PO19 8SQ, UK

Editorial offices: 9600 Garsington Road, Oxford, OX4 2DQ, UK
The Atrium, Southern Gate, Chichester, West Sussex, PO19 8SQ, UK
2121 State Avenue, Ames, Iowa 50014-8300, USA

For details of our global editorial offices, for customer services and for information about how to apply for permission to reuse the copyright material in this book please see our website at www.wiley.com/wiley-blackwell.

Library of Congress Cataloging-in-Publication Data

Toothwear : The ABC of the worn dentition / edited by Dr Farid Khan and Professor William George Young.
       p.   ;   cm.
   Includes bibliographical references and index.
   ISBN 978-1-4443-3655-9 (paperback : alk. paper)
   1. Teeth–Abrasion.   I. Khan, Farid, editor.   II. Young, William George, 1939- editor.
   [DNLM: 1. Tooth Wear–diagnosis.   2. Dental Restoration, Permanent–methods.   3. Tooth Wear–prevention & control.
4. Tooth Wear–rehabilitation. WU 210]
   RK307.T66 2011
   617.6′075–dc22   2010047726

A catalogue record for this book is available from the British Library.

This book is published in the following electronic formats: ePDF 9781444341119; ePub 9781444341126; Mobi 9781444341133

Set in 9.5/12 pt Palatino by Aptara® Inc., New Delhi, India

Printed in Singapore by Markono Print Media Pte Ltd

1   2011

Contents

Contributors   ix

Foreword: *Adrian Lussi*   xi

1   The multifactorial nature of toothwear   1
Farid Khan and William G. Young

Toothwear processes   1
Saliva protection   4
Intrinsic and extrinsic acids   4
Examination of facial, extraoral and intraoral soft tissues   4
Toothwear in children   9
Toothwear and dental caries   9
Toothwear – A multifactorial process   12
References   14

2   Diagnosis and management of toothwear in children   16
W. Kim Seow and Sue Taji

Clinical presentations of toothwear in children   16
History-taking, assessment and diagnosis   20
Children at increased risk for toothwear   21
Management of toothwear in children   25
The global perspective   32
References   32

3   Childhood diet and dental erosion   34
Louise Brearley Messer and William G. Young

Dental erosion in children, adolescents and teenagers   34
Concerns of patients and parents   34

Clinical appearance of dental erosion   35
Dietary findings in dental erosion   35
Dental erosion as a lifestyle issue   37
Recommendations for patients to reduce erosion   39
Dental erosion and dental caries compared   41
Dietary counselling for children and adolescents   42
The key messages   48
References   48

4   The oral presentation of toothwear in adults   50
Farid Khan and William G. Young

Diagnostic modalities   50
Surface susceptibility of toothwear and site specificity of dental caries   52
The clinical presentation of toothwear   53
Charting toothwear   65
Application of *The Stages of Wear* to diagnosing toothwear   71
Utilising the charted odontogram to assess patient risk   72
Summary   73
References   73

5   Salivary protection against toothwear and dental caries   75
Colin Dawes

Factors causing toothwear   75
Factors causing dental caries   75
Why does a tooth dissolve in acid?   77
Sources and components of saliva relevant to toothwear and caries   78
Conclusions   86
References   87

6   Dental diagnosis and the oral medicine of toothwear   89
William G. Young and Colin Dawes

The approach   89
Mild, moderate or severe toothwear   89
Complaint/discovery   90
Development   90
Attrition   91
Abrasion   92
Toothbrushing   92
Oral hygiene   93
Diet erosion   93
Gastric erosion   94
Sports and social   94
Medical   95
Addictions, fixations and confidentiality   95
The cases   96

	Summary	108
	References	108

7	**Preventive and management strategies against toothwear**	**111**
	Farid Khan and William G. Young	
	Aiming prevention at all ages	111
	Lifestyle, health and environmental risk factors	114
	The *WATCH* strategy	117
	Adjunctive products	117
	Diet diaries and review	126
	Patient's reporting sensitivity	126
	Treatment planning	128
	The review appointment	129
	Summary	130
	References	131

8	**Measurement of severity and progression of toothwear**	**134**
	William H. Douglas and William G. Young	
	Non-parametric or semi-parametric approaches	134
	Parametric measurement of toothwear	135
	Reporting toothwear	137
	The cases	145
	References	151

9	**Biomaterials**	**153**
	Stephen C. Bayne	
	Introduction	153
	Overview of biomaterials wear	157
	Clinical wear performance of biomaterials	161
	Comments on special wear situations	165
	References	167

10	**The role of toothwear in occlusion**	**168**
	Anders Johansson and Gunnar E. Carlsson	
	Development of occlusion	170
	Patterns of toothwear on anterior palatal and posterior occlusal surfaces and Angle's classification	176
	Conclusion	179
	References	180

11	**Restoration of the worn dentition**	**182**
	Ian Meyers and Farid Khan	
	To restore or not to restore is a central question	182
	Pre-restorative treatment – preparation and planning	183

Restorative challenges   184
Restoring the stages of wear   184
Patient demands, aspirations, aesthetics and case selection   187
Conservative restorative options for partial or full-mouth occlusal reconstruction 188
Summary   202
References   202

12 Rehabilitation of the worn dentition   **205**
Ridwaan Omar and Ann-Katrin Johansson

Principles and strategies for rehabilitating worn dentitions   206
Conclusion   226
References   226

Index   **229**

Contributors

Stephen C. Bayne
Professor and Chair
Cariology, Restorative Sciences, and
    Endodontics
School of Dentistry
University of Michigan
Ann Arbor, MI, USA

Gunnar E. Carlsson
Emeritus Professor
Department of Prosthetic Dentistry
Institute of Odontology
The Sahlgrenska Academy
University of Gothenburg
Göteborg, SE, Sweden

Colin Dawes
Emeritus Professor
Department of Oral Biology
Faculty of Dentistry
University of Manitoba
Winnipeg, MB, Canada

William H. Douglas
Emeritus Professor
School of Dentistry
University of Minnesota
Minneapolis, MN, USA

Anders Johansson
Professor
Department of Clinical Dentistry –
    Prosthodontics
Faculty of Medicine and Dentistry
University of Bergen
Bergen, Norway

Ann-Katrin Johansson
Associate Professor
Specialist in Pediatric Dentistry
Chairman
Department of Clinical Dentistry – Cariology
Faculty of Medicine and Dentistry
University of Bergen
Bergen, Norway

Farid Khan
Director
Queensland Dental Group™
Indooroopilly
Brisbane, Queensland, Australia

Adrian Lussi
Professor
Director
Department of Preventive, Restorative, and
    Pediatric Dentistry

University of Bern
Freiburgstrasse, Bern, Switzerland

Louise Brearley Messer
Emeritus Professor
Paediatric Dentistry
Melbourne Dental School
University of Melbourne
Victoria, Australia

Ian Meyers
Professor
School of Dentistry
University of Queensland
Brisbane, Queensland, Australia

Ridwaan Omar
Professor
Department of Restorative Sciences
Head of Prosthodontics
Faculty of Dentistry
Kuwait University
Safat, Kuwait

W. Kim Seow
Professor
Director
Centre for Paediatric Dentistry Research
    and Training
School of Dentistry
University of Queensland
Brisbane, Queensland, Australia

Sue Taji
Specialist in Paediatric Dentistry
Brisbane, Queensland, Australia

William G. Young
Associate Professor
Oral Pathologist
Brisbane, Queensland, Australia

Foreword

In recent decades there has been a remarkable caries decline in developed countries. This is mainly due to improved oral hygiene and fluorides. During the same period, people with high awareness of health have changed their dietary habits. Nowadays, more acidic drinks and juices are consumed compared with a few decades ago. These changes and other factors have led to an increased loss of dental hard tissue such as toothwear.

Toothwear is a multifactorial condition of growing concern to the clinician. Only a few books have been published, collecting comprehensive knowledge about this subject. The present book is one of them.

The 12 chapters of the book cover important aspects of toothwear, from childhood to adults. It covers not only the multifactorial nature of toothwear but also the diagnosis and prevention of it. Four chapters are dedicated to restorative aspects, dental materials, occlusal problems and rehabilitation procedures.

The task of bringing together the current knowledge of toothwear is not easy, but has been perfectly accomplished in this book. It gives guidelines to practitioners, dental students and teachers.

Professor Adrian Lussi
University of Bern
Switzerland

The multifactorial nature of toothwear

Farid Khan and William G. Young

TOOTHWEAR PROCESSES

Attrition, erosion and abrasion describe wear processes (Fig. 1.1). Attrition involves two-surface (tooth-to-tooth) wear. Erosion, less commonly referred to as corrosion, results from acidic dissolution of mineralised tooth structure. Abrasion on a surface comprises wear from externally applied particles or objects.

When a patient presents with a heavily worn dentition (Fig. 1.2), the clinician considers whether the toothwear processes have involved elements of attrition, erosion or abrasion. Whilst the wear facets identified on the lower anterior teeth suggest attrition, numerous high margins on restorations point to involvement of erosion, removing tooth structure adjacent to these restorations. Demineralisation of tooth structure further predisposes to abrasion as evident in cervical regions, many of which have previously been restored. Since placement of these restorations, toothwear processes have continued. This case highlights that interrelationships exist between toothwear processes which potentiate one another.

Although the processes of attrition, erosion and abrasion can be simulated under laboratory conditions, clinically these processes do not occur independently (Fig. 1.3). The coarse particles of foods in primitive diets potentiated the wear facets (Young 1998) of attrition by abrasion (Fig. 1.3a). Modern diets lack such abrasives; however, oral acids that cause erosion demineralise enamel and dentine, potentiating attrition and abrasion (Figs. 1.3b & c). A recent literature review on erosion noted that dietary acids are considered by many researchers probably to be the most common cause of acid erosion (Bartlett 2009). Exaggerated wear facets are the first sign of erosion-potentiated attrition in young adults' permanent teeth. Toothbrush and toothpaste combinations are important considerations, particularly in patients in whom dental erosion has also been identified, for abrasiveness becomes potentiated when tooth structure is demineralised. A combination of these two

Toothwear: The ABC of the Worn Dentition, First Edition. Edited by Farid Khan and William George Young.
© 2011 John Wiley & Sons, Ltd. Published 2011 by John Wiley & Sons, Ltd.

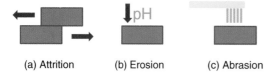

(a) Attrition   (b) Erosion   (c) Abrasion

Figure 1.1   The processes of attrition, erosion and abrasion: (a) Attrition is wear between two tooth surfaces. (b) Erosion is tooth surface loss from acids. (c) Abrasion is loss of tooth surface from a foreign body.

processes can lead to severe toothwear (Fig. 1.4). When used on demineralised tooth structure, abrasion from routine use of standard toothbrushes and toothpaste formulations is significant, whilst in the absence of erosion, it is considered to be minimal (Addy 2005). Attritional facets and cuspal-cupped lesions can be found on the same tooth (Fig. 1.5). This suggests that the wear facet worn by the mesiobuccal cusp of the upper first molar has been potentiated or exaggerated by occlusal erosion that has produced the cuspal-cupped lesions.

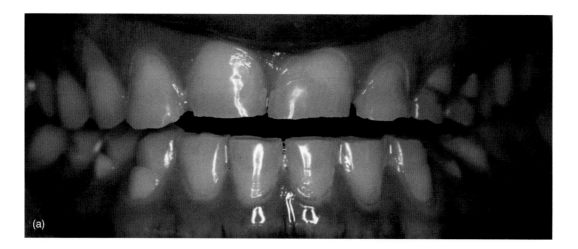

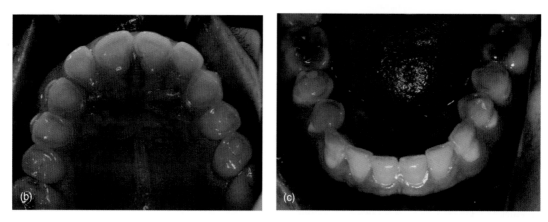

Figure 1.2   Three processes of toothwear are reported in this case: (a) Incisal attrition on incisors. (b) Occlusal erosion on premolars and molars and around amalgam restorations. (c) Various cervical regions have been restored previously, with further loss of tooth structure since the time of restoration. (From Young, 2001, with permission of Dentil Pty Ltd.)

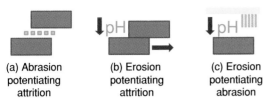

(a) Abrasion potentiating attrition

(b) Erosion potentiating attrition

(c) Erosion potentiating abrasion

Figure 1.3 Interactions of abrasion, attrition and erosion in toothwear: (a) Acids soften surfaces potentiating attrition. (b) Acids soften surfaces potentiating abrasion. (c) Abrasion from particles harder than enamel and dentine potentiates attritional wear.

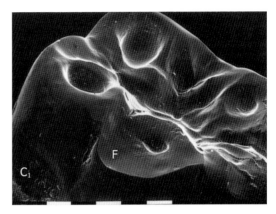

Figure 1.5 An attritional wear facet (F) on a buccal cusp of a lower first permanent molar. On all cusps are the cupped lesions of erosion not necessarily associated with attrition. A shallow buccal cervical lesion (C1) is also present on this tooth (Bar = 1 mm). (From Young & Khan, 2009, with permission from Erosion Watch Pty Ltd.)

Moreover, erosion has produced the shallow cervical lesion on the buccal surface of this tooth possibly potentiated by toothbrush abrasion.

These interrelationships between attrition, erosion and abrasion highlight that multifactorial processes create a worn dentition (Fig. 1.6). Each patient has a variation in the involvement of attrition, erosion and abrasion. In many patients, it is predominantly underlying erosion that potentiates the secondary effects of attrition and abrasion. Appreciating that different processes are working concurrently allows

the clinician to focus diagnostic, preventive and management strategies on all three aetiologies. Thus, tooth tissue loss will continue if its multifactorial nature is not recognised and addressed.

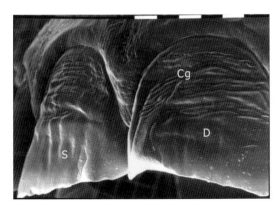

Figure 1.4 Facial surfaces of the central incisors are devoid of enamel in a 31-year-old female gymnast. The dentine is deeply grooved by toothbrush abrasion. The approximal enamel is remarkably intact. Scanning electron microscopy (SEM) (Bar = 1 mm). (From Khan et al., 1999, with permission from the *Australian Dental Journal*.)

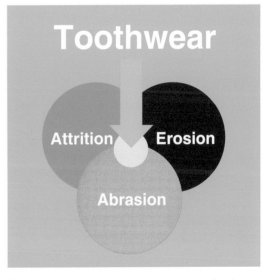

Figure 1.6 Toothwear is best conceptualised as a combination of erosion, attrition and abrasion.

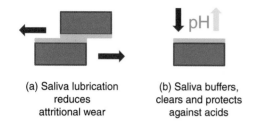

(a) Saliva lubrication reduces attritional wear

(b) Saliva buffers, clears and protects against acids

Figure 1.7 Saliva offers protection against attritional wear (a) through lubrication and (b) by raising the pH through buffering and clearance of acids that produce erosion.

SALIVA PROTECTION

Saliva is central in counteracting and balancing toothwear processes, and tooth surfaces are protected against toothwear by salivary buffering capacity, salivary pellicle, acid clearance and washing of the dentition (Dawes 2008). The unstimulated flow rate of saliva and salivary buffering capacity have been directly associated with dental erosion (Zero & Lussi 2005). Both mucous and serous saliva protect against attritional wear through lubrication of the teeth and areas of interarch contact, as well as neutralise acids within the oral environment. Saliva also reduces demineralisation by its content of calcium and phosphate (Fig. 1.7).

INTRINSIC AND EXTRINSIC ACIDS

Acids that demineralise teeth are extrinsic dietary or intrinsic, gastric or plaque in origin. Dietary acids most commonly implicated are ascorbic acid (vitamin C), citric acid, sodium citrate and orthophosphoric acid, because these are used as flavours and preservatives in most acidic beverages. So, soft (Johansson et al. 2002), sports (Milosevic 1997) and energy drinks are sources, with other acids in wines. Hydrochloric acid from gastric juice is the usual intrinsic acid implicated in dental erosion and toothwear

(Scheutzel 1996). A study examining 19 professional wine tasters found mild-to-severe dental erosion and found the subjects with severe dental erosion also to have had a history of gastritis or reduced salivary flow rate and/or buffering capacity (Wiktorsson et al. 1997).

The case presented in Fig. 1.8 shows the toothwear of an elite athlete, 24 years of age. His lifestyle placed him at risk of developing severe toothwear. His rigorous training regimes reduced the salivary protection of his dentition. Subsequent rehydration with acidic sports drinks at times of dehydration affected his dentition. Acidic beverages and foods are important contributors to erosive toothwear in many individuals (see Chapter 3), given their common availability, and yet the pH alone is insufficient to determine their erosive potential, which is instead influenced by a large range of variables including consumption patterns, adhesion and chelating properties of salivary protection, and swallowing and clearance patterns (Lussi et al. 2004). Frequent episodes of reduced saliva protection and acid drinks resulted in severe loss of enamel and dentine in this young adult, principally from dental erosion. Dental erosion in athletes is a growing concern (Sirimaharaj et al. 2002); however, many children and young adults also frequently consume such beverages. Increased consumption of sports drinks and acidic beverages, during the day and also during heavy exercise, is likely contributing to the increasing dental erosion prevalence (ten Cate & Imfeld 1996), particularly in young individuals.

EXAMINATION OF FACIAL, EXTRAORAL AND INTRAORAL SOFT TISSUES

The multifactorial nature of toothwear is further highlighted by benefits from identifying facial, extraoral and intraoral soft tissue features even before a worn dentition is assessed.

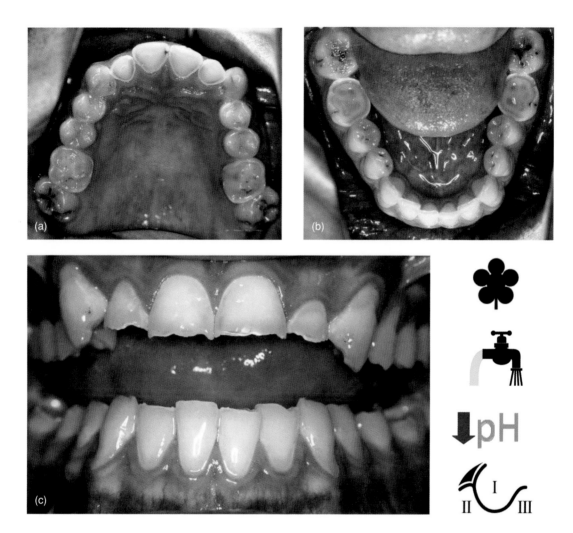

Figure 1.8 A 24-year-old male patient with a long history of athletic training at a professional level. Acidic beverage rehydration frequently occurred subsequent to intense physical training sessions, at times of dehydration and low salivary protection. This allowed rapid loss of tooth structure to occur. (a) Near exposures of the pulpal tissues are evident on the lingual surfaces of the maxillary anterior teeth. (b) Extensive areas of erosion have notably affected his first molar teeth. (c) Cervical lesions are evident on the maxillary and mandibular buccal surfaces of canine and lateral incisor teeth. (From Young, 2003b, with permission of Dentil Pty Ltd.)

Much can be learned of lifestyles, general medical conditions, temporomandibular joint (TMJ) disorders and salivary gland pathology by considering signs and symptoms relevant to toothwear. For the clinician, a schematic approach for examination of facial, extraoral and intraoral features adds diagnostic information relevant to the aetiology of the patient's condition. Icons applicable to these features are included to trigger the clinician's mind during the examination (Fig. 1.9). These icons are used throughout this text alongside clinical photographs of interesting cases to indicate additional findings. Visual inspection and manual palpation are all

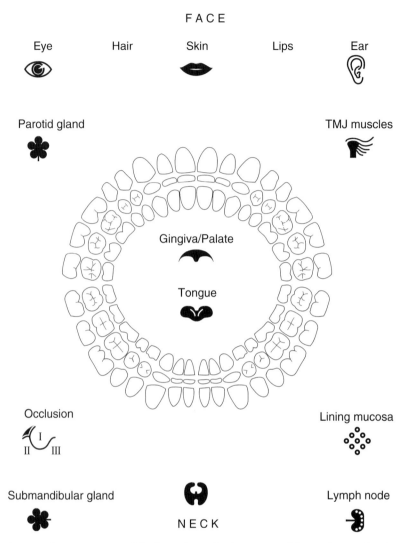

FACE

Eye   Hair   Skin   Lips   Ear

Parotid gland   TMJ muscles

Gingiva/Palate

Tongue

Occlusion   Lining mucosa

Submandibular gland   Lymph node

NECK

Figure 1.9 The icons for examination of the face, the oral soft tissues and the teeth, as utilised on standardised examination sheets applied clinically for patients with worn dentitions. (From Young & Khan, 2009, with permission of Erosion Watch Pty Ltd.)

the clinical skills the clinician needs to make additional important observations. The icons remind us to record the relevant ones. The odontogram (Fig. 1.9, centre) describes each tooth as an icon. Three surfaces of each tooth are represented, as approximal surfaces are almost never significantly affected by toothwear and consequently the clinician need only record

the severity of wear on the occlusal and cervical surfaces illustrated. Detailed methods for examination of the worn dentition are provided in Chapter 4.

 Eye contact is the first event of examination. Trust and empathy are established and concern is communicated between the patient and the

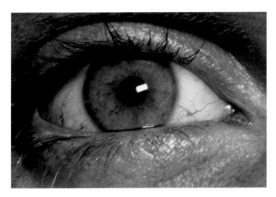

Figure 1.10 Lacrimal duct aplasia with epiphora in congenital dysfunction of major salivary glands. (From Young et al., 2001, with permission of *Oral Surgery, Oral Medicine, Oral Pathology*.)

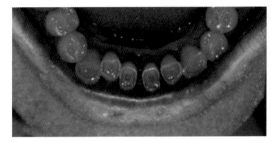

Figure 1.11 Sun-affected damaged lip from a lifetime of dehydrating outdoor work in a 60-year-old construction worker with a heavily worn dentition.

clinician. Yet, for the clinician concerned with toothwear, the patient's eyes can communicate insights into medical conditions and syndromes that explain why the patient is at risk. The lacrimal glands produce tears which have many similarities to saliva. Hence, conjunctivitis and dry mouth in Sjögren's syndrome are obvious examples wherein both lacrimal glands and saliva fail to protect mucosal surfaces. Examination of the eye and discussion with the patient might reveal lacrimal duct aplasia with epiphora (Fig. 1.10), as found in this patient with congenital dysfunction of major salivary glands, who experienced severe dental erosion (Young et al. 2001).

 The skin of the lower lip is particularly susceptible to sun damage, as the vermilion border is usually not pigmented in Caucasian people in the subtropics. Outdoor work frequently damages the patient's skin (Fig. 1.11). Actinic cheilosis is often identified on the lower lips of patients who are regularly exposed to the sun in their sports activities and outdoor occupations. This may indicate a lifestyle involving frequent work-related dehydration, which by reducing saliva protection against acids in the mouth, puts patients at risk of toothwear.

The patient's facial hair gives clues to hormonal status. Thus, *lanugo* – a fine, fair, facial hair – is noticed at puberty in both boys and girls. It is also found in patients with the hormonal upsets of *anorexia nervosa* and as a result of hormone replacement therapy at the menopause. Thus, lanugo may alert the clinician to consider this further when compiling a clinical history.

Evidence of skin irritation or presence of eczema (Fig. 1.12) may be evident periauricularly or on any part of the body and may suggest syndromic associations as in cases of hereditary ectodermal dysplasia. Hearing loss in young patients may be part of a syndrome. In congenital rubella syndrome, the patient has glaucoma, bilateral hearing aids, and a congenital heart defect as a triad (Young et al. 2001). This triad of signs has considerable relevance to dental treatment, as considered further in Chapter 6.

The TMJ can click, or even lock, when the patient opens and closes their mouth. The muscles of mastication may be painful to palpation in TMJ pain–dysfunction syndrome. When the teeth are clenched, the masseter muscles tense and become prominent. Behind this muscle and in front of the ear lies the preauricular crease (Fig. 1.12).

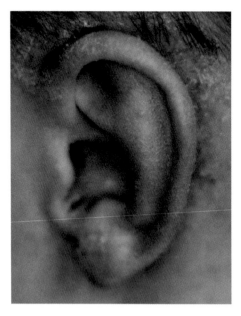

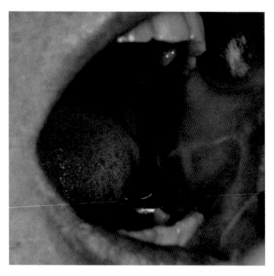

Figure 1.13 White lines on the buccal mucosa (*linea alba*) and lateral indentations of the tongue indicate parafunctional habits. (From Young, 2001b, with permission of Dentil Pty Ltd.)

Figure 1.12 Eczema around and behind the ear of a patient with ectodermal dysplasia.

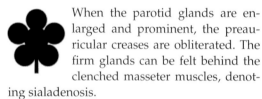 When the parotid glands are enlarged and prominent, the preauricular creases are obliterated. The firm glands can be felt behind the clenched masseter muscles, denoting sialadenosis.

Indentations of the lateral borders of the tongue indicate that the patient presses their tongue against the lingual surfaces of the teeth during parafunctional habits (Fig. 1.13).

 The lining mucosae are studded with minor mucous glands. Lining mucosae cover the undersurfaces of the tongue, the floor of the mouth, the labial sulci and the soft palate. When saliva covering these surfaces is viscous, frothy and white, it is slow-flowing saliva. When thrush (*Candida albicans*) is found on these surfaces, it indicates loss of immunity conferred by saliva against this microorganism. *Linea alba*, white calluses on the buc-

cal mucosae along the occlusal plane, occurs in patients who have parafunctional habits, such as bruxism (Fig. 1.13).

Gingivitis and gingival recession may indicate poor oral hygiene and periodontal changes or toothbrush trauma. The gingivae and the hard palate contain virtually no salivary gland tissue, except at the back of the vault where the hard palate joins the soft palate.

Occlusion of the teeth may show deep overbite, overjet or open bite between the anterior teeth. Crossbite may be found in the posterior quadrants. Angle's class I, II or III malocclusion is delineated from the relationship of the mesiobuccal cusp of the maxillary first molar to the mesio- and distobuccal cusps of the mandibular first molar. All variations in occlusion have significance for finding exaggerated wear facets.

 The submandibular glands, when enlarged, are best appreciated by bimanual palpation. The fingers of one hand are placed below the lower border of the mandible and pressed into the submandibular triangle of the neck. A finger of the other hand feels along the lingual sulcus in the floor of the mouth. Normal salivary glands are difficult to feel, but the volume of enlarged, slightly firm submandibular glands can be appreciated both in the floor of the mouth, behind the mylohyoid muscle, and in the submandibular triangle. This enlargement is sialadenosis. It is neither a lumpy tumour nor a tender inflammation. A tender lump may be an inflamed lymph node within the gland.

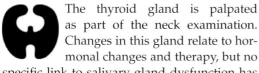 The lymph nodes of the neck are palpated to rule out inflammation or tumour. In sialadenosis, the lymph nodes are normal.

The thyroid gland is palpated as part of the neck examination. Changes in this gland relate to hormonal changes and therapy, but no specific link to salivary gland dysfunction has been made.

TOOTHWEAR IN CHILDREN

Few of these facial features and salivary gland or soft tissue changes observed in adults are found during the examination of the child-patient with toothwear. Eye and ear changes are rare. The skin of the face and lips may show lanugo found at puberty in boys and girls. The major salivary glands are underdeveloped in young children. They may be affected at puberty, but are more usually normal. The temporomandibular joints and muscles of mastication are affected only if severe trauma has altered their growth. Tongue indentations and linea alba are rarely found, even in children whose parents give testimony of night grinding habits. Rarely oral thrush may be found on the tongue, palate and gingivae.

Consequently, the best indicator of excessive toothwear in children is a reduction in occlusal vertical dimension within the deciduous dentition. As shown in Fig. 1.14, the patient's perma-

nent anterior teeth and permanent first molars are relatively unaffected by wear. However, the deciduous canines and molars attest to occlusal surface loss from erosion potentiated by attrition. On the upper teeth, the surfaces most affected are the occlusal and palatal slopes. On the lower teeth, it is the occlusal and buccal surfaces that are most worn. When the clinician encounters this clinical presentation in the mixed dentition, caution must be exercised before concluding that the pattern of wear is the result of bruxism. This 11-year-old patient gave a history of early childhood gastric reflux and ongoing asthma with long-term medications, which reduced saliva protection against intrinsic acids and those in frequently consumed soft drinks and other acidic beverages. Patients of all ages may be affected by intrinsic acids, and 60% of the population may experience reflux at some stage in their lives (ten Cate & Imfeld 1996). However, longer term exposure to intrinsic acids is required to result in significant toothwear. As conceptualised in Fig. 1.15, the most severe lesions on the deciduous teeth are on surfaces least protected by saliva from the major glands. Intrinsic and extrinsic acids would further affect certain parts of the dentition and particular tooth surfaces more than others. Further investigation is warranted to identify multifactorial aetiology. The presentation of and reasons for toothwear in children and appropriate management approaches are further considered in Chapters 2 and 3.

TOOTHWEAR AND DENTAL CARIES

It is rare for the clinician to encounter active dental caries in patients with worn dentitions. This is because erosion, attrition and abrasion are not caused by bacteria. In fact, the metabolic activities of cariogenic organisms that convert simple sugars to acids are inhibited by the low pH found on the surfaces susceptible to dental erosion, as key enzymes in *Streptococcus*

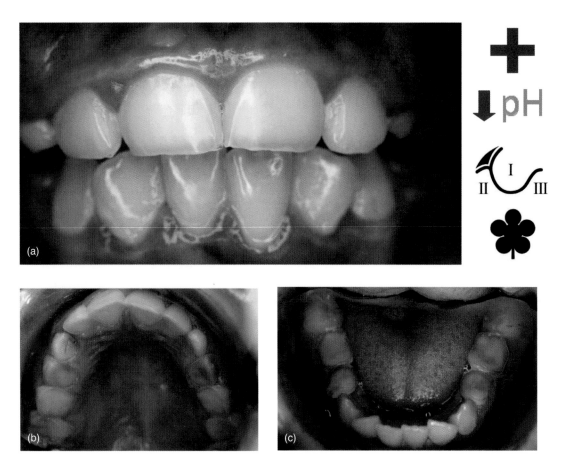

Figure 1.14 This 11-year-old male patient has (a) incisal attrition, chipping and mild thinning of enamel across the anterior teeth. (b) The maxillary teeth show heavily worn surfaces on deciduous canine and molar teeth with near exposures of the pulp. (c) The lower permanent canine and incisor teeth have erupted, but as yet were unworn. Near exposures on the heavily worn lower deciduous molar teeth are evident. (From Young, 2001a, with permission from the *Australian Dental Journal*.)

mutans cease to metabolise at pH values of 4.2 or below at which they become increasingly unviable (Meurman & ten Cate 1996). In the case illustrated in Fig. 1.16, the astute clinician would have no problem discriminating buccal cervical lesions on the lower anterior teeth with undermined enamel edges as arrested caries of dentine from shallow cervical erosions. This 19-year-old female patient was a professional dancer, who consumed fluoridated water in the first 12 years of her life and had no other active caries lesions. In her early teenage years,

the patient commenced binge eating of sugary snacks between ballet rehearsals. This presumably caused the observed dental caries. However, a few years subsequently, attacks of self-induced vomiting and high consumption of soft drinks increased the higher influence of intrinsic and extrinsic acid consumption. This changed the nature of her oral pathology.

The distribution of both the lesions of erosion and caries (Fig. 1.17) can in part be explained by loss of saliva protection from dehydration. Acids from sugars, produced by dental

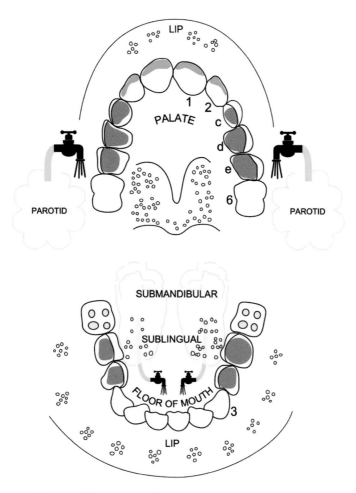

Figure 1.15 Conceptualisation of the 11-year-old patient shown in Fig. 1.14. Mild attrition is present on his incisors (green). Two deciduous canines and eight molar teeth are severely worn (orange). The two permanent lower molars show the amount of erosion (yellow) that occurred since age 6, when they erupted into his mouth. Mucous is secreted from the inner surfaces of the lips, cheeks, back of the palate, and sublingual glands. Serous saliva flows from the parotid glands through ducts that open on the inner surface of the cheeks (taps). In the floor of the mouth serous and mucous saliva are mixed from the submandibular ducts (taps) with mucous from the sublingual gland. (From Young, 2003a, with permission of Erosion Watch Pty Ltd.)

plaque bacteria at sites of caries, usually do not contribute to demineralisation on surfaces susceptible to dental erosion. Also, these surfaces are normally protected by saliva. Reduced saliva flow in anorexia nervosa and bulimia (Milosevic & Dawson 1996) placed this patient, in recent years, at risk of both gastric and dietary acids that cause erosion but not dental caries. Patients with poor oral hygiene are at greater risk of developing dental caries and/or periodontal disease. Most patients with moderate or severe toothwear, however, present with good oral hygiene and low levels of plaque accumulation. Dental erosion from intrinsic acids involves the strongest acids with a pH as low as 1, whilst soft drinks and fruit juices may

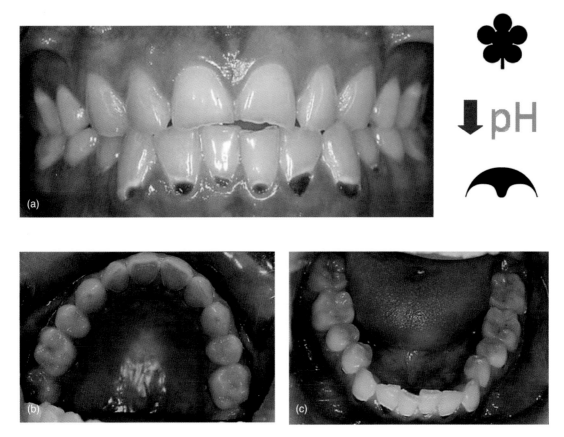

Figure 1.16 A 19-year-old female ballet dancer with bulimia, whose (a) incisal edges and (b) palatal surfaces show evidence of erosion. Occlusal erosion was present on her (c) canine, premolar and molar teeth. Arrested caries is evident at the cervical margins of her lower anterior teeth (a & c). (From Young, 2001a, with permission from the *Australian Dental Journal*.)

have a range around pH 3, but the critical pH at which teeth dissolve should be more appropriately considered a range (Dawes 2003) depending on the concentration of calcium and phosphate in saliva (see Chapter 5). The pH ranges involved in dental caries are higher than those in dental erosion, and these processes are generally independent and significant lesions of both are infrequently found in the one dentition. When found, careful history-taking may reveal changes in diet, health or lifestyle that account for the presence of both dental erosion and dental caries within a patient's mouth, having occurred at different stages in the pa-

tient's life. Oral health promotion internationally has reinforced the risk of dental caries due to high sugar consumption across most populations. However, public awareness of dental erosion is still limited (Lussi et al. 2006).

TOOTHWEAR – A MULTIFACTORIAL PROCESS

Toothwear is best considered a multifactorial process (Fig. 1.18) involving significant variation from one individual to the next (Khan

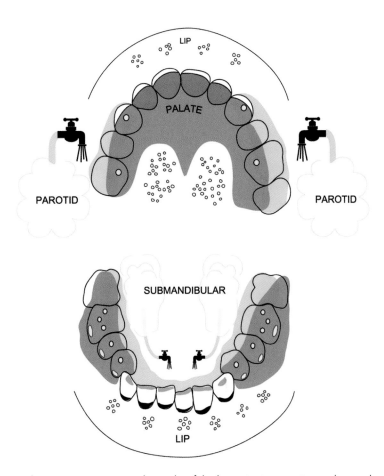

Figure 1.17 Dental caries was present at the necks of the lower incisor, canine and premolar teeth. The lower premolars and molars had erosion on their cusp and shallow erosions cervically (yellow). The upper front teeth were chipped on their edges and denuded of enamel on their palatal surfaces (orange). Mucous from minor salivary glands has failed to protect against decay or erosion, as it contains no bicarbonate buffer. Serous salivary (blue) contains buffer and flows from the parotid and submandibular ducts (taps) to mix with mucous and to neutralise acids. Poor flow of serous saliva fails to neutralise acids on the palatal and buccal surfaces of lower teeth. (From Young, 2003a, with permission of Erosion Watch Pty Ltd.)

et al. 1998). Identifying and understanding the relative involvement of a broad range of contributing factors ensures the clinician will succeed in any restorative or rehabilitative efforts. The interplay of intrinsic and extrinsic acids, of saliva protection, of health and lifestyle issues potentiates attrition, erosion and abrasion, creating lesions in a site-specific manner (Young & Khan 2002). Toothwear starts and can be prevented from early on in life. Identification

and management of toothwear in children is a priority, particularly when the deciduous teeth are eroded, although the permanent teeth appear only mildly worn by attrition. This is the early warning sign for the clinician. Prevention must start early on to prevent possible immense restorative challenges in later life. Although progression of toothwear is generally slow, some individuals will experience rapid tooth structure loss (Bartlett 2005), and monitoring

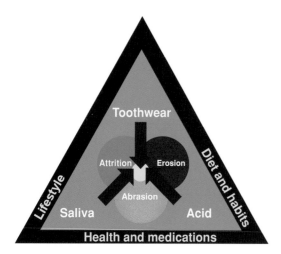

Figure 1.18 Toothwear can be conceptualised as a combination of erosion, attrition and abrasion over considerable time, interplaying with varying levels of extrinsic acid, intrinsic acid and salivary protection, each affected by lifestyle, diet, habits, health and medications.

toothwear over time with diagnostic study models is important to provide a reference baseline for subsequent comparisons (see Chapter 8). Those at risk need to be identified and managed comprehensively with dietary, lifestyle and preventive strategies, using adjuncts where appropriate. Focus must continue on prevention and control of all toothwear processes and aim to limit influence of potential accelerating factors to avoid, in later life, the development of a dentition in need of comprehensive rehabilitation, which remains a complex clinical challenge (Johansson et al. 2008).

References

Addy, M. (2005) Tooth brushing, tooth wear and dentine hypersensitivity – are they associated. *International Dental Journal*, **55**(4 Suppl 1), 261–267.

Bartlett, D. (2005) The role of erosion in tooth wear: aetiology, prevention and management. *International Dental Journal*, **55**(4 Suppl 1), 77–284.

Bartlett, D. (2009) Etiology and prevention of acid erosion. *Compendium*, **30**, 616–620.

Dawes, C. (2003) What is the critical pH and why does a tooth dissolve in acid? *Journal of the Canadian Dental Association*, **69**, 722–724.

Dawes, C. (2008) Salivary flow patterns and the health of hard and soft oral tissues. *Journal of the American Dental Association*, **139**, s18–s24.

Johansson, A., Johansson, A.K., Omar, R., et al. (2008) Rehabilitation of the worn dentition. *Journal of Oral Rehabilitation*, **35**, 548–566.

Johansson, A.K., Lingström, P., Birkhed, D. (2002) Comparison of factors potentially related to the occurrence of dental erosion in high- and low-erosion groups. *European Journal of Oral Sciences*, **110**, 204–211.

Khan, F., Young, W.G., Daley, T.J. (1998) Dental erosion and bruxism. A tooth wear analysis from South East Queensland. *Australian Dental Journal*, **43**, 117–127.

Khan, F., Young, W.G., Shahabi, S., et al. (1999) Dental cervical lesions associated with occlusal erosion and attrition. *Australian Dental Journal*, **44**, 176–186.

Lussi, A., Hellwig, E., Zero, D., et al. (2006) Erosive tooth wear: diagnosis, risk factors and prevention. *American Journal of Dentistry*, **19**, 319–325.

Lussi, A., Jaeggi, T., Zero, D. (2004) The role of diet in the aetiology of dental erosion. *Caries Research*, **38**(Suppl 1), 34–44.

Meurman, J.H., ten Cate, J.M. (1996) Pathogenesis and modifying factors of dental erosion. *European Journal of Oral Sciences*, **104**, 199–206.

Milosevic, A. (1997) Sports drinks hazard to teeth. *British Journal of Sports Medicine*, **31**, 28–30.

Milosevic, A., Dawson, L.J. (1996) Salivary factors in vomiting bulimics with and without pathological tooth wear. *Caries Research*, **30**, 361–366.

Scheutzel, P. (1996) Etiology of dental erosion–intrinsic factors. *European Journal of Oral Sciences*, **104**, 78–190.

Sirimaharaj, V., Brearley Messer, L., Morgan, M.V. (2002) Acidic diet and dental erosion among athletes. *Australian Dental Journal*, **47**, 228–236.

ten Cate, J.M., Imfeld, T. (1996) Dental erosion, summary. *European Journal of Oral Sciences*, **104**, 241–244.

Wiktorsson, A.-M., Zimmerman, M., Angmar-Månsson, B. (1997) Erosive toothwear: prevalence and severity in Swedish winetasters. *European Journal of Oral Sciences*, **105**, 544–550.

Young, W.G. (1998) Anthropology, tooth wear and occlusion *ab origine*. *Journal of Dental Research*, **77**, 860–1863.

Young, W.G. (2001a) Oral medicine of toothwear. *Australian Dental Journal*, **46**(4), 236–250.

Young, W.G. (2001b) *Oral Medicine of Toothwear CD Rom*. Dentil Pty Ltd. Queensland, Australia.

Young, W.G. (2003a) *Teeth on Edge*. Erosion Watch Pty Ltd. Queensland, Australia.

Young, W.G. (2003b) *What Colour Is Your Sports Drink CD Rom*. Dentil Pty Ltd. Queensland, Australia.

Young, W.G., Khan, F. (2002) Sites of dental erosion are saliva-dependent. *Journal of Oral Rehabilitation*, **29**, 35–43.

Young, W.G., Khan, F. (2009) *By the Skin of Our Teeth*. Erosion Watch Pty Ltd. Queensland, Australia.

Young, W.G., Khan, F., Brandt, R., et al. (2001) Syndromes with salivary dysfunction predispose to tooth wear: case reports of congenital dysfunction of major salivary glands, Prader-Willi syndrome, congenital rubella, and Sjögren's syndrome. *Oral Surgery Oral Pathology Oral Medicine Oral Radiology Endodontology*, **92**, 38–48.

Zero, D.T., Lussi, A. (2005) Erosion – chemical and biological factors of importance to the dental practitioner. *International Dental Journal*, **55**, 285–290.

Diagnosis and management of toothwear in children

W. Kim Seow and Sue Taji

Toothwear in children and adolescents is a common condition with a prevalence rate severalfold that of caries. It may begin in the primary dentition of a young child and persist to involve the permanent dentition in adulthood. As many children with mild-to-moderate toothwear do not complain of symptoms, by the time of presentation the condition can be associated with extensive destruction of the primary and young permanent dentition, loss of aesthetics and masticatory function, pulpal exposure and abscess formation (Linnett & Seow 2001). In children, toothwear usually results from a combination of attrition, abrasion and erosion (Fig. 2.1). Of these, dental erosion is usually the predominant underlying mechanism, and involves extrinsic acids from dietary intake (Fig. 2.2) or intrinsic gastric acids.

The influence of abrasion is usually minimal. As toothwear in children has traditionally not been well recognised clinically, the condition is often undiagnosed until extensive tooth structure has been lost and poses a restorative challenge (Fig. 2.3).

CLINICAL PRESENTATIONS OF TOOTHWEAR IN CHILDREN

Primary teeth are more susceptible to toothwear compared to permanent teeth due to structural differences such as lower degrees of crystallite arrangement and mineralisation, greater amounts of water and increased permeability (Johansson et al. 2001). Also, the thinner enamel and dentine layers in primary teeth together with larger pulp chambers can lead to more rapid pulpal inflammation and exposures from toothwear. Furthermore, immaturity of the salivary glands in children may be associated with less salivary protection from erosion due to relatively low flow rates and less secretory capacity compared to adults (Watanabe & Dawes 1990).

In the primary dentition, it is often difficult to discriminate between the individual effects of erosion, attrition and abrasion as all these processes usually occur concurrently and contribute to the overall clinical appearance of

Toothwear: The ABC of the Worn Dentition, First Edition. Edited by Farid Khan and William George Young.
© 2011 John Wiley & Sons, Ltd. Published 2011 by John Wiley & Sons, Ltd.

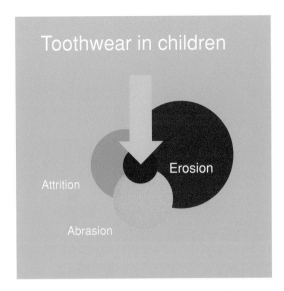

Figure 2.1   Erosion is usually the predominant contributing aetiology in toothwear in most children, with attrition playing a secondary role and abrasion a minimal role.

the lesions. It is notable that cervical toothwear lesions are rare in children, probably due to the relatively short time the primary teeth are present in the mouth and the fact that gingival recession and exposure of cementum surfaces are uncommon in children. Toothwear is

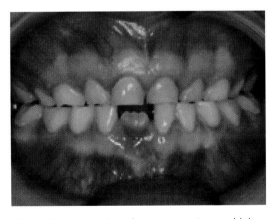

Figure 2.2   Incisal toothwear in a 5-year-old boy with a history of frequent soft drink consumption. His mother reported occasional night-time grinding of teeth.

thus predominantly observed in the occlusal surfaces of the primary, mixed and early permanent dentitions.

Toothwear facets in the primary and permanent dentitions which result from normal occlusal contacts can be found in most dentitions, and in milder forms, they can be considered physiological. Facets resulting from physiological toothwear usually appear as well-demarcated regions on occlusal surfaces and cuspal inclines. The processes of dental erosion can underlie these facets to result in rapid loss of tooth structure. In the late mixed dentition, differences in wear of the primary teeth and the permanent successors are readily discernible (see Fig. 1.14). These differences result from the length of time of exposure to toothwear processes as well as differences in structural composition of primary and permanent teeth. Effects of loss of vertical dimension occur with advanced toothwear, and these are further detailed in Chapter 10. Erosion lesions may often be distinguished by their characteristic appearance. In the earliest stages, an erosion lesion usually presents as a smooth, glazed surface with increased incisal translucency, loss of surface anatomy and chipping of the incisal edges (Ganss & Lussi 2006). With further attack from acid, the cusps, grooves and incisal edges often become rounded, there is loss of occlusal morphology (Figs. 2.4a & b), and the smooth surfaces appear concave, dished out or cup shaped (Khan et al. 2001).

Exposure time, patterns of consumption as well as clearance of acidic foods and beverages are important contributing variables which influence the site specificity of erosion lesions. The parts of the dentition which are most susceptible to dental erosion compared to those affected by dental caries are contrasted in Table 2.1.

As with adults, the common sites for erosion lesions in children are also heavily influenced by salivary flow and clearance patterns. The locations of the parotid gland openings on the buccal surfaces of the maxillary molars and the

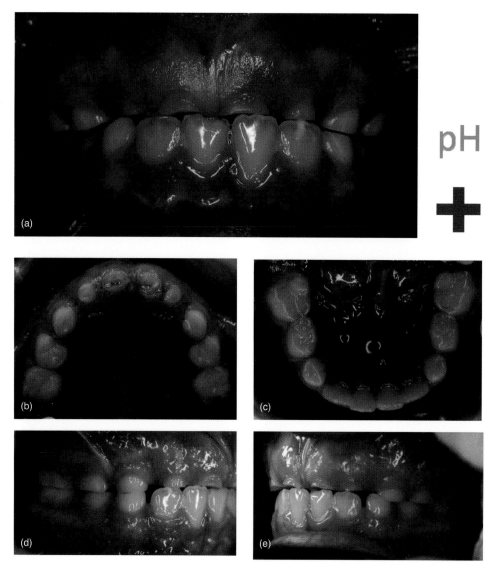

Figure 2.3 Anterior view of a 6-year-old boy with a history of gastro-oesophageal reflux disease, showing severe toothwear in the primary anterior teeth (a). The maxillary teeth are severely affected by erosive toothwear (b). Whilst the recently erupted mandibular teeth show minimal wear, the primary molars and canines are moderately worn (c). Left- and right-sided buccal views of the teeth in occlusion highlight the severe loss of occlusal vertical dimension (d) and (e).

submandibular and sublingual glands openings on the lingual surfaces of the mandibular teeth allow the tooth surfaces approximating these sites to be better protected in relation to the other surfaces.

As shown in Figs. 2.4a and b, erosion lesions in children are characteristically first noticed on the buccal and occlusal aspects of the primary mandibular molars, the occlusal and palatal aspects of the maxillary primary molars, and

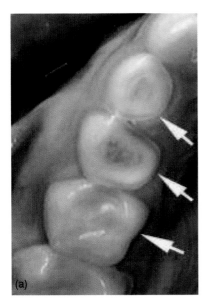
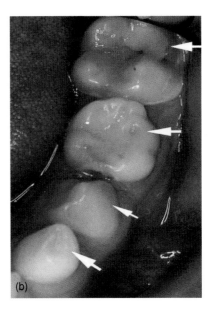

Figure 2.4 Sites of toothwear in maxillary teeth are commonly found on the palatal aspects (a), whereas those of the mandibular teeth are usually located on the buccal aspects (b).

the incisal surfaces of the maxillary primary incisors. Furthermore, in cases where the source of acid is external, the location of the erosion lesions may vary according to whether the drink is consumed through a straw (minimal lesions) or gulped and swished in the mouth prior to swallowing (extensive lesions) or suckled through a baby bottle (mainly on the palatal aspects). The frequency of exposure and duration of the acid drink held in contact with teeth may also affect the severity of the lesions (Zero 1996).

Although both erosion and caries result from acid attack on the teeth, the involvement of a bacterial biofilm in the caries process results in caries lesions being different in presentation and site specificity compared to erosion lesions (Table 2.2). These differences help to distinguish erosion lesions from carious lesions and provide an explanation for the involvement of

Table 2.1 Predominant sites of toothwear and dental caries in paediatric patients.

Age group (y)	Dentition	Toothwear sites	Dental caries
0–3	Primary	Maxillary anteriors – palatal Mandibular anteriors – incisal	Early childhood caries Maxillary anterior teeth Maxillary and mandibular first molars
3–6	Primary to early mixed	Occlusal surfaces of mandibular and maxillary primary teeth	Fissural and proximal caries in primary molars
6–12	Mixed	Primary and first permanent molars occlusally	Fissural and proximal caries in primary and first permanent molars
Teenage	Permanent	Maxillary anteriors – palatal First permanent molars –occlusal	Fissural and proximal caries

Table 2.2 Site involvement of toothwear and dental caries in the primary and mixed dentition.

Teeth	Surfaces	Toothwear	Dental caries
Anterior	Incisal/palatal	Common	Minimal unless caries is rampant
	Cervical	Minimal	Common
	Interproximal	Nil	Common
Posterior	Cusps	Common	Uncommon unless caries is rampant
	Fissures	Minimal unless severe	Common
	Cervical	Minimal	Uncommon unless caries is rampant
	Interproximal	Nil	Common

the proximal lesions in caries but not in erosion. Early childhood caries (Fig. 2.5), for example, affects different surfaces compared to erosion in young children (see Fig. 2.2). Importantly, children are predisposed to both caries and erosion in the presence of enamel hypoplasia (Seow et al. 2009). Teeth with structural defects of enamel and dentine are also at risk for rapid toothwear and are further considered later in this chapter.

The extent of toothwear and loss of vertical dimension is highly variable in children at any particular age. When assessing children, it is important to consider the length of time a particular tooth has been in the mouth to appreciate the risk for toothwear. For example, in the early and late mixed dentitions, care must be exercised in diagnosing erosion as the newly erupted permanent incisors and first

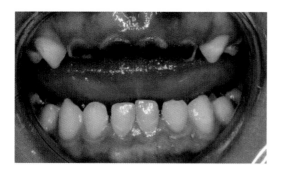

Figure 2.5 Early childhood caries in a 3-year-old boy. Note location of dental caries on maxillary anterior teeth, whilst the mandibular anterior teeth are relatively protected.

molars may show only minimal wear. On the other hand, wear observed on the primary canines and first and second molars should be carefully assessed for signs of toothwear processes that may continue to affect the new permanent dentition.

HISTORY-TAKING, ASSESSMENT AND DIAGNOSIS

A child's dentition contains a record of past toothwear activity, and the results of a single examination are insufficient to determine the risk for further toothwear. It is prudent to obtain thorough medical, dietary and dental histories to help diagnose the aetiology of the toothwear.

Medical history

The clinician should check the medical history for conditions that can place a child at risk for toothwear and erosion, including the following:

* Gastro-oesophageal reflux, rumination or chronic vomiting which exposes the teeth to direct contact with gastric acid
* Symptoms of undiagnosed gastro-oesophageal reflux such as epigastric pain or regurgitation
* Asthma therapy using beta-adrenergic bronchodilators which are associated with reduced salivary flow, and increased risk of erosion from oral inhalation of aerosols

containing acidic particles of drug being in direct contact with the teeth
- Conditions with abnormal neuromuscular activity and severe bruxism such as cerebral palsy and Down syndrome

Dietary history

Taking a thorough dietary history is further discussed in Chapter 3, and should include the following:

- A 6-day diet diary documenting all foods and beverages consumed
- Enquiry about the method, the frequency of consumption and the length of time the acidic foods and beverages are in the mouth
- Questioning with regard to possible grazing habits such as constant sipping of fruit juices from a drink bottle

Dental history

The enquiry of toothwear risk factors in a child's dental history should include the following:

- History of grinding or clenching of teeth during the day or at night
- Excessive toothbrushing in children and adolescents with psychological problems
- History of pica or eating of non-food substances such as soil, sand and hair
- Oral habits including frequently biting on hard objects such as pencils

CHILDREN AT INCREASED RISK FOR TOOTHWEAR

In assessing and diagnosing the aetiology of toothwear, an understanding of risk factors for toothwear in children is critical. Table 2.3 provides the groups of children who are at increased risk for toothwear. A high frequency of consumption of beverages and foods with erosive potential is the most common risk factor for toothwear in children. In addition, children who have gastro-oesophageal reflux conditions, oral habits such as bruxing and reduced salivary function, as well as developmental abnormalities of enamel and dentine

Table 2.3 Risk conditions for toothwear in children.

Risk condition	Example
High frequency of acidic beverage consumption	Soft drinks, fruit juices, sports drinks Falling asleep with nursing bottle
Children with gastro-oesophageal reflux condition	Gastro-oesophageal reflux disease Bulimia
Oral habits, e.g. bruxism or clenching	Neurological abnormalities, e.g. cerebral palsy Psychological stress
Reduced or absent salivary function	Drug-induced xerostomia Inherited conditions, e.g. salivary gland aplasia Acquired conditions, e.g. radiation-induced xerostomia
Structural defects of enamel	Inherited disorders of enamel, e.g. amelogenesis imperfecta Acquired defects of enamel e.g. systemic conditions
Structural defects of dentine	Inherited disorders of dentine, e.g. dentinogenesis imperfecta

structure, are also predisposed to increased risk for toothwear.

Children who frequently consume beverages and foods with erosive potential

Extrinsic acids derived from soft drinks, fruit juices and carbonated beverages are currently the most common cause of erosion in children and adolescents. There has been a recent global increase in the consumption of carbonated beverages, particularly among children and adolescents of all ages. The effects of erosion on the teeth may be direct or enhanced by secondary attrition of demineralised tooth structure (Fig. 2.6). Children who habitually consume acidic drinks during times of reduced salivary flow, such as during or after strenuous physical activity, are at increased risk for dental erosion. The severe toothwear reported in athletes is often attributed to consumption of acidic sports drinks during times of dehydration and low salivary flow (Milosevic 1997).

Less common extrinsic sources of acid which have been reported to cause erosive toothwear include medications in the form of liquid and effervescent acidic tablets formulated for children. Many oral drug preparations are rendered acidic in order to facilitate drug dispersion and improve palatability and patient compliance. Children who constantly consume such oral medications for chronic diseases are at increased risk for erosion. For example, effervescent citric acid tablets are common preparations for drugs which are prescribed on a long-term basis for children with chronic renal diseases (Nunn et al. 2001). Other acidic oral preparations which are increasingly consumed by children are vitamin C tablets and aspirin, which may be taken frequently and left in direct contact with the teeth (Young 2005). Patients who chew vitamin C tablets have been reported to have up to fivefold increased risk of toothwear from erosion (Al-Malik et al. 2001).

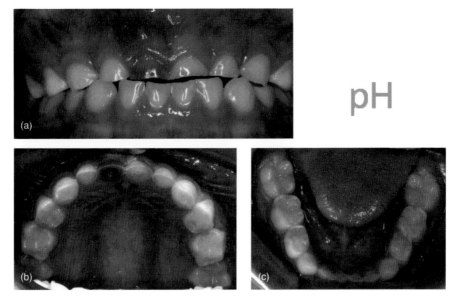

Figure 2.6   Anterior view of a 5-year-old girl with a history of frequent consumption of soft drinks, showing severe toothwear in the primary anterior teeth (a). The maxillary anterior teeth show severe erosive toothwear, and the right primary central incisor is darkened and non-vital due to exposure of the pulp from toothwear (b). Incisal and occlusal wear is evident on the mandibular primary incisors, canines and molars (c).

Children who have gastro-oesophageal reflux conditions

Gastric acid, which has a high erosive potential, may enter the oral cavity as a result of pyloric sphincter incompetence, gastro-oesophageal reflux, eating disorders, chronic vomiting, persistent regurgitation or rumination. Several studies have shown that children with gastro-oesophageal reflux or the involuntary passage of gastric contents into the oesophagus are at risk for erosive toothwear (Linnett et al. 2002). Reflux which occurs during sleep usually causes the greatest amount of tooth structure loss, presumably due to the greatly reduced levels of saliva produced during sleep. The effect on the dentition can be severe even from a young age (see Figs. 1.14 & 2.3).

Children who have reduced saliva flow

Saliva has a major protective role in erosive toothwear through its pellicle, oral clearance of dietary acids and buffering capacity (Young & Khan 2002). Children who have congenital abnormalities, including salivary gland aplasia, and acquired hypofunction of the salivary glands such as radiation-induced xerostomia, are thus at high risk for erosive toothwear in addition to other well-recognised oral health problems and notably rampant caries (Taji et al. 2010).

Salivary flow rates in children can be further reduced by medications such as antihistamines and beta-2 agonist antiasthmatic drugs, such as salbutamol and terbutaline (Dugmore & Rock 2003). Although the majority of research studies have not established a direct link between these drugs and dental erosion, children on these medications are potentially at risk for erosive toothwear due to reduced oral clearance and lowered buffering capacity of acids due to reduced amounts of saliva. In addition, the acidic nature of some oral aerosols which contact the teeth directly may also cause dental erosion in asthmatic children (Dugmore & Rock 2003). The protective role of saliva in toothwear and dental caries is further discussed in Chapter 5.

Children who have oral habits

Children with bruxing habits are at risk for toothwear from attrition. Although some children may grind their teeth at night, this is commonly transient and self-limiting. In rare situations, neurological conditions or psychological stress may be associated with grinding of the teeth. Children with abnormal neuromuscular activity such as cerebral palsy often have sustained bruxing habits, which can lead to severe toothwear through attrition. As gastro-oesophageal reflux is commonly associated with these conditions, further damage to the teeth can result from erosion (Pope 1991). Figure 2.7 depicts the severe toothwear in a 6-year-old child with a bruxing habit. The lesions found on the palatal aspects of the incisors and canines are suggestive of erosion as a contributory mechanism in the destructive process. Children with unusual oral habits, such as pica (eating of non-food items), may chew on materials with rough surfaces, such as sand, which can cause rapid removal of tooth structure by abrasion (Barker 2005).

Children who have structural defects of enamel and dentine

Clinical reports of children affected by structural defects of enamel and dentine suggest that their teeth are less resistant to physical wear and chemical dissolution. Developmental enamel defects are common in children, and may be inherited or acquired. They can present as enamel opacities (changes in the translucency) or enamel hypoplasia (reduced or lack of enamel formation; Seow 1997a). Inherited enamel defects, such as amelogenesis imperfecta (Fig. 2.8), are uncommon, and may present

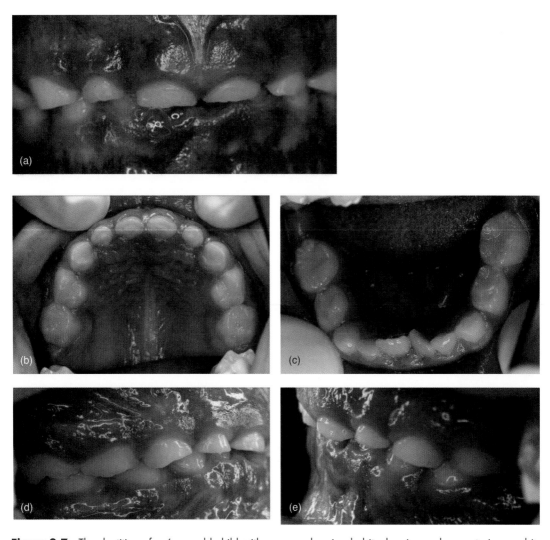

Figure 2.7 The dentition of a 6-year-old child with a severe bruxing habit, showing a deep anterior overbite due to loss of vertical height of the molars (a). Severe toothwear of the palatal surfaces of the incisors and canines is suggestive of the significant contribution of dental erosion (b). Flattening of the cusp tips and cup-like lesions are evident on the occlusal surfaces of the mandibular primary molars (c). Left- and right-sided views of the teeth show the extensive loss of occlusal vertical dimension (d) and (e).

clinically as reduction in thickness (hypoplastic) or decrease in mineralisation (hypomineralised) or altered maturation (hypomature; Witkop, Jr 1988).

The mode of inheritance may be autosomal dominant or -recessive or X-linked, and several abnormal genes coding for enamel pro-

teins have been identified for amelogenesis imperfecta (Seow 1994; Wright 2006). Both primary and permanent dentitions are affected, although the defects may be less obvious in the primary teeth due to the thinner enamel (Seow 1994). Enamel defects can also result from many systemic insults to the developing enamel, the

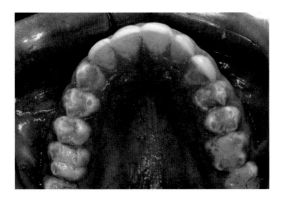

Figure 2.8 The maxillary teeth of a 14-year-old boy affected by amelogenesis imperfecta. The teeth show thin hypoplastic enamel and extensive toothwear.

most common being childhood infections (Ford et al. 2009) and birth prematurity (Seow 1997b). Excessive fluoride associated with inadvertent ingestion of toothpaste in young children is another common cause of enamel hypoplasia. In contrast to amelogenesis imperfecta, acquired defects of enamel can affect a single tooth or groups of teeth that are developing at the time of the systemic insult. The structural and mineralisation changes found in the teeth with enamel defects predispose them to higher risk for toothwear.

As is the case with amelogenesis imperfecta, inherited structural defects of dentine also predispose the teeth to high risk of toothwear. The most common developmental dentine defect is dentinogenesis imperfecta, also known as hereditary opalescent dentine, which can occur as a primary defect of dentine or in association with osteogenesis imperfecta (Hart & Hart 2007). Dentinogenesis imperfecta results from mutations in the dentin sialoprotein 1 gene, and is usually inherited in an autosomal-dominant manner (Hart & Hart 2007). Although osteogenesis imperfecta results from a different genetic defect, the clinical presentations and structural changes in dentine are similar. Teeth affected by dentinogenesis imperfecta are at high risk for toothwear, as the abnormally mineralised dentine does not support the enamel which

fractures and exposes the dentine. There is usually rapid wear of the exposed dentine, and the crowns of the teeth can be reduced to the gingival level within a few years of eruption (Fig. 2.9). Protection of affected molars with stainless steel crowns soon after eruption is recommended.

MANAGEMENT OF TOOTHWEAR IN CHILDREN

General guidelines for management of toothwear in children must include education and prevention, early diagnosis and intervention, monitoring of toothwear and restorative treatment. Developmental considerations in the management of paediatric patients should also be taken into consideration (Table 2.4).

(I) Education of parents and caregivers using an anticipatory guidance approach

The prevention of dental erosion in children may be incorporated as part of general dental education of parents/caregivers using an age-related framework of anticipatory guidance. Anticipatory guidance is the provision of appropriate health care information to parents/caregivers in anticipation of staged physical, emotional and psychological development of children. Thus, from the time of eruption of the primary incisors at approximately 6 months of age to full function of the permanent dentition in the teenage years, prevention and monitoring of toothwear can be included in the general anticipatory guidance framework for children's dental health. Prevention of toothwear in children should focus on education of parents and children regarding the dental risks of frequent consumption of acidic beverages and foods. This is discussed in detail in Chapter 3. Public oral health education should target children, parents, teachers and sports coaches at schools

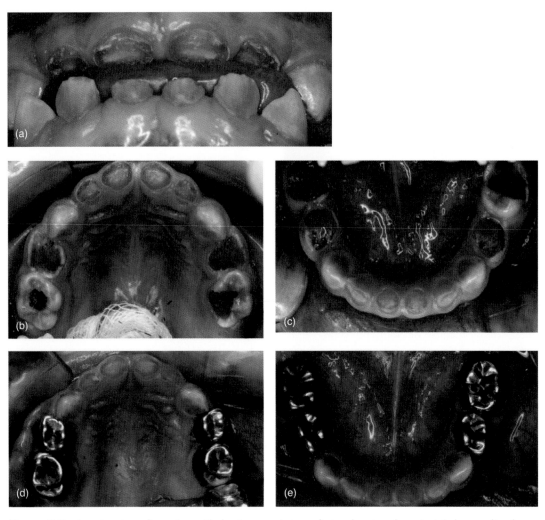

Figure 2.9 Anterior view of a patient with dentinogenesis imperfecta, showing characteristic brown discolouration and shortened incisor crowns due to extensive toothwear (a). Both the maxillary and mandibular primary teeth show extensive toothwear (b) and (c). The worn maxillary and mandibular primary molars were restored with stainless steel crowns (d) and (e).

Table 2.4 Developmental considerations for management of paediatric patients.

Age group (y)	Parent's influence on diet	Child's ability to brush own teeth
0–3	Exclusive	None
3–6	Moderate	Limited
6–12	Partial	Manual dexterity limited until age 8 y
Teenage	Restricted	Capable, but may need encouragement

and colleges, and may be performed by dental and other health professionals.

Zero- to three-year-olds (emerging primary dentition)

This is the period when newly erupted tooth surfaces are highly vulnerable to colonisation by cariogenic bacteria and attack by extrinsic acids. As infants are highly dependent on their caregivers, counselling of parents and guardians is central to preventing toothwear and other dental problems in this age group:

- Toothbrushing with a soft toothbrush should commence as soon as the new teeth erupt. A 'smear' amount of child toothpaste with low-dose fluoride should be used.
- Breastfeeding should be encouraged for young infants.
- Cow's milk should be consumed without added flavourings and sugar.
- Acidic beverages – particularly soft drinks, vitamin C syrups and cordials – should be eliminated as they can be both acidic and cariogenic.
- Fruit juices should be restricted to meal times.
- Children should not be given a nursing bottle filled with fruit juice, syrup or cordials to take to sleep.
- Weaning diets should be non-cariogenic and non-acidic, such as cheese and milk products.
- Infants commonly have oesophageal reflux in the first few months of life, which may persist in a few children. Medical treatment may be necessary for some infants who have gastro-oesophageal disease.
- Plain water can be given to the infants after reflux to reduce the erosive damage from intrinsic acids.

Three- to six-year-olds (primary to early mixed dentition)

At this stage, prevention of caries and dental erosion may be achieved by good nutrition, oral hygiene and preventive care products.

As with infants, parents and guardians should be given guidance for prevention of dental erosion and caries in this age group:

- Toothbrushing should be performed twice daily with a 'smear' amount of child's toothpaste.
- Selective preventive topical agents may be applied daily on defective primary enamel.
- Dietary advice is further considered in Chapter 3, but should include promoting consumption of fresh fruit – such as bananas and apples – and cheese and avoiding acidic beverages and processed fruit bars that are often sticky and contain sugar and acids. Plain milk should be encouraged.

Six- to twelve-year-olds (early mixed to permanent dentition)

From about the age of 6 years, most children are in primary schools and have some independence with regard to purchasing their own food and drinks. Children at these ages are highly receptive to education regarding food choices and healthy eating habits. However, they can be influenced by peer pressure, and often model their behaviours on influential peers. Health promotion regarding preventing dental erosion in this age group may be taught at the dental chairside or in the classroom. In addition to behaviours recommended for the younger age groups, the following points are pertinent for 6- to 12-year-olds:

- Newly erupting permanent teeth are highly susceptible to damage from acids from beverages.
- Hypoplastic molars may need to be capped with steel crowns or restored with composite resins.
- Fluoride rinses and other preventive topical agents may be applied to teeth with enamel hypoplasia.
- Teeth should be cleaned twice daily with a soft toothbrush and fluoride toothpaste.
- Healthy snacking with plain milk, cheese and fresh fruit should be promoted.

Teenagers (permanent dentition)

Although most teenage children have achieved adult-level cognitive ability, their behaviours are often under the influence of peers and the media. Previous compliance and good behaviours regarding healthy eating may be challenged by new influences during adolescence. Points that are relevant to education of teenagers include the following:

- Discussion of the causes and effects of behaviour, habits, diet and hygiene and their implications on the current and future oral health of the patient with the patient.
- Increased peer pressure for consumption of acidic beverages, including sports drinks.
- Oral care may be neglected due to other interests and pressures.
- Suspected cases of anorexia nervosa or bulimia often require sensitive handling and involvement of a medical team and parents.

(II) Intervention

Upon diagnosing toothwear and identifying the risk factors, the clinician should intervene to prevent further damage to the teeth. In most cases, in children who frequently consume beverages and foods with erosive potential, intervention includes dietary modifications to prevent further erosion and oral care to prevent further damage: For children with gastro-oesophageal reflux conditions, medical consultation for further assessment and management may be recommended. General recommendations for intervention management of toothwear are detailed in Chapter 7.

Ingestion of acidic medicines

Wherever possible, acidic oral medicines should be changed to neutral syrup preparations. If alternatives are unavailable, the acidic medicines should be ingested with water and if possible, at meal times when salivary flow is high.

Children who have oral habits, e.g. bruxing and pica

In children with severe bruxing habits, acrylic occlusal splints may be prescribed to protect the teeth and help break the habit. The underlying causes of bruxing in children are unknown, and the majority who brux do not require any intervention. Referral to medical specialists may be required if psychological or medical reasons are thought to be associated with the bruxism. Children who give a history of pica should be referred for medical management as pica may be associated with other complications and developmental problems.

Children who have structural defects of enamel and dentine

Teeth affected with amelogenesis imperfecta or dentinogenesis imperfecta require early institution of preventive procedures due to the high risk of toothwear of the altered tooth structure. Affected primary and permanent molars often require restoration with stainless steel crowns soon after emergence to prevent excessive destruction of tooth structure. The anterior teeth should be regularly reviewed, and when signs of toothwear become evident, composite resin restorations should be placed.

Dietary modifications

Dietary modification and preventive advice should be based on information obtained from a 6-day diet diary as detailed in Chapter 3. Foods and beverages which are known to pose risks for erosion in children – such as carbonated soft drinks, sports drinks and acidic fruit juices – should be identified. These should be replaced with non-acidic substitutes – such as cheese and milk – where possible or limited to meal times when there is good salivary flow.

Therapeutic products

In some children, the application of preventive adjuncts containing therapeutic agents may help to reharden the enamel surface and decrease tooth sensitivity. The efficacy of therapeutic agents for toothwear is discussed in Chapter 7. Current agents available include traditional desensitising compounds, such as potassium nitrate, which form protective barriers on the tooth surface, as well as fluoride varnish. Promising compounds which are suitable for children are undergoing further research and evaluation include casein phosphopeptide-amorphous calcium phosphate (CPP-ACP), which has demonstrated effectiveness in reducing the dental erosion potential caused by citric acid and acidic sports drinks. In addition, sugar-free chewing gums may be useful for older children who have been identified as having reduced salivary protection.

(III) Monitoring toothwear

Monitoring is essential to determine if the toothwear process is ongoing or has ceased. It may be achieved using dental impressions, study casts and photographs. In adolescents, monitoring of dental sensitivity could also be employed to determine if the patient has been compliant in carrying out recommended preventive behaviours such as avoiding sports drinks. Monitoring of the toothwear is covered in detail in Chapter 8.

(IV) Restorative management

Although attrition in the primary dentition is often self-limiting and does not require restoration (Fig. 2.10), teeth affected by moderate-to-severe erosion will usually need to be restored to protect the exposed tooth surfaces from further destruction. In addition, restorative treatment is often indicated when erosive toothwear is associated with discomfort or loss of aesthetics or reduced occlusal vertical dimensions. In the primary dentition, as erosion removes the thin enamel quickly and the dentine and pulp can be exposed within a relatively short period of time, primary teeth which are not due to exfoliate within a period of 9–12 months and show moderate-sized lesions will require restorations. Furthermore, in children who have lost significant amounts of posterior vertical dimension, regaining the occlusal height will help restore normal occlusal development.

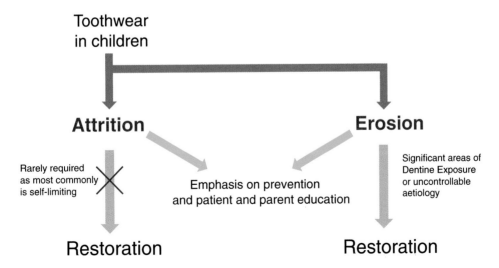

Figure 2.10 Decision pathways for restorative management of toothwear in children.

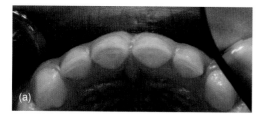 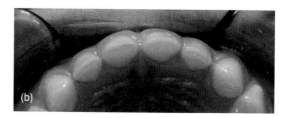

Figure 2.11   Severe palatal erosion on the maxillary primary central incisors resulted in near-exposure of pulp (a). Conservative restoration utilising the sandwich technique with glass ionomer cement lining and composite resin was provided to protect the pulp (b).

Restoration of anterior teeth

Erosive toothwear lesions on the labial and palatal surfaces of the incisors are best restored using composite resins in the young permanent incisors as these teeth are not suitable for full coverage with permanent porcelain crowns. Even on palatal surfaces of primary maxillary incisors, such restorations are appropriate particularly in cases of near pulpal exposure to offer protection to the underlying tooth structures (Fig. 2.11).

If there is sufficient space, the sandwich technique with a glass ionomer lining may be applied. Where there has been a reduction in occlusal vertical dimension from the toothwear, the anterior restorations are usually placed after regaining the occlusal height with posterior crowns, so that optimal anterior crown length and maximum aesthetics may be achieved. Figure 2.12 shows the restoration of the maxillary permanent central incisors of a young athlete affected by erosive toothwear with composite resins. These restorations were placed after regaining vertical occlusal height with stainless steel crowns.

Restoration of posterior teeth

In primary molars, medium-sized cup lesions on the occlusal surfaces may be restored using glass ionomer cements in the deeper parts of the cavity followed by composite resins on the occlusal aspects. Properties of these materials and material selection are further discussed in

Chapter 9. For the more extensive lesions, stainless steel crowns inserted using the conservative technique are probably the best restorative option as these are durable and can restore and maintain arch length and occlusal height. Stainless steel crowns also achieve complete crown coverage, reduce dentine sensitivity and protect the teeth from further erosive damage.

The conservative technique for stainless steel crowns (see Fig. 2.12) is appropriate for management of moderately to severely worn primary molars and permanent first molars in children, as this method utilises minimal tooth preparation (Seow 1984; Seow & Latham 1986). In this technique, the proximal contacts are separated with orthodontic separators between 1 and 7 days prior to crown insertion (Fig. 2.13). When the separators are removed at the operative visit, sufficient interproximal spaces are present, which lessen or eliminate the need for proximal tooth reduction. In contrast to conventional techniques, there is usually minimal need for occlusal reduction as the cusps of the teeth are often severely worn by toothwear. In most cases, when preparing worn teeth for stainless steel crowns, only minimal preparation is required, such as smoothening of the surface line angles with a tapered fine diamond bur. Caries remaining on the teeth should be removed using high- and slow-speed preparation and hand instruments for deeper cavities, which may be lined with a glass ionomer base before luting the stainless steel crowns with a glass ionomer cement.

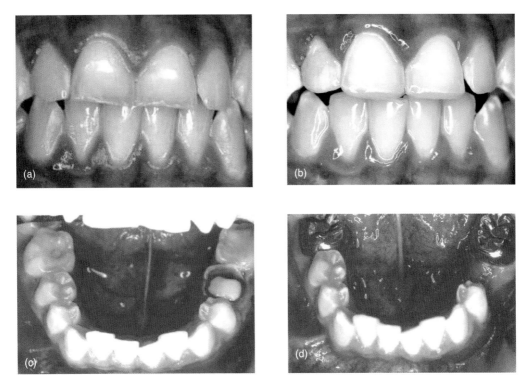

Figure 2.12 The anterior dentition of a 13-year-old athlete who habitually consumed sports drinks during sporting activities was affected by dental erosion, thinning enamel facially and incisally (a). Bonded composite resin facings offered an aesthetic protection of affected surfaces (b). The mandibular first molars were moderately eroded across the occlusal surface with loss of cuspal contours (c). Stainless steel crowns were placed on the mandibular first permanent molars using the conservative technique and the heavily worn and previously restored primary left second molar tooth was extracted (d).

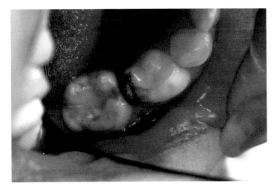

Figure 2.13 Orthodontic tooth separators can be used to create proximal spaces, which facilitate the conservative placement of stainless steel crowns.

Although the occlusal height is usually restored after crown placements, the conservative technique may result in a slight increase in vertical dimension immediately after crown insertion. However, the vertical occlusal height usually returns to its original dimensions within a week or two in the majority of cases. To avoid discomfort associated with slight increases in occlusal height, bilateral crown placements of each arch are recommended, with an intervening period of approximately 4–6 weeks between the treatment of each arch to allow the occlusion to settle before restoring the opposing arch.

THE GLOBAL PERSPECTIVE

High prevalence rates of toothwear in the primary dentition have been reported from various countries. Reports from the United Kingdom have found toothwear reaching dentine on the palatal surfaces of primary teeth to be 8% in 2-year-old and 24% in 5-year-old children (O'Brien 1993). In a recent review of literature, prevalence of toothwear in the primary dentition was reported to range from 6% (China) and 12% (Brazil), to 71% (Germany) and as high as 78% (Australia) (Taji & Seow 2010). In the adolescent permanent dentition, a worldwide prevalence rate of approximately 10–70% has been documented (Taji & Seow 2010). The relatively high prevalence of toothwear in children justifies the recommendation that examining for toothwear lesions be an integral part of the routine paediatric dental examination and that prevention of toothwear be incorporated into the general preventative regime for children. Timely management of toothwear in the primary or mixed dentition prevents the destructive processes continuing into the permanent dentition.

References

Al-Malik, M.I., Holt, R.D., Bedi R. (2001) The relationship between erosion, caries and rampant caries and dietary habits in preschool children in Saudi Arabia. *International Journal of Paediatric Dentistry*, **11**, 430–439.

Barker, D. (2005) Tooth wear as a result of pica. *British Dental Journal*, **199**(5), 271–273.

Dugmore, C.R., Rock, W.P. (2003) Asthma and tooth erosion: is there an association? *International Journal of Paediatric Dentistry*, **13**, 417–424.

Ford, D., Seow, W.K., Newman B., et al. (2009) A controlled study of risk factors for enamel hypoplasia in the permanent dentition. *Pediatric Dentistry*, **31**(5), 382–388.

Ganss, C., Lussi, A. (2006) Diagnosis of erosive tooth wear. *Monorgraphs in Oral Sciences*, **20**, 32–43.

Hart, P.Z., Hart, T.C. (2007) Disorders of Human Dentin. *Cells Tissues Organs*, **186**, 70–77.

Johansson, A.K., Sorvari, R., Birkhed D., et al. (2001) Dental erosion in deciduous teeth – an in vivo and in vitro study. *Journal of Dentistry*, **29**, 333–340.

Khan, F., Young, W.G., Law V., et al. (2001) Cupped lesions of early onset dental erosion in young southeast Queensland adults. *Australian Dental Journal*, **46**, 100–107.

Linnett, V., Seow, W.K. (2001) Dental erosion in children: a literature review. *Pediatric Dentistry*, **23**, 37–43.

Linnett, V., Seow, W.K., Connor F., et al. (2002) Oral health of children with gastroesophageal reflux disease: a controlled study. *Australian Dental Journal*, **47**(2), 156–162.

Milosevic, A. (1997) Sports drinks hazard to teeth. *British Journal of Sports Medicine*, **31**, 28–30.

Nunn, J.H., Ng, S.K., Coulthard M., et al. (2001) The dental implications of chronic use of acidic medicines in medically compromised children. *Pharmacy World and Science*, **23**, 118–119.

O'Brien, M. (1993) *Children's Dental Health in the United Kingdom*. HMSO, London.

Pope, J.E.C. (1991) The dental status of cerbral palsied children. *Pediatric Dentistry*, **13**(3), 156–162.

Seow, W.K. (1984) The application of tooth-separation in clinical pedodontics. *Journal of Dentistry for Children*, **51**(6), 428–430.

Seow, W.K. (1994) Clinical diagnosis and management strategies of amelogenesis imperfecta variants. *Pediatric Dentistry*, **15**(6), 384–393.

Seow, W.K. (1997a) Clinical diagnosis of enamel defects: pitfalls and practical guidelines. *International Dental Journal*, **47**(3), 173–182.

Seow, W.K. (1997b) Effects of preterm birth on oral growth and development. *Australian Dental Journal*, **42**, 85–91.

Seow, W.K., Clifford, H., Battistutta D., et al. (2009) Case-control study of early childhood caries in Australia. *Caries Research*, **43**(1), 25–35.

Seow, W.K., Latham, S.C. (1986) The spectrum of dental manifestation in vitamin D-resistant rickets: implications for management. *Pediatric Dentistry*, **8**(3), 245–250.

Taji, S.S., Savage, N., et al. (2010) Congenital aplasia of the major salivary glands: literature review and case report. *Pediatric Dentistry*, (in press).

Taji, S.S., Seow, W.K. (2010) A review of the literature on dental erosion in children. *Australian Dental Journal*, **55**(4), 358–367.

Watanabe, S., Dawes, C. (1990) Salivary flow rates and salivary film thickness in five year old children. *Journal of Dental Research*, **69**(5), 1150–1153.

Witkop, Jr, C.J. (1988) Ameolgenesis imperfecta, dentinogenesis imperfecta and dentin dysplasia revisited: problems in classification. *Journal of Oral Pathololgy*, **17**, 547–553.

Wright, J.T. (2006) Research review: the molecular etiologies and associated phenotypes of amelogenesis imperfecta. *American Journal of Medical Genetics*, **A**(140A), 2547–2555.

Young, W.G. (2005) Tooth wear: diet analysis and advice. *International Dental Journal*, **55**(2), 68–72.

Young, W.G., Khan, F. (2002) Sites of dental erosion are saliva-dependent. *Journal of Oral Rehabilitation*, **29**, 35–43.

Zero, D.T. (1996) Etiology of dental erosion: extrinsic factors. *European Journal of Oral Science*, **104**, 162–177.

Childhood diet and dental erosion

3

Louise Brearley Messer and William G. Young

The two most common dental diseases in children and adolescents, dental caries and erosion both have strong dietary components in their causation. Dental caries is increasing even in long-term fluoridated communities in Western society, and dental erosion is manifesting as the new disorder resulting in toothwear. Dental erosion is increasing in children, adolescents and teenagers, and in many cases, it is a lifestyle issue where specific causation related to dietary intake and conditions producing dehydration can be identified. Dietary counselling in dental practice can have a major impact on addressing both dental erosion and dental caries.

DENTAL EROSION IN CHILDREN, ADOLESCENTS AND TEENAGERS

Dental erosion is commonly found in these age groups. The extent of the problem was described more than 15 years ago when over 17 000 children were assessed in the UK 1993 National Survey of Children's Dental Health: 52% of 5- to 6-year-olds were found to have one or more eroded primary incisors and 24% of these lesions extended into the dentine; 27% of 12-year-olds showed signs of erosion with 1% of the erosive lesions involving dentine (O'Brien 1994). More recent studies in various countries have made similar observations.

CONCERNS OF PATIENTS AND PARENTS

In the young child, the parents may become concerned when the child resists oral hygiene because the teeth are sensitive to hot or cold water, toothpaste and toothbrushing. Closer inspection of the teeth by the parents may reveal some loss of tooth structure and discolouration. On occasion, the parents may notice that the teeth, especially primary incisors, appear to have become shorter in length and worn down. A change in the child's smile and smile line

Toothwear: The ABC of the Worn Dentition, First Edition. Edited by Farid Khan and William George Young.
© 2011 John Wiley & Sons, Ltd. Published 2011 by John Wiley & Sons, Ltd.

may be noticed, with a reduction in the amount of tooth surface that is visible. Concerned that the permanent incisors may become similarly affected, the parents seek professional dental advice.

CLINICAL APPEARANCE OF DENTAL EROSION

Initially, erosion may appear as a glazed enamel surface with loss of surface features such as perikymata. Early lesions are usually coronal, and the enamel at the gingival margin remains intact, perhaps protected by saliva and gingival crevicular fluid. However, it is difficult to show the patient and the parents that saliva from the major glands protects the surfaces of the deciduous teeth due to absence of cervical lesions (Young & Khan 2002). The patient may present complaining of tooth sensitivity associated with loss of tooth structure. Maxillary anterior teeth of affected primary dentitions show reduction in vertical height and thin, chipped incisal edges. The incisal edges of primary incisors and canines become worn down fully into dentine, and a concave surface is formed as the less mineralised dentine erodes more rapidly than the surrounding enamel. In older children, the palatal surfaces of permanent incisors may show loss of enamel with sharply defined gingival margins. Grey or brown coronal colour changes, visible particularly on the palatal surfaces, may indicate pulpal pathology. The enamel is thinned, and the underlying dentine is visible as yellow or brown. Oval lesions representing pulpal proximity may be visible and the lesions may progress to pulpal exposure.

Primary posterior teeth show flattened convex surfaces or concavities which develop in cusp tips, becoming hollowed out ('cuspal cupping'). Margins of existing restorations (particularly amalgam) may appear raised or 'proud', due to erosive loss of surrounding enamel. More extensive erosion of occlusal surfaces ap-

pears as flattened cuspal inclines or shallow saucer-shaped facets. The facets typically show sharply defined 'leading edges' and more indistinct 'trailing edges', respectively, representing the direction of the occlusal stroke across the enamel surface and patterns of salivary flow (Khan et al. 1998).

DIETARY FINDINGS IN DENTAL EROSION

A number of dietary findings are common in the histories of individuals with erosion. High intakes, both in frequency and in volume, of acidic drinks in particular are noted. These include carbonated soft drinks, fruit juices, juice-flavoured drinks, citrus-flavoured mineral waters, citrus-flavoured cordials and sports drinks. Citrus fruits and spicy snack foods (such as Asian or Mexican snacks) are also reported frequently. Histories may also include medications taken orally that can linger in the mouth and be retained on the teeth, such as asthma powder inhalants, and prolonged holding of vitamin C tablets in the mouth, slowly chewing and swishing them before swallowing.

Consumption of acidic drinks

Most sweet drinks, including diet soft drinks, contain orthophosphoric, carbonic and citric acids; malic, tartaric and other organic acids may also be present. Fruit drinks typically contain 20–30% juice, and food acids may be added during manufacture of both regular sugared and diet soft drinks. Preservatives and food acids, including organic and inorganic acids, are added commonly during manufacture to increase the sharp tang or zesty flavour, and thereby promote the palatability, of citric drinks. These acids supplement the natural acidity of citrus juice and considerably increase the erosive potential of acidic drinks. Examples of such acids are 300 ascorbic acid, 330 citric acid, 331 sodium citrates (mono-, di- and trisodium citrate), 334 tartaric acid, 338 phosphoric acid, 260 acetic acid, 270 lactic acid, 296 malic acid and 297 fumaric acid coded numerically by food industry standards. Sports drinks contain citric acid. Supplemented fruit juices contain organic acids from fruit concentrates, such as citric acid from oranges, malic acid from apples and guarana extract.

Soft drinks have little nutritional value, contain high amounts of sugar and are classified as an 'extrafood' to be consumed only occasionally or in small amounts (National Health and Medical Research Council [NHMRC] Australian Government 2005). In addition to acids, soft drinks contain simple sugars (glucose, fructose, sucrose, maltose and lactose) which can serve as metabolic substrates for cariogenic bacteria. A can (375 mL) of soft drink in Australia may contain 10 teaspoons of sugar, while in the United States, a can (345 mL) of regular soft drink is labelled to contain up to 11 teaspoons of sugar.

Consumption of sports drinks

Sports drinks are recommended widely by organisations for athletes as sources of carbohydrates, electrolytes and water for energy and rehydration and are consumed frequently during or following athletic events. During strenuous exercise, salivary gland function is unable to meet the metabolic demands and the oral mucosa becomes dehydrated. The enamel is then largely unprotected by saliva and is susceptible to erosive risk from acidic sports drinks. A study of Australian university students participating in a variety of athletic clubs found significant associations between their reported dental erosion, tooth sensitivity and age and their frequency of drinking juices and sports drinks (Sirimaharaj et al. 2002).

Sports drink consumption is no longer solely the habit of high-performance athletes; such drinks are consumed frequently following less demanding exercise, such as gardening, or as recreational or social drinks. Erosion from sports drinks is therefore no longer limited to elite athletes.

Erosive potential of acidic drinks

Juices, regular sugared soft drinks, diet soft drinks, fruit-flavoured drinks and sports drinks can all erode enamel. The enamel dissolution by soft drink acids can exceed the effects of bacterial acids from metabolism of sugars in the drink. The pH range of most fruit juices, soft drinks and sports drinks is 2.5–4.5, which is below the critical pH range associated with demineralisation of enamel under ambient concentrations of salivary calcium and phosphate (see Chapter 5). Of importance in dietary counselling, regular sugared and diet soft drinks have similar erosive potential. Sports drinks and cola drinks have an immediate erosive potential tenfold higher than that of fruit juices (Jensdottir et al. 2006).

Regular sugared and diet soft drinks have high titratable acidity (TA). TA is deemed more important than pH in determining the erosive potential of a drink. TA determines the amount of hydrogen ions available to interact with the enamel surface. Foods and drinks can have similar pH values, but vary in erosive potential due to differing values for TA. In the laboratory, TA is measured as the volume of base (e.g. sodium hydroxide) required to neutralise the acidity to a given pH (typically 7). For example, a greater volume of base may be required for orange juice than for a cola drink. Therefore, the TA of the orange juice is greater than that of the cola drink, indicating a greater potential for erosivity. In addition, acids have pK_a values, which describe how readily hydrogen ions can dissociate from compounds, indicating the amount of acid available. Relatively low pK_a values, e.g. for citric acid, indicate that hydrogen ions can readily dissociate in this acid.

Diluting an acidic drink with water reduces the erosivity of the drink by lowering the TA, but has little effect on pH. Diluting fruit drinks with water up to a ratio of 1:15 has been found to raise pH values significantly, but even greater dilution is required to reduce overall acidity. This approach is impractical for it diminishes the palatability of the drink (Hunter et al. 2008). At higher temperatures the erosivity of acidic drinks is increased, associated with decreased pH, decreased enamel hardness and increased depth of erosive lesions (Barbour et al. 2006). Of importance then in dietary counselling, individuals choosing to consume acidic drinks should be advised to drink these chilled.

Sports drinks have low pH values and high TA values. Laboratory studies of the effect of sports drinks on enamel have shown that the initial erosive effect is demineralisation, apparent as a pre-softening of the surface enamel. The processes of oral hygiene and masticatory forces on the enamel then lead to attrition with loss of superficial enamel. Repeated application of a sports drink produces deeper enamel loss. An *in vitro* study has shown that adding low concentrations of casein phosphopeptide-amorphous calcium phosphate (CPP-ACP, 0.1–0.2% w/v) to four citric-flavoured soft drinks significantly decreased erosive depths of enamel (Manton et al. 2008). Adding CPP-ACP to a sports drink decreased the erosion potential, attributed to raising the pH and decreasing the TA of the modified drink (Ramalingam et al. 2005). Preliminary studies have shown that supplementing sports drinks with CPP-ACP had no discernible effect on the taste of the product as determined by a taste panel (Ramalingam et al. 2005).

DENTAL EROSION AS A LIFESTYLE ISSUE

Changes in societal behaviours over the last 30 years have increased availability and access to fast food, processed foods and drinks. Today in Western societies, fewer meals are eaten together in families and there is increasing reliance on meals eaten away from home. A great increase in availability and consumption of acidic drinks has occurred – including carbonated soft drinks, fruit juices, juice-flavoured drinks, citrus-flavoured mineral waters and sports drinks – by children, adolescents and teenagers. This has been accompanied by advertising and promotion, much of which is directed towards young people.

Erosive risk factors

Erosion is considered a lifestyle issue, with both dietary selection and intake habits combining as risk factors. From a clinical study in the United Kingdom, the relative erosive risk of popular acidic drinks has been formulated into simple clinical recommendations for patients as follows: holding or swishing acidic drinks in the mouth increases the risk of erosion by 25-fold; having more than one 'fizzy' drink per day increases the risk of erosion by 6-fold; having more than one glass of fruit juice per day increases the risk of erosion by 3-fold; and not drinking water increases the risk of erosion by 11-fold (O'Sullivan & Curzon 2000). Confirming these observations, a recent Australian study of primary-school children, based on a parent questionnaire and a clinical examination, reported statistically significant risk factors for erosion in terms of odds ratios (ORs): drinking two to four cups of soft drink per day (9.5); drinking two to four cups of fruit juice per day (3.2); and consuming citrus sweets once or more per day (5.1; Fung 2009).

Asthma and erosion

The clinical presentation of a child with asthma is illustrated in Fig. 3.1. Asthma is a common condition in children, adolescents and teenagers, and poses particular erosive risk. Both erosion and asthma appear to be increasing in Western societies. The child with asthma is often thirsty, and the acidic anti-inflammatory aerosol medications used in treatment may be dispersed onto the teeth and soft tissues in addition to the pharynx. Wanting to immediately overcome the taste of the

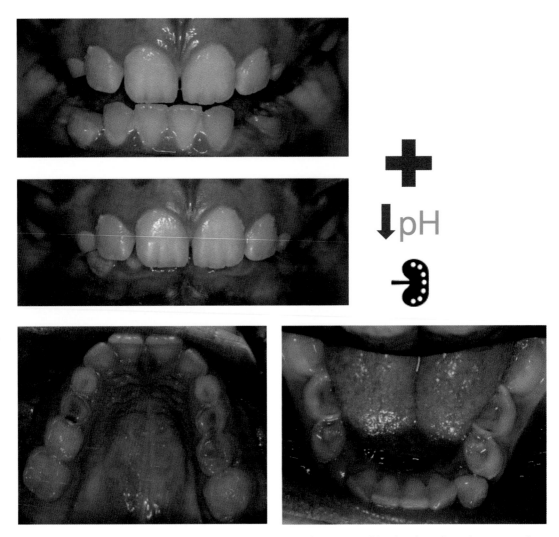

Figure 3.1 Severe dental erosion on the primary dentition of a 10-year-old girl with moderately severe asthma controlled twice daily with corticosteroids and long-acting beta-2 agonists and relieved with 5 mL of salbutamol nebuliser as required. Her cervical lymph nodes were tender secondary to an upper respiratory infection. Near pulp exposures on her maxillary primary canines and first molar. The second primary molars were less affected and the margins of the restoration on tooth 74 were elevated. Wear on her permanent teeth was negligible.

medication and reduce their dehydration, the child with asthma favours drinking acidic drinks in preference to water.

The beta-2 adrenoceptor agonists used in asthma management reduce salivary flow and thereby reduce its acid-buffering capacity, so the acidic drink is not well buffered in the mouth. Instead of reaching for acidic drinks after using these medications, the individual with asthma should be encouraged to drink water for rehydration and rinse thoroughly with water to minimise the erosive potential of the medications. To further complicate matters, one of possible side effects of asthma medications is gastric reflux and hence intrinsic acids.

Diabetes mellitus and erosion

One of the key presentations of diabetes mellitus in a child is constant thirst. Children are more likely to be recommended sugar-free drinks than water, with the consequent risk of erosion. Alternatively, sweet drinks may have been recommended by other health professionals to address the child's need to prevent hypoglycaemic episodes. Thus consultation with the child's physician, diabetic nurse, dietitian and parents is necessary to formulate a health care plan which addresses both the patient's metabolic and dental concerns.

Overweight and obesity

Clear associations between soft drink intake, increased energy intake and increased body weight have been found, and there is now strong evidence linking the intake of sweet drinks, particularly soft drinks, to childhood weight gain and obesity. As a health intervention to combat obesity, sales of sweet drinks in government schools in Victoria, Australia, were banned in 2007; regular sugared soft drinks can no longer be sold or consumed in these schools. Diet (low- or no-sugar alternative) soft drinks are permitted, as are fruit juices (no added sugar) and milk. In the United States, the American Association of Pediatrics and the American Academy of Pediatric Dentistry have also recommended eliminating sweet drinks access in elementary schools to prevent health problems related to overconsumption (AAP 2004; AAPD 2007–2008).

Relationships between increasing obesity and soft drink consumption of children have been shown in the United States and Australia. A prospective study of American children found sweet drink intake was associated with obesity in 11- to 12-year-olds, with the obesity risk estimated to increase 60% for each can of soft drink consumed daily (Ludwig

et al. 2001). A 2-year longitudinal, cross-sectional study of grade 3–5 children residing in Nebraska, United States, found increased diet soft drink intake was associated with increased body mass index scores (Blum et al. 2005). Amongst Australian children, similar associations have been noted between sweet drink intake and increasing body weight. In 1995 the Australian Bureau of Statistics (ABS) National Nutrition Survey investigated fluid intakes of 5- to 12-year-olds and found that overweight or obese children tended to obtain more energy from drinks other than milk or water than those in a healthy weight range (Australian Bureau of Statistics 1998). A longitudinal study of Australian children found soft drink or cordial consumption at age 8 years was associated statistically with excess weight gain 5 years later (Tam et al. 2006), and a study of 4- to 12-year-olds in Victoria, Australia, found those regularly drinking sweet drinks, and those who had drunk more than two serves of juice, cordial or soft drink on the day prior to the survey day, were twice as likely to be overweight or obese (Sanigorski et al. 2007).

Concerning general health, obese children and adolescents are at increased risk of sleep apnoea, mobility impairment, diabetes type II, early development of cardiovascular disease risk factors, greater risk of adult obesity and associated health risks. Concerning dental health, the increased consumption of acidic sugared drinks has clear correlations with both dental erosion and dental caries.

RECOMMENDATIONS FOR PATIENTS TO REDUCE EROSION

Frequency and timing of consumption of acidic drinks

Frequent between-meal consumption of acidic drinks presents a major erosive risk for the dentition. Individuals with erosion, or those at risk for erosion, and who want to continue consuming acidic drinks should be encouraged to have these *with* meals, rather than *between* meals. The best between-meal drink to encourage is water. Consuming acidic drinks at meals reduces the potential for erosion as the effects are diluted by the presence of other substances in the mouth at the same time, which may counteract the acidity.

Drinking habits that allow slow consumption, such as swishing, slow sipping, and from pop-tops and spout cups, should be avoided. If straws are used, they should be placed towards the back of the mouth, so that acidic fluids are not delivered directly onto the tooth surfaces. A popular habit among adolescents and teenagers is to hold the carbonated soft drink in the mouth for a prolonged period, enjoying the sensation of the carbonation bubbles 'popping' on the mucosa. Swishing of soft drinks around the mouth so that the teeth and soft tissues become bathed in the acidic fluid for extended periods is also popular. The erosive risk of these habits should be explained to the individual and more favourable drinking patterns established (Table 3.1).

Guidelines for safe use of acidic soft drinks

Sound guidelines for dentally 'safe use' of acidic soft drinks have now been established and are implemented readily by parents and patients (Tahmassebi et al. 2006). These guidelines are as follows: limit consumption of acidic drinks to mealtimes; keep drinking times short; do not use soft drink in an infant's nursing bottle; consume soft drink chilled using a straw; do not swish or hold a soft drink in the mouth, and avoid toothbrushing immediately after consumption. Acidic drinks should be avoided at bedtime. Recommendations for safer consumption of acidic drinks must be advocated by all health professionals and promoted to the community to educate and benefit those who regularly consume these drinks (Tahmassebi et al. 2006).

Individuals using asthma medications should drink water rather than acidic drinks for rehydration and should rinse thoroughly with water after taking aerosol medications to minimise the erosive risk. Athletes should manage their dehydration during sports events

Table 3.1 Clinical recommendations for prevention of dental erosion.

Condition	Recommendations
Eroded enamel	Avoid acidic drinks or limit intake to meal times Avoid holding and swishing acidic drinks in the mouth Drink acidic drinks through a straw placed to back of mouth Avoid toothbrushing for an hour after acidic drinks Use a fluoride gel toothpaste instead of an abrasive toothpaste Apply a remineralising casein phosphopeptide-amorphous calcium phosphate crème
Asthma	Rinse with water after taking aerosol medications Avoid acidic drinks or limit intake to meal times
Athletes	Drink water before and after athletic events to reduce dehydration Rinse with water after consuming sports drinks
Vomiting	Avoid toothbrushing after vomiting Rinse with a neutral pH fluoride mouthrinse Use a fluoride gel toothpaste or desensitising toothpaste instead of an abrasive toothpaste Apply a remineralising casein phosphopeptide-amorphous calcium phosphate crème

by drinking 2 L of water 2 h before, or 1 L of water 1 h before, the session. If sports drinks are consumed for energy and electrolyte balance during the athletic event, water should also be included and the athlete should rehydrate with water and rinse with water following the event. Concentrated acidic products designed for rapid energy boosts should be avoided when saliva is reduced and the oral mucosa is dehydrated.

While increasing water consumption is strongly recommended for all patients, particularly those with erosion or at risk for erosion, it is important to also recognise that many individuals choose bottled water preferentially over fluoridated tap water. Bottled waters have become very popular worldwide. Bottled waters typically do not contain fluoride at optimal levels for caries prevention, although legislation in some countries (e.g. Australia and United States) now permits manufacturers to add fluoride and suitably label and market these products as containing fluoride for caries prevention. Individuals choosing to drink bottled water only may then be at risk of not receiving the caries-preventing benefits of community water fluoridation. Individuals at risk for dental erosion should be reminded that the preferred water source is one containing an optimal level of fluoride.

Oral hygiene advice

Patients with erosion, or those at risk of erosion, should be encouraged to delay toothbrushing for about an hour after consuming acidic drinks. This is to allow the natural remineralising processes of saliva to occur, i.e. to avoid 'disturbing' the tooth surface. The pre-softened enamel is readily brushed away if a period of remineralisation is not allowed. Instead of immediate toothbrushing, a water rinse is recommended. For the same reasons, toothbrushing immediately after vomiting should be avoided. Instead, a non-alcoholic, neutral pH fluoride mouthrinse or a basic sodium bicarbonate

mouthrinse should be used to counteract the gastric acidity in the mouth and to refresh the mouth (see Table 3.1).

Toothbrushing should be performed using a fluoride gel toothpaste or a desensitising toothpaste, rather than an abrasive toothpaste, as once again the pre-softened enamel can be removed by the abrasive particles. A daily or weekly non-alcoholic, neutral pH fluoride mouthrinse can be recommended to promote remineralisation. A cream containing CPP-ACP (with or without added fluoride, Tooth Mousse™) can also be recommended.

DENTAL EROSION AND DENTAL CARIES COMPARED

Dental caries is a multifactorial disease in which diet is a primary risk factor, although other factors such as suboptimal fluoride exposure, past caries, sociodemographics, saliva and medical conditions are implicated. Dietary risk factors include the amount of sugars consumed, manner of consumption, frequency of exposure and retentiveness of fermentable carbohydrates in dental plaque. Following widespread introduction of community water fluoridation, the cariogenicity of sugar is weaker due to the protective influence of fluoride from multiple sources. Fluoride has raised the threshold of sugar exposure required to promote caries progression to cavitation in fluoridated communities. Common fermentable carbohydrates in Western diets are simple sugars (glucose, fructose, sucrose, maltose and lactose) found in sweet drinks and sweet foods; these can be metabolic substrates for cariogenic bacteria. Between-meal consumption, high frequency of intake and plaque retention all increase the cariogenic potential of sweet foods and sweet drinks.

Dental erosion appears to be increasing in all age groups, and in many cases, it is a lifestyle issue where specific causation related to dietary intake and conditions producing dehydration can be identified. Between-meal consumption increases the frequency of acid exposure; the more often the dentition is recoated with dietary acids, the more severe the dental erosion and subsequent toothwear will become. Concerning dental caries, retention and bacterial metabolism of sugars within plaque allow slow and sustained demineralisation to occur over a period of just under 1 h. Conversely, dental erosion is associated with rapid periods of acidic demineralisation. Hence, the modes of consumption, whether through a straw, bottle or cup, sipped slowly or swished, or drunk all at once, are pertinent in accelerating the erosive processes. Effective dietary advice aimed at preventing erosion must, therefore, address drinking habits in addition to amount and frequency of consumption.

DIETARY COUNSELLING FOR CHILDREN AND ADOLESCENTS

Indications in dental practice

In dental practice, all patients should be alerted to the importance of diet in oral health. Dietary counselling by dental staff is indicated particularly in individuals where teeth show erosion or a high caries experience. Moreover, referral to a dietitian may be indicated where existing diabetic management of a patient's diet calls for collaboration between health professionals. Children with type I diabetes, placed on low-sugar diets, rarely experience dental caries.

Current basis and national guidelines

The current basis for dietary counselling in Australia is the dietary guidelines published by the National Health and Medical Research Council (NHMRC) (2005), which provide Recommended Daily Amounts (RDAs) in five food groups for different ages, with additional general recommendations for healthy dietary selections (NHMRC Australian Government 2005). Comparable to dietary guidelines promulgated in the United Kingdom and United States, the five food groups described by the NHMRC are breads and cereals, fruit and vegetables, meat and meat alternatives, milk and dairy products, and fluids. As numbers of servings per day for different age groups, RDAs are as follows: breads and cereals: four or more; meat and meat alternatives: one or more; milk and milk products: three or more (more for teenagers and pregnant and lactating women); fruit and vegetables: 4- to 7-year-olds: one fruit plus two vegetables, 8- to 11-year-olds: one fruit plus three vegetables, 12- to 18-year-olds: four fruit plus four vegetables, adults: two fruit plus five vegetables; water: eight cups of non-alcoholic fluids (NHMRC Australian Government 2005).

Recent information suggests that many Australian children and adolescents are failing to meet these guidelines. The current inadequacies in their diets were demonstrated recently in an Australian National Children's Nutrition and Physical Activity Survey (2007). This survey found that only 61% of 4- to 8-year-old children met the RDA for fruit consumption (one to three serves), increasing to 93% if juices were included. Only 3% met the RDA for vegetable consumption (two to four serves), increasing to 22% if potatoes were included. Among 9- to 13-year-olds, only 51% met the RDA for fruit consumption (one to three serves), increasing to 90% if juices were included. And only 2% met the RDA for vegetable intake (two to four serves), increasing to 14% if potatoes were included. Clearly, children and adolescents are at risk of inadequate intake of fruit sufficient to meet their RDAs unless juice is included, which can pose an erosive risk. Moreover, the marked inadequacy in vegetable intake is a major concern for nutritional adequacy and also has relevance for dental erosion since chewing the fibre in fresh fruit and vegetables promotes salivation. This pattern appears to be occurring in other developed countries, including the United Kingdom and

United States, reflecting a substitution of fruit, vegetables and dairy products with processed foods and drinks.

Low intake of milk and milk products by children is also a concern as acidic drinks may be displacing milk as well as water in the diets of many children. A parent questionnaire conducted in 2009 of primary-school children in fluoridated Melbourne, Australia, found that 35% of 4- to 7-year-olds and 26% of 8- to 12-year-olds had not consumed any milk on the day previous to the study day (Lee & Messer 2010). Similar inadequacies in diets of children and adolescents in other Western countries may well be occurring. As dairy produce and fresh green vegetables are major sources of dietary calcium, the RDA of calcium for growing children may not presently be adequate.

A clinical approach to dietary counselling

Dietary counselling can be performed informally by discussing the patient's favourite foods and drinks or formally using a food frequency list (Table 3.2) or a diet diary recorded over several days. The informal food approach includes asking the patient open-ended questions about their preferred foods and drinks, perhaps including pamphlets from the local dental association or nutrition groups concerning healthy eating for oral health. This approach can often identify an adverse habit of dental importance, e.g. consuming acidic drinks or foods at bedtime.

Using a food frequency list

The food frequency list is an assembly of common foods and drinks, including local popular items. The patient 'ticks and tallies, counts and plots' these on a healthy eating plan, e.g. on the Healthy Eating Pyramid (available from the Australian Nutrition Foundation, www.nutritionaustralia.org), shown in Fig. 3.2. The Healthy Eating Pyramid is three tiered, with foods to be eaten most (e.g. fruit, veg-

etables, breads, cereals and pasta) in the base, foods to be eaten moderately (e.g. meat, fish, eggs and dairy products) in the middle, and foods to be eaten in small amounts (e.g. spreads, oils, butter and margarine) in the top tier. Alongside is a tap, promoting water consumption, and a crossed-out salt shaker, advising salt avoidance. Running figures around the pyramid encourage physical activity. A quick comparison of their preferences can show the clinician and the patient if their overall diet is in balance.

Using a diet diary

The diet diary requires the patient to keep a daily record of everything they eat and drink for several days, including any medications taken. Since weekday and weekend diets usually vary, a 6- or 7-day diet diary (Table 3.3) gives the best representation of intakes. The patient or parents records everything consumed, concentrating on servings or exposures, rather than portion sizes.

The distribution of servings in each of the five food groups is then tabulated on a worksheet (Table 3.4). The frequency and timing of fluid intake is particularly relevant to erosion. The recommended RDAs are one to one and a half litre of non-alcoholic fluids per day, and attention should be paid to the types of fluids consumed, as well as the timing and frequency of intake.

The first consideration in discussing the diet is nutritional adequacy, i.e. does the diet meet the RDAs for the patient's age and energy needs? Only secondarily should the diet be discussed in relation to the dental condition which prompted the dietary counselling. This sequence is important because the dental condition may well be occurring when overall diet is nutritionally inadequate. For example, a child may be snacking frequently on acidic drinks and spicy snacks because their energy needs are not being met by regular meals. Increasing food intake at main meals should then lead to reduced between-meal snacks and improved

Table 3.2 A sample food frequency list.

Name: _____ Age: _____ Male: _____ Female: _____

In the list below, tick the box that best describes how frequently you usually have these foods and drinks.

Foods and drinks	Never have this √	Have this sometimes √	Have this frequently √
Breads			
Cereals			
Rice			
Pasta			
Noodles			
Crackers (add local items)			
Potatoes			
Carrots			
Peas			
Beans			
Tomatoes			
Zucchini			
Broccoli (add local items)			
Apples			
Oranges			
Bananas			
Grapes			
Plums (add local items)			
Milk			
Yogurt			
Cheese			
Milk alternatives (add local items)			
Meat			
Chicken			
Fish			
Nuts			
Legumes (add local items)			
Cakes			
Pies			
Sweet biscuits			
Soft drinks			
Sweets			
Chocolate (add local items)			

energy balance, leading to reduced erosivity of the diet. It is important to address the individual dietary preferences and habits as adverse patterns established in childhood can persist into adulthood with detrimental long-term effects on general and dental health.

Discussing the diet diary

The diet diary should be discussed in a neutral environment, such as a consultation room, as the dental surgery may be an emotionally charged environment for the patient. The diet is

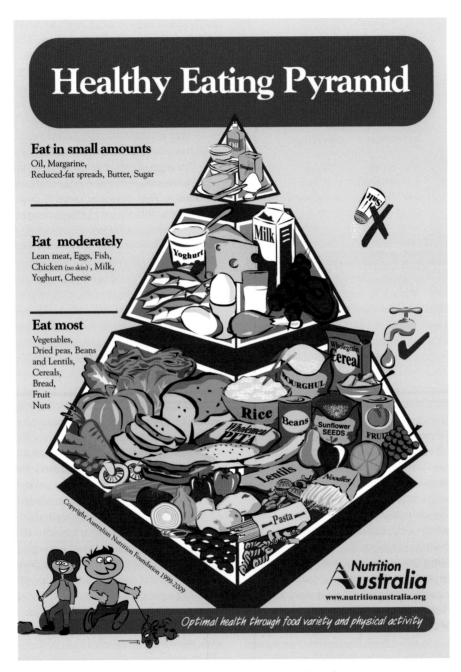

Figure 3.2 The Healthy Eating Pyramid. (By permission of Nutrition Australia.)

Table 3.3   A sample diet diary.

Name: _____ Age: _____ Male: _____ Female: _____
Record everything you eat and drink during the coming week and include any medications you take. Don't worry about portion sizes, just record all the different items and when you eat or drink them.

Days	Breakfast	Mid-morning	Lunch	Mid-afternoon	Dinner	Evening and night-time
Example	One bowl oatmeal and milk, one glass orange juice, one slice toast with butter and honey	One cup choc milk, one vitamin tablet	One cheese sandwich, two choc chip cookies, one glass milk	One glass fizzy orange drink, one box raisins	One plain hamburger, French fries, one glass coke	One glass fizzy orange drink, one handful small snack crackers
Day 1						
Day 2						
Day 3						
Day 4						
Day 5						
Day 6						
Day 7						

discussed (rather than 'reviewed' or 'assessed') empathetically in the context of the family and social history, noting that foods and drinks can have deep emotional and cultural significance. Many social groups preserve identity by traditional strongly held eating habits and dietary beliefs. Today's lifestyles should be acknowledged, noting an increase in meals consumed away from home and takeaway meals, multi-snacks instead of regular meals, peer pressure for 'designer' foods and drinks, and less weekly but more daily food shopping.

The erosive risk assessment

After discussing the patient's overall nutritional adequacy from tabulating the diet diary, the key considerations in conducting an erosive risk assessment are as follows: Are the age-relevant RDAs for intake of fruit and vegetables met? Is the RDA for fluid intake met, and is it met based primarily by consuming water and milk? To what extent are other fluids such as acidic drinks contributing to the fluid intake? To what extent are acidic drinks contributing to the total energy intake? Are acidic drinks recognised as occasional drinks or are they consumed regularly? At what time of the day are acidic drinks consumed? What kinds of snacks are consumed regularly? Are these dry and spicy in nature? Is the RDA for milk and milk products being met?

On the basis of observations from the diet diary, the overall erosive risk is then classified as low, moderate or high. Clinical experience indicates that managing erosion in children, adolescents and teenagers often focuses on increasing water intake, reducing acidic

Table 3.4 Tally sheet for diet diary.

Tally up all the foods and drinks consumed by the patient under the food groups. Then add up all the exposures and calculate their average daily exposure to each food group over the week and compare this with the Recommended Daily Amounts (RDAs) shown at the top of each food group column.

Age groups (y)	Breads, cereals, rice, pasta, noodles (RDA)	Vegetables (RDA)	Fruit (RDA)	Milk, yogurt, cheese (RDA)	Lean meat, fish, poultry, nuts, legumes (RDA)	Extras (e.g. cakes, pies, soft drinks, sweets, etc.) (RDA)
4–7	5–7	2	1	2	$\frac{1}{2}$	1–2
8–11	6–9	3	1	2	1	1–2
12–18	5–11	4	4	3	1	1–3
Example from Table 3.3	IIIII	I	I	III	I	IIIII
Day 1						
Day 2						
Day 3						
Day 4						
Day 5						
Day 6						
Day 7						
Average intake						

Source: NHMRC 2005.

drink consumption, eating more fresh fruit and vegetables, and increasing intake of calcium-containing foods and drinks (Young 2005). Patients and parents should be advised that foods and drinks can be categorised based on their relative acidity and sugar contents. A simple classification published recently in a popular Australian consumer magazine classifies foods and drinks by brand names as those with higher sugar and higher acidity (e.g. brand-named sour candies, honey and no-added-sugar fruit juices); higher sugar and lower acidity (e.g. brand-named sweetened cereals, muesli bars and low-acid fruit juices); lower sugar and higher acidity (e.g. brand-named spicy snacks, sugar-free candies, sports drinks, high-energy drinks and no-added-sugar cordials); and lower sugar and lower acidity (e.g. low-sugar cereals, milk and water; Oakenfull & Cochrane 2010).

Simple approaches to preventing erosion

Emphasis on increasing the nutritional intake (food volume) at main meals, instead of multiple eating episodes throughout the day ('grazing'), can be effective in promoting good nutrition, reducing erosive and cariogenic snacks, and allowing saliva to maintain enamel mineralisation.

In motivating dietary changes, the clinician must talk in simple terms, *with* rather than *at* the patient or parent, leading them to suggest feasible changes they can make. The clinician's attitudes should be enthusiastic and non-judgemental, believing that change is possible and rewarding dietary changes with praise, no matter how small the accomplishment. For example, in reducing acidic drink consumption, the frequency of intake could be halved in the first week, halved again in the second week, and so on, until the habit has been eliminated and replaced with more favourable drinking patterns. Information overload should be avoided, e.g. not giving dietary recommendations and teaching toothbrushing and flossing, all in one appointment. A stepwise approach is recommended for achieving realistic goals.

THE KEY MESSAGES

The dietary factors in erosion and dental caries are similar, and the oral health promotion messages for each overlap fully. Dietary counselling can be an effective approach to managing both the conditions in children, adolescents and teenagers. The consumption of fruit, vegetables and dairy products is decreasing, while the consumption of acidic drinks is increasing, with associated erosive and cariogenic risks to the dentition. Adverse dietary patterns established during childhood can persist into later years, with detrimental long-term effects on dental and general health.

The frequency and timing of consumption of acidic drinks should be included in discussing dietary risk factors for both dental erosion and dental caries with patients and parents. Recommendations for safer consumption of acidic drinks must be advocated by health professionals and promoted to the community in order to educate and benefit regular con-

sumers of these drinks. Public health information should increase awareness that intake of acidic drinks can have deleterious effects on the dentition, as well as the potential for promoting systemic diseases. Restricting sales of sweet drinks and sweet foods and providing healthy food and drinks for purchase in schools is paramount. Sporting children should be encouraged to drink water before sports events and avoid sports drinks and soft drinks when dehydrated after sports. Especially for older children and adults, it is ideal to drink water before sports events, 2 L 2 h before, 1 L 1 h before.

References

AAP (2004) American Academy of Pediatrics, Committee on School Health. Soft drinks in schools. *Pediatrics*, **113**, 152–154.

AAPD (2007–2008) American Academy of Paediatric Dentistry, Council on Clinical Affairs. Policy on beverage vending machines in schools. *Pediatric Dentistry*, **29**, 47–48.

Australian Bureau of Statistics (1998) *National Nutrition Survey of Nutrient Intakes and Physical Measurements (1995)*. Canberra, Australia.

Barbour, M.E., Finke, M., Parker, D.M., et al. (2006) The relationship between enamel softening and erosion caused by soft drinks at a range of temperatures. *Journal of Dentistry*, **34**, 207–213.

Blum, J.W., Jacobsen, D.J., Donnelly, J.E. (2005) Beverage consumption patterns in elementary school aged children across a two-year period. *Journal of the American College of Nutrition*, **24**, 93–98.

Fung, A. (2009) Tooth wear: prevalence and risk factors in a sample of primary school aged children. DCD thesis, University of Melbourne, Australia.

Hunter, M.L., Patel, R., Loyn, T., et al. (2008) The effect of dilution on the in vitro erosive potential of a range of dilutable fruit drinks. *International Journal of Paediatric Dentistry*, **18**, 251–255.

Jensdottir, T., Holbrook, P., Nauntofte, B., et al. (2006) Immediate erosive potential of cola drinks and orange juices. *Journal of Dental Research*, **85**, 226–230.

Khan, F., Young, W.G., Daley, T.J. (1998) Dental erosion and bruxism. A tooth wear analysis from South East Queensland. *Australian Dental Journal*, **43**, 117–127.

Lee, J.G., Messer, L.B. (2010) Intake of sweet drinks and sweet treats versus reported and observed caries experience. *European Archives of Paediatric Dentistry*, **11**, 5–17.

Ludwig, D.S., Peterson, K.E., Gortmaker, S.L. (2001) Relationship between consumption of sugar-sweetened drinks and childhood obesity: a prospective, observational analysis. *Lancet*, **357**, 505–508.

Manton, D.C., Cai, F., Yuen, Y., et al. (2008) The effect of adding casein phosphopeptide-amorphous calcium phosphate complexes to soft drinks on enamel erosion in vitro. Caries Research *(Abstract)*, **42**, 188.

National Health and Medical Research Council, Department of Health and Aging, Australian Government (2005) *Dietary Guidelines for Australians. A Guide to Healthy Eating*. National Health and Medical Research Council, Canberra.

Oakenfull, D., Cochrane, N. (2010) Eating away your teeth. *Choice*, July 24. Available at: www.choice.com.au. Last accessed August 2, 2010.

O'Brien, M. (1994) *Children's Dental Health in the United Kingdom 1993*. Her Majesty's Stationery Office, London.

O'Sullivan, E.A., Curzon, M.E. (2000) A comparison of acidic dietary factors in children with and without dental erosion. *American Society of Dentistry for Children*, **67**, 186–192.

Ramalingam, L., Messer, L.B., Reynolds, E.C. (2005) Adding casein phosphopeptide-amorphous calcium to sports drinks to eliminate in vitro erosion. *Pediatric Dentistry*, **27**, 61–67.

Sanigorski, A.M., Bell, A.C, Swinburn, B.A. (2007) Association of key foods and beverages with obesity in Australian schoolchildren. *Public Health Nutrition*, **10**, 152–157.

Sirimaharaj, V., Messer, L.B., Morgan, M.V. (2002) Acidic diet and dental erosion among athletes. *Australian Dental Journal*, **47**, 228–236.

Tahmassebi, J.F., Duggal, M.S., Malik-Kotru, G, et al. (2006) Soft drinks and dental health: a review of the current literature. *Journal of Dentistry*, **34**, 2–11.

Tam, C.S., Garnett, S.P., Cowell, C.T., et al. (2006) Soft drink consumption and excess weight gain in Australian school students: results from the Nepean Study. *International Journal of Obesity*, **30**, 1091–1093.

Young, W.G. (2005) Tooth wear: diet analysis and advice. *International Dental Journal*, **55**, 68–72.

Young, W.G., Khan, F. (2002) Sites of dental erosion are saliva-dependent. *Journal of Oral Rehabilitation*, **29**, 35–43.

The oral presentation of toothwear in adults

4

Farid Khan and William G. Young

Toothwear processes are active at different times in the life of an individual and differ from person to person. As considered in the preceding chapters, some patients may have a large amount of tooth structure loss occurring early in life, whilst others do so at a later stage. In either case, all patients with toothwear have alternating stages of stability and progression throughout their lifespan. The presentation of toothwear in adults is thus a cumulative result of all the events leading to the state of the dentition at the time of presentation. The case shown in Fig. 4.1 highlights how progression of toothwear processes challenges even the most technically sound restorations, when patient compliance is lacking, their lifestyles continue to challenge their dentition and when the underlying aetiology may not have been fully appreciated during the assessment and diagnostic stages.

DIAGNOSTIC MODALITIES

For correct prevention, management and possibly restorative intervention, if required, to be implemented, correct identification of toothwear lesions, toothwear processes and underlying aetiology is paramount. Diagnostic and assessment modalities used to identify dental caries are inappropriate and differ substantially from those applied to toothwear (Table 4.1).

Diagnostically, no one tool exists to detect dental erosion or toothwear, making visual identification and evaluation of clinical appearance essential (Lussi et al. 2009). Those diagnostic modalities useful in the detection of dental caries have limited application in the assessment of toothwear and are more applicable to general patient examination to exclude other dental anomalies. Radiographs are of benefit to identify or exclude the presence

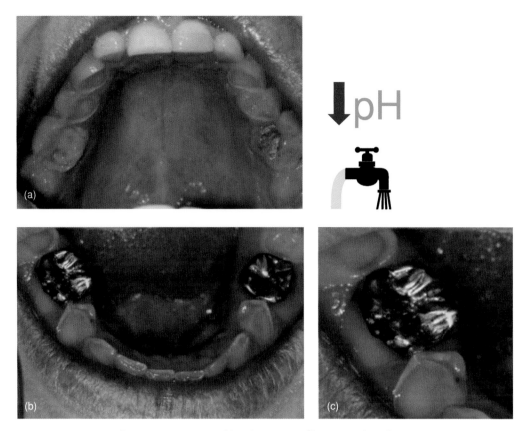

Figure 4.1   Severe toothwear in a 22-year-old male patient affecting tooth surfaces across the dentition. The patient reported a partygoing lifestyle, regular binge drinking, frequent vomiting and high volumes of acidic beverage consumption over the past 5 years. He admitted drinking no water throughout the day and instead resorted to acidic beverages. He was aware of a severely dry mouth particularly at rave parties when resorting to recreational drugs. Severe erosion affected the palatal surfaces of the maxillary teeth (a). Gold onlays were placed on the mandibular first molar teeth (b) at the age of 17 years as his dentist suspected a bruxism habit and had a splint made, which he has worn every night since fabrication. Since placement, severe erosion processes have undermined the gold onlays, (c) and the adjacent premolar has lost extensive tooth structure. (From Young, 2003a, with permission of Erosion Watch Pty Ltd.)

of interproximal caries or assess the state of periodontal bone support across the dentition. Transillumination and laser diagnostic modalities are of assistance in the diagnosis of dental caries. The worn dentition however requires a different approach based on assessment of the hard and soft tissues, examination of the dentition and charting of toothwear (Table 4.2). The examination of extraoral and soft tissue features detailed in Chapter 1 is paramount,

often providing valuable insight and diagnostic information in elucidating the multifactorial aetiology underlying toothwear processes in an individual. Hence, even prior to examination of the dentition, the astute clinician may identify extraoral or soft tissue signs relevant to the diagnostic assessment process. A good clinical history will further assist in identifying contributing dietary, health and lifestyle factors. Whilst clinical photographs provide

Table 4.1   Diagnostic modalities for toothwear and dental caries.

Diagnostics	Toothwear	Dental caries
Tactile probing	Of little significance	May further damage porous enamel or fissures and only limited sources still recommend probing
Transillumination, laser diagnostics	Of little application	Useful for detecting decay in interproximal, pit and fissure regions
Radiographs	Of little significance other than excluding other pathologies	Important to check for interproximal lesions and ascertain depth of decay
Presence of plaque and tartar	Is encouraging as it is suggestive of salivary remineralisation potential	Important to identify presence at surfaces at risk of decay
Saliva tests: Flow rate, buffering capacity, pH, bacterial counts	Toothwear patients often in good health but suffer sports- or work-related dehydration. Confirms medically induced xerostomia.	Beneficial to ascertain at-risk status
Study models	Important for most cases to assess worn surfaces and consider vertical dimension	Of little benefit unless rampant decay requires complex rehabilitation
Clinical photography	Appropriate in all cases with significant aesthetic bearing	Appropriate in all cases with significant aesthetic bearing
Existing restorations	High margins provide a record of dental erosion since placement	Record of past caries experience Check marginal leakage
Clinical history	Very important	Less important
Pulp testing	Rarely required	Frequently indicated

Table 4.2   Examination of toothwear and dental caries.

Diagnostics	Toothwear	Dental caries
Extraoral examination	Facial features: eyes, ears Complexion of skin, lips, hair Parotid regions, TMJ	Of little significance except subcutaneous abscesses or sinuses
Intraoral soft tissue examination	Sialadenosis Linea alba Salivary glands Tongue indentations	Of little significance Dento-alveolar abscesses
Intraoral hard tissue examination	Visual inspection of: Incisal/occlusal, buccal/palatal surfaces for wear Charting of toothwear	Visual inspection for white-spot lesions, staining and cavitation DMFS or DMFT charting of dentition

some aesthetic reference points, study models provide an important and appropriate baseline reference point that may be compared to at subsequent recall appointments over time or when new study models are taken every 2 years.

SURFACE SUSCEPTIBILITY OF TOOTHWEAR AND SITE SPECIFICITY OF DENTAL CARIES

Lesions of toothwear affect the dentition in a surface-specific manner (Khan et al. 1998, 1999, 2001). Lesions occur in certain areas more than others, not so by chance, but for reasons of variations in exposure levels of different surfaces to extrinsic and intrinsic acids, elements of abrasion, attrition and salivary protection (Young & Khan 2002). Appreciating how these elements affect certain parts of the dentition more so than others helps in understanding how the worn dentition a patient presents with has developed and what processes may be involved. Identifying toothwear on particular teeth across the dentition and more specifically on different tooth surfaces assists in conceptualising thought processes to elucidate the underlying aetiologies (Fig. 4.2).

Tooth surfaces are differently affected by toothwear and dental caries. Interproximal regions are almost never affected by attrition and erosion, yet are susceptible to develop dental caries. Whilst considerable wear on approximal surfaces has been documented in aboriginal dentitions (Kaidonis et al. 1992), toothwear in modern-day societies is different from that experienced in historic civilisations (Young 1998). Modern dietary trends do not promote such excessive wear on approximal surfaces, and in the majority of cases, they can be considered negligible. On maxillary anterior teeth, wear facets develop on incisal edges, marginal ridges and cingula as the palatal

surfaces are also occluding surfaces (Fig. 4.3). As severity of erosion and attrition increases further, tooth structure on the palatal surfaces is lost. Maxillary anterior teeth are often found devoid of enamel surface palatally in patients with high exposure to dietary or intrinsic acids. Dental caries, however, does not affect the occluding surfaces and instead may form in any deep palatal pits or fissures. It is rare to see decay on wear facets, even if dentine is exposed, as plaque has limited opportunity to evolve and develop on occluding surfaces. Mandibular anterior teeth may develop wear facets chipped and worn regions of dental erosion incisally, but are rarely affected by caries on these surfaces. Further, given the salivary protection offered by the submandibular glands, toothwear on lingual surfaces of the mandibular anterior teeth is rare.

In molar teeth, the regions of the occlusal surfaces affected by attrition and erosion also vary from those affected by dental caries (Fig. 4.4). Attrition affects the cuspal inclines and tips. Erosion results in cup- or bowl-shaped lesions on the cuspal apices and inclines. Caries affects fissures on the occlusal surface and buccal pits. Similar to anterior incisal surfaces, attrition facets are sites that are not prone to dental caries, and interproximal regions susceptible to dental caries are rarely affected by toothwear. Such surface- and site-specific differences further highlight the different processes resulting in the various types of tooth structure loss. Toothwear and dental caries are clearly different processes. The patterns by which tooth structure is lost vary by segment of teeth and site across the dentition and even on individual surfaces (see Figs. 4.3 & 4.4). This surface specificity has restorative and dental material selection implications discussed in later chapters and also requires different approaches to the charting of such lesions. Application of caries assessment techniques to areas of toothwear to characterise the different lesions of non-carious tooth surface loss is inappropriate.

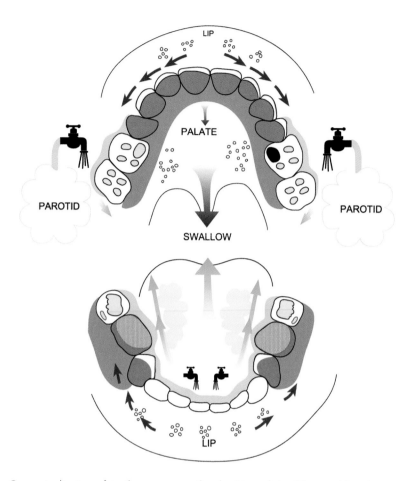

Figure 4.2 Conceptualisation of toothwear across the dentition of the 22-year-old male patient depicted in Fig. 4.1. States of repeated dehydration, use of recreational drugs, frequent vomiting and high acidic beverage consumption combined to result in severe dental erosion in this patient. Whilst lingual surfaces of the mandibular teeth have been protected, the minimal saliva available afforded little protection against the highly acidic and repeated insults on the dentition for the maxillary anterior palatal and mandibular posterior buccal surfaces, which have been severely affected by dental erosion. (From Young, 2003a, with permission of Erosion Watch Pty Ltd.)

THE CLINICAL PRESENTATION OF TOOTHWEAR

Having introduced the differences in surface specificity, consideration is next given to the clinical presentation of toothwear across the dentition. Clinically, given the limited diagnostic modalities available, in the assessment of toothwear heavy emphasis is placed on visual identification. A strategy for identifying toothwear is detailed based on morphology of toothwear lesions of different surfaces. Scanning electron microscopy techniques have offered valuable insight into the descriptive parameters required to characterise lesions, describe subtle changes on the tooth surface and form the basis from which the identification strategy presented has been developed over the past decade. High-magnification microscopy techniques allow detailed visualisation of

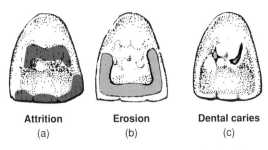

Attrition	Erosion	Dental caries
(a)	(b)	(c)

Figure 4.3 The incisal edges and palatal surfaces affected by attrition (a) or erosion (b) are contrasted with sites susceptible to caries (c) on an upper first permanent incisor. Wear facets on the incisal edge, marginal ridges and cingulum characterise attrition. The incisal edge and marginal ridges are hollowed out in cases of erosion. Palatal pits are sites susceptible to dental caries. (From Young & Khan, 2009, with permission from Erosion Watch Pty Ltd.)

ultrastructural components, whilst lower magnification microscopy techniques provide type specimens for occlusal and incisal attrition and erosion, cervical lesions, and areas of lesion fusion, involving both occlusal and cervical surfaces.

Attrition

Facets of attrition by definition are flat, well defined and demarcated (Fig. 4.5). They appear shiny to visual inspection, especially following recent active progression. Matching facets are often identified in opposing teeth, as wear progresses from tooth-to-tooth interaction. Whilst identification may be easier on a set of study models, when examining a patient's dentition directly, it is important to dry the tooth surface fully to allow better visualisation. Matching facets can also be identified by asking the patient to lightly occlude on a piece of articulating paper. Facets on the palatal slopes of maxillary anterior teeth often extend in an incisal-to-apical direction due to the upward and backward movement of the lower incisor teeth in normal occlusion. Whilst wear of the mamelons of newly erupted incisor teeth in children is physiologic, multiple wear facets across the dentition are the first sign of a patient being at risk of developing significant toothwear. Well-marked mesial and/or distal facets on the

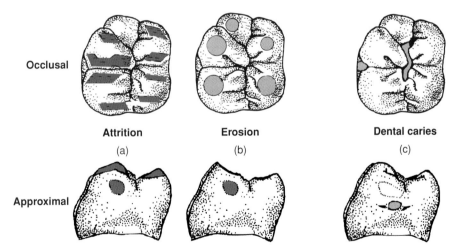

Figure 4.4 The five cusps of a lower first permanent molar, surfaces affected by attrition (a) or erosion (b), are contrasted with sites of pit and fissure caries (c). Wear facets on the cusp slopes and marginal ridges characterise attrition. Cusp apices develop bowl-shaped lesions through processes of erosion. Buccal pits and occlusal fissures are sites prone to the development of dental caries. (From Young & Khan, 2009, with permission from Erosion Watch Pty Ltd.)

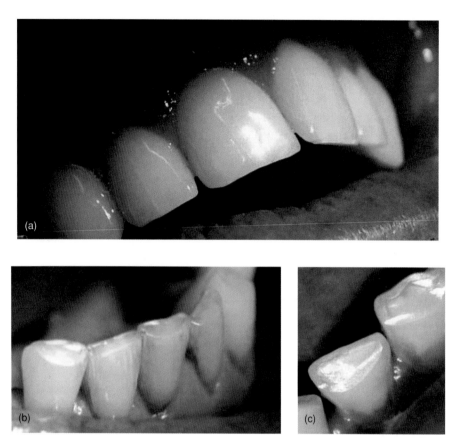

Figure 4.5   Mild attrition on the incisal edges of maxillary anterior teeth (a). Lower anterior teeth with moderate attrition on the incisal edges (b) exposing dentine. Facets are shiny, flat, highly polished and well demarcated (c).

incisal edges of canine teeth reflect the more anterior indentation of the lower on the upper canine. In premolar and molar teeth, the mesial and distal slopes of the cusps and the marginal ridges are the common surfaces where facets usually develop. The mesiobuccal cusp of the upper first permanent molar teeth develops a facet over the central fissure between the mesio- and distobuccal cusps of its lower counterpart in normal occlusion (Angle class I malocclusion). Attrition involves the earliest forms of tooth structure loss and often simultaneously the least amount volumetrically. Teeth in contact undergo physiologic wear throughout their lifetime. Areas of heavy contact wear gradually. The physiologic balance across the dentition is

hence maintained over a lifetime and is not a static process.

In areas of attrition, as shown in Fig. 4.6, dentine is exposed in accordance with the Greaves effect (1973). The leading-edge enamel protects the adjacent dentine and a shallow slope is formed. Dentine is scooped out in front of the trailing-edge enamel. This describes the Greaves effect, which has been used to deduce the direction of the chewing stroke on fossil teeth (Greaves 1973). These shallow differences in contour can be seen on the incisal edge wear facet of the incisor illustrated in Fig. 4.6a. The literature will continue to debate the limited role of bruxism in some cases of toothwear and the sometimes-severe attrition that may result

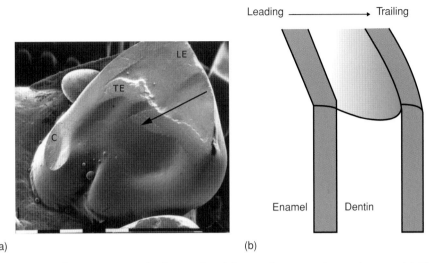

Figure 4.6   Scanning electron micrograph of a maxillary left second incisor with incisal attrition (a). The shallow leading edge (LE) enamel-to-dentine interface contrasts with the hollowed and chipped dentine-to-enamel interface of the trailing edge (TE). The arrow on the incisal edge indicates the orientations of striae. The cingulum (C) shows compression pits consistent with wear in centric occlusion. When an opposing tooth produces a wear facet that penetrates to dentine, the direction of travel of the opposing tooth can be deduced from the contours on the dentine within the facet (b), as leading-edge enamel (LE) protects the adjacent dentine and a shallow slope is formed. Dentine is scooped out in front of the trailing-edge enamel (TE). This is termed 'Greaves effect' (Greaves 1973). (From Young & Khan, 2009, with permission from Erosion Watch Pty Ltd.)

and a detailed consideration of the literature on the topic is presented in Chapter 10.

Erosion

The appearance of dental erosion differs markedly from attrition. On the incisal edges of the incisor teeth, thin enamel margins and peripheries are prone to chipping (Fig. 4.7). The dentine is deeply scooped out and lesions are not as well defined. On maxillary incisor teeth, in addition to thinning of the incisal edge, the palatal surface is susceptible to erosion (Fig. 4.8).

Dental erosion on the molar and premolar teeth characteristically involves cup- or bowl-shaped lesions. Cup-shaped lesions are symmetrical dentine exposures affecting the cuspal apices and inclines (Fig. 4.9). Margins of existing restorations may stand proud of surrounding tooth structure. Progression of occlusal

dental erosion results in merger of cup-shaped lesions across the oblique and marginal ridges to ultimately affect the entire occlusal surface and form a bowl-shaped lesion (see Fig. 1.8b). Unlike facets, cuspal-cupped lesions do not match where the upper and lower teeth meet in occlusion. The mandibular molar teeth are far more severely affected compared to the opposing maxillary molar teeth and are an important indicator of early-onset dental erosion in children (Khan et al. 2001).

Microscopy helps explain why cup-shaped lesions are symmetrical. Figure 4.10a shows rods of enamel run in bands parallel to one another. One band, the parazone, cuts across another zone, the diazone. Parazones and diazones are alternating Hunter–Schreger bands within enamel (Osborn 1990). This complex arrangement of enamel rods gives the cusp tip its high-impact strength to resist the high forces of chewing and prevents it cracking under stress

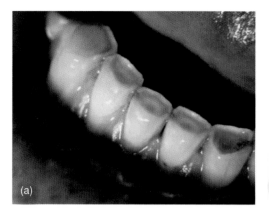
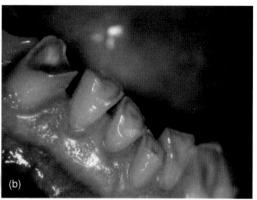

Figure 4.7 Mandibular anterior teeth with moderate dental erosion. Cupping or scooping of dentine on the incisal edges is notable, and the lower right canine has been restored previously with high restorative margins and further loss of surrounding tooth structure since placement of the restoration is evident (a). Sharp enamel peripheries and chipping are common as erosion progresses (b).

over the tip of the crown dentine (D). As shown in Fig. 4.10b, these alternating bands spiral down from the very tip of the cusp. When the spirals are cut in longitudinal section, their complexity results in the gnarled appearance to the enamel on the tip. Whilst the cusp tips are highly resistant to masticatory forces, when sustained acids etch the gnarled enamel, the symmetry of the spirals is revealed and the dentine becomes exposed, forming cup-shaped lesions.

Cervical lesions

Three types of non-carious cervical lesions are easily discernible, namely a shallow cervical

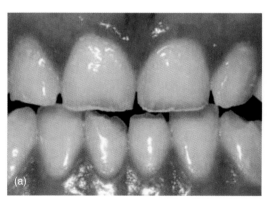
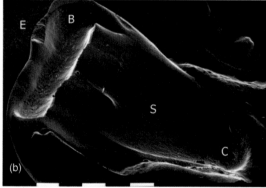

Figure 4.8 Dental erosion on the incisal edges of maxillary incisor teeth is visible from the facial perspective as bluish-grey regions of translucency through the thinned enamel shell remaining (a). (From Young & Messer, 2002, with permission of Dentil Pty Ltd.) Scanning electron micrograph of a maxillary left lateral incisor with erosion of the incisal edge (B) and palatal surface (C) extending to the gingival margin (b). The facial enamel is chipped (E) due to softening and lack of support from the hollowed-out incisal dentine (B). Striations (S) on the palatal surface indicate attrition and abrasion of softened dentine. The cingulum is lost and erosion extends into the gingival crevice (C) (Bar = 1 mm). (From Khan et al., 1998, with permission from the *Australian Dental Journal*.)

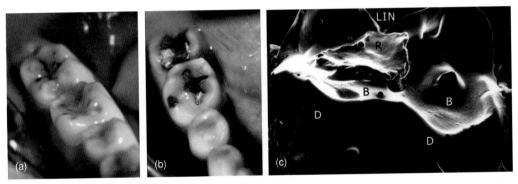

Figure 4.9 Cup-shaped lesions on the cuspal inclines and apices indicate dental erosion on these mandibular molar teeth (a). Previously placed restorations, such as the amalgam restorations on the lower right first molar (b), stand notably higher of the surrounding tooth structure as erosion processes have occurred or continued since their placement. Proud amalgam restorative margins are evident on this lower right first molar tooth, severely affected by occlusion erosion (B), which has fused with cervical toothwear (c), resulting in degradation (D), severely eroding both buccal cusps. The lingual cusps (LIN), occlusal fissures and marginal ridges are eroded on all sides of the occlusal amalgam restoration (R). (From Teo et al., 1997, with permission from the *Australian Dental Journal*.)

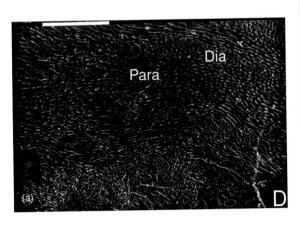

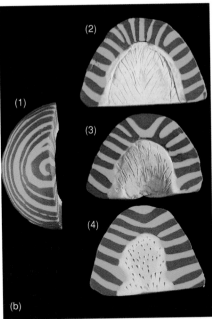

Figure 4.10 (a) Enamel within the apex of a molar cusp consists of parazones (Para) and diazones (Dia), alternating to form a pattern termed Hunter–Schreger bands (b). This complexity above the tip of the cuspal dentine (D) has given it the name gnarled enamel. (b) This series of models represent how alternating Hunter–Schreger bands (red and green PLASTICINE™) spiral down from the tip of the cusp (1). Three longitudinal sections (1–4) show how Hunter–Schreger bands cut in different orientations at the tip give rise to the appearance called 'gnarled enamel'. The cuspal-cupped lesion evolves by progressive involvement of the spirals of Hunter–Schreger bands of the gnarled enamel and exposes the dentine (yellow). (From Young & Khan, 2009, with permission of Erosion Watch.)

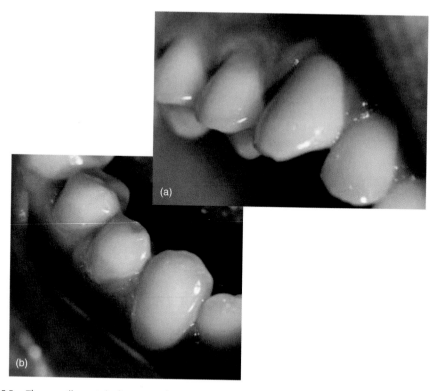

Figure 4.11   The maxillary right first premolar (a) and mandibular left canine and both premolar teeth (b) are all affected buccally by shallow cervical lesions.

lesion, grooved cervical lesion and wedge-shaped cervical lesion (Khan et al. 1999). Out of the three types, the shallow cervical erosion is the most common, which is found in association with both occlusal attrition (Fig. 4.11) and occlusal erosion (Fig. 4.12). The enamel slopes gently across the dentinoenamel junction and into a shallow dentine concavity. The lesions are predominantly found in the cervical third of the tooth and have peripheries that are not as easily definable as the other two types. The enamel peripheral to the lesion is thinned and the Hunter–Schreger bands may be accentuated by etching and show as fine furrows. More aprismatic enamel is found within the cervical third of the tooth and the margins of the shallow cervical lesions are generally within the aprismatic enamel, which is more acid resistant

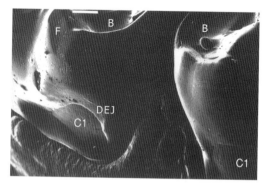

Figure 4.12   Lower right first molar and second premolar teeth affected by cup-shaped lesions and occlusal erosion (B) and shallow cervical lesions on the buccal surface (C1). The margins of the shallow cervical lesions dentinoenamel junction are indicated (DEJ). (From Khan et al., 1999, with permission from the *Australian Dental Journal*.)

than prismatic enamel. However, when etching exposes the Hunter–Schreger bands deeper into the surface, their pattern becomes revealed at the microscopic level. Thus, the interactions between the oral acids, the surface aprismatic and subsurface enamel rod and rod sheaths influence the form of the shallow cervical lesion in the relative absence of saliva protection.

Incisor, canine and premolar teeth are the most common sites for facial or buccal cervical non-carious lesions. The buccal aspects of the upper molar teeth are more rarely affected as they are opposite the parotid duct orifices. Serous (watery) saliva, from the parotid and submandibular major salivary glands, neutralises and clears acids from the teeth, preventing erosion. Serous saliva is also supersaturated with respect to tooth mineral which prevents demineralisation. It is rare to find any cervical lesions on the lingual aspects of the lower teeth as this region is well protected being located opposite the submandibular gland duct openings. If cervical lesions are found on the lingual aspects of the lower teeth, the patient would be considered at high risk of further toothwear and would deserve further investigation for the underlying saliva deficiencies and high exposure to acids, likely intrinsic in nature.

In rare cases, and especially in patients with high exposure to acids and secondary toothbrush abrasion, grooved cervical lesions may be found (Fig. 4.13; see also Fig. 1.4). Upon finding these lesions, the clinician should be alerted to offering strong preventive advice to avoid brushing immediately subsequent to the dentition being exposed to acids. The grooves are predominantly horizontal and evidence that toothbrush abrasion exacerbates cervical erosion. Horizontal toothbrush strokes have finely abraded the softened enamel and accentuated the Hunter–Schreger bands visible on the proximal enamel. Accordingly for all patients with any form of non-carious cervical lesions, it should be reinforced preventively that a soft toothbrush with a gentle circular brushing mo-

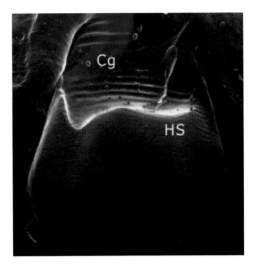

Figure 4.13 Maxillary left canine with a grooved facial cervical lesions (Cg). The grooves in dentine extend horizontally above the marginal gingiva. Toothbrushing has abraded softened dentine and accentuated Hunter–Schreger bands (HS) of the etched enamel. (From Teo et al., 1997, with permission from the *Australian Dental Journal*.)

tion is indicated and brushing immediately after acidic exposure is avoided.

Wedge-shaped lesions form the third significant type and are found in older adults whose teeth show either severe occlusal attrition or equally severe occlusal erosion. At the apical extent of the lesion, the floor is often horizontal with an oblique planar face obliquely extending in a coronal and buccal direction. The junction of the horizontal floor and oblique planar face occurs at the deepest zone of dentine exposure (Fig. 4.14). These lesions occur, in dentine, associated with either occlusal attrition or erosion and develop slowly evolving from shallower cervical lesions, occurring most commonly on surfaces lubricated by mucous and rarely at sites protected by serous saliva, thus forming more regularly where saliva does not buffer or clear acids effectively (Young & Khan 2002). Interestingly, teeth are not found with wedge-shaped cervical lesions on both their buccal and lingual surfaces, and as opposed

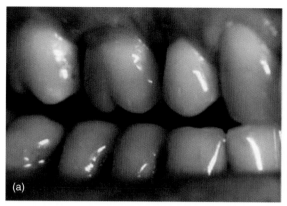 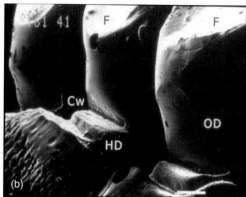

Figure 4.14   Wedge-shaped cervical lesions on upper right first molar and second premolar teeth with no associated occlusal toothwear on these teeth (a). Incisal attrition is notable on the canine teeth. (From Khan et al., 2010, with permission of Copyright Publishing.) Mandibular anterior teeth (b) with incisal attritional facets (F) and buccal wedge-shaped cervical lesions (Cw) with an oblique dentine planar face extending coronally from the horizontal dentine floor (HD). (From Khan et al., 1999, with permission from the *Australian Dental Journal*.)

to carious lesions, non-carious cervical lesions do not occur on approximal surfaces or join up circumferentially.

Paediatric patients and adolescents may present with extensive occlusal toothwear, but rarely present with non-carious cervical lesions. Cervical lesions require more time to develop and appear to form at a later stage, and while sometimes found on teeth with no obvious occlusal or incisal toothwear, they are generally found in dentitions where occlusal toothwear is already established (Khan et al. 1999).

A recent review of non-carious lesions considered a large volume of teeth that were archival material, having been extracted more than 60 years ago, and suggested classifications of cervical lesions to also include two further categories of concave cervical lesions and secondly irregular cervical lesions to describe those that were not describable in any other category (Michael et al. 2010).

Just under two decades ago, it was proposed that stress corrosion on the tooth should be termed 'abfraction' (Grippo 1991) and that this process was of central importance in the formation of cervical lesions, termed 'abfraction lesions' in parts of the literature. Occlusal stress

can indeed be shown to be translated as strain to enamel and dentine where the 'fulcrum' is artificially stimulated at the amelocemental junction *in vitro* (Rees 1998). There is, however, no evidence that the crestal fibres of the periodontium constitute a fulcrum *in vivo*. The consensus in the literature suggests that 'corrosion' (dental erosion) is the most important mechanism in the formation of the cervical lesion than the physiologic stresses and strain on enamel and dentine.

Research has shown that wedge-shaped cervical lesions were found as commonly on teeth with occlusal attrition as on teeth with occlusal erosion (Khan et al. 1999). Interestingly, sites were identified with wedge-shaped cervical lesions, but no discernible occlusal wear, further suggesting factors other than occlusion and stress transmission to be important in development of these lesions. Moreover, the most common sites, where wedge-shaped lesions occur, are those least protected by serous saliva.

In a different study, Daley et al. (2009) considered ten heavily worn lower incisor and canine teeth with non-carious cervical lesions, sectioning and further assessing them with light microscopy (Fig. 4.15) and scanning

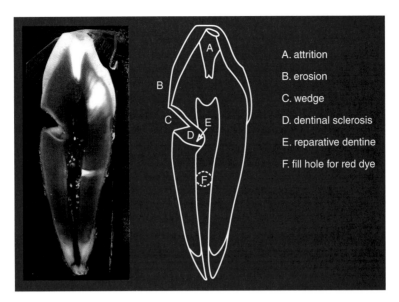

Figure 4.15 Longitudinal section of a canine impregnated with red dye in resin through patent tubules from the pulp. A tract of white sclerotic tubules extends beneath the occlusal attrition (A). The facial (B) enamel is thinned to a knife edge above the wedge-shaped cervical lesion (C). Sclerotic dentine (D) constitutes both the 'ceiling' and the 'floor' of the wedge-shaped lesion. Reparative dentine (E) was present on the pulpal wall. Red dye infiltrated the pulp through the hole drilled at (F). (From Young & Khan, 2009, with permission from Erosion Watch Pty Ltd.)

electron microscopy. Utilising ground sections of the teeth, which in life had occlusal attrition and facial wedge-shaped cervical lesions, five important clinical implications were derived from this dye infiltration experiment:

1. Dentine beneath occlusal wear facets is sclerotic.
2. If enamel surface is thinned by erosion, but is intact, the dentine is not sclerotic.
3. The form of the wedge-shaped lesion is determined by the curvature of dentinal tubules in the 'ceiling'.
4. The 'floor' of the lesion is sclerotic dentine.
5. Reparative dentine forms on the pulpal wall of the wedge.

Non-carious cervical lesions appear to evolve with age through a series of grades from the shallow to the grooved or to the wedge shaped. Wood et al. (2008), in a review of the literature on non-carious cervical lesions,

noted that the older the population considered, the greater the percentage of lesions found per patient. Figure 4.16 illustrates that as incisal or occlusal toothwear and cervical lesions progressively increase in size, fusion of the two zones ultimately occurs resulting in degradation, as considered in the next section.

Lesion development and surface morphology is influenced initially by erosion of aprismatic and prismatic enamel. Toothbrush abrasion accentuates the Hunter–Schreger bands in the enamel and scores the dentine in the grooved lesion. It is not known to what extent abrasion contributes to the clinical progression towards the wedge-shaped lesion. What is certain, microscopically, is that where the enamel is still intact above the wedge in dentine, the dentinal tubules remain patent. The aprismatic and prismatic enamel are thinned by erosion or abrasion. When dentine is exposed, it undergoes sclerosis and sclerotic tubules involved in their long axes form the ceiling of the lesion,

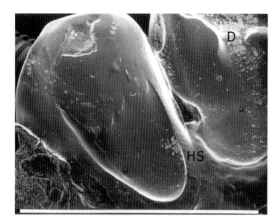

Figure 4.16 The maxillary left canine tooth has a large cervical lesion palatally, leaving a thin collar of enamel following the gingival margin, with Hunter–Schreger (HS) bands of the etched enamel. Fusion of occlusal and cervical toothwear on the neighbouring first premolar tooth has resulted in degradation. (From Young & Khan, 2002, with permission of the *Journal of Oral Rehabilitation*.)

whilst the tubules at the base of the lesion cut across the floor. It is probable that both serous and mucous saliva normally protect the lingual, approximal and buccal cervical surfaces, with formation of salivary pellicle. Addy (2005) discussed the relationship of dentine hypersensitivity, toothwear and toothbrushing, and concluded that the available evidence suggests that cervical wear will reach pathological proportions only when combined with the dominant process of erosion, unless the patient is extremely vigorous with brushing and oral hygiene measures.

It has been suggested that salivary pellicle protects cervical surfaces from toothwear. Collins and Dawes (1987) mapped the thickness of salivary pellicle across the dentition, and Dawes (2008) concluded that the salivary pellicle affords only a small degree of protection given its thickness of 1 μm or less. However, when the thickness of salivary pellicle (Amechi et al. 1999) on these surfaces is compared with the percentages of surfaces affected by noncarious cervical lesions (Young & Khan 2002), at the clinical level cervical surfaces are best pro-

tected by serous saliva from the major glands. Parotid saliva from Stenson's ducts and submandibular saliva from Wharton's ducts are the principal sources of the protective properties of saliva.

Non-carious cervical lesions are:

- Common on the facial and palatal surfaces of the maxillary anterior teeth
- Common on the buccal surfaces of the maxillary premolar teeth
- Common on the buccal aspect of the mandibular premolar teeth
- Uncommon on the lingual aspect of all mandibular teeth
- Uncommon on the buccal aspects of the maxillary molar teeth

Degradation

Degradation describes the fusion of toothwear on occlusal or incisal surfaces with a noncarious cervical lesion (see Fig. 4.16) and occurs at a later stage. Teeth susceptible to cervical lesions are also those that progress to develop degradation. These teeth have considerable loss of tooth structure and create a restorative challenge, given the scarcity of enamel remaining and predominant dentine surface available for bonding. Maxillary anterior teeth are affected on incisal and palatal surfaces (Fig. 4.17), sometimes even extending to involve the facial surface. In the rare instances in which the lingual surfaces of the mandibular anterior teeth are affected, remaining enamel is found to follow the gingival contour (Fig. 4.18a). Posteriorly, proud restorations and loss of cuspal tooth structure are noted in the premolar (Fig. 4.18b) and more rarely the molar teeth.

Near and frank exposures

In severe cases of toothwear, lesions may encroach close to pulpal structures (Fig. 4.19). Briggs et al. (1998) reported 14 cases of pulp exposure beneath regions of labial cervical erosion. In the primary dentition, frank exposures

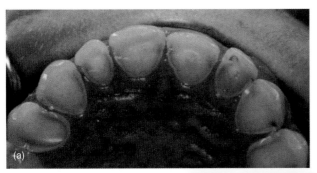

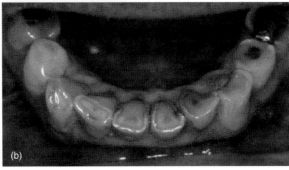

Figure 4.17 Fusion of incisal and palatal wear in the maxillary anterior teeth has resulted in degradation on the palatal surfaces of maxillary premolar, canine and incisor teeth (a) Close proximity of the pulp is evident on all incisor teeth. Degradation of the lingual aspects of lower anterior teeth is rare (b) as submandibular and sublingual salivary glands normally offer good protection to these sites. (From Young, 2001a, with permission from the *Australian Dental Journal*.)

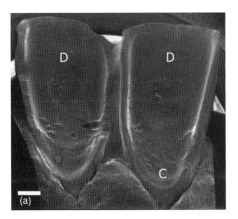

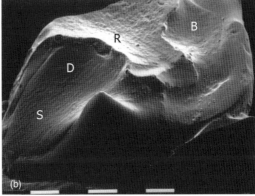

Figure 4.18 (a) All enamel has been eroded from the lingual surfaces of these mandibular central incisor teeth except in gingival margin areas, likely protected by crevicular fluid. The cingulum is lost (C) and degradation (D) affects the entire lingual surface in these teeth (Bar = 1 mm). (From Teo et al., 1997, with permission from the *Australian Dental Journal*.) (b) This maxillary right first premolar tooth shows an existing amalgam restoration (R) proud of surrounding tooth structure that has been eroded over time to result in degradation (D) as a result of fusion of occlusal erosion (B) and cervical toothwear lesions with striations in the dentine (S). (From Teo et al., 1997, with permission from the *Australian Dental Journal*.)

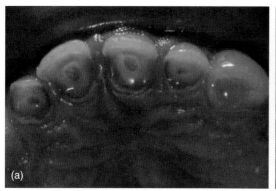
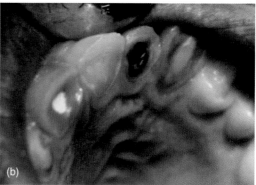

Figure 4.19 (a) Near-exposures on the palatal surfaces of maxillary central and lateral incisor teeth in a patient with severe dental erosion. Toothwear extends to the gingival margin regions with only a minimal collar of enamel remaining in these areas. (By courtesy of Professor Ian Meyers.) (b) By time of presentation, this 21-year-old male patient had root canal treatments commenced or completed on all maxillary teeth. The referring dentist had trialled various materials and fabricated a splint for this patient, whilst underlying erosive processes continued uncontrolled.

are found more commonly from the occlusal surfaces on incisor and molar teeth. Figure 4.19 shows extreme cases of toothwear, where multifactorial aetiologies have lead to rapid tooth structure loss.

Near and frank exposures of the pulp due to erosion are more common on the occlusal surfaces of primary teeth of children. In adults, toothwear is rarely the cause of a frank exposure or of root canal therapy being required. Such exposures may occur in cases of severe toothwear involving rapid progression. In permanent teeth, whilst dental pulp exposures from toothwear are rare, exposures from dentinal infection are relatively frequent due to dental caries. The rate of dentine destruction by attrition and erosion is sufficiently slow and sporadic, allowing sclerotic dentine and reparative dentine to be formed. In cases of fast-progressing and severe dental erosion, upon closer examination of the palatal surfaces of severely degraded maxillary incisor and canine teeth, the pulps of the teeth may be seen shining pink through the thinned dentine. Where dentinal tubules are patent, the pulp can show through as a pink point. However, vital pulp is rarely seen through the occlusal surface of a premolar or permanent molar. Restoratively, in-

direct pulp capping should still be attempted and 'elective' endodontics should be avoided given the differences to the dental caries infection process.

CHARTING TOOTHWEAR

An odontogram allows accurate description and recording of tooth surfaces. The odontogram introduced in Chapter 1 forms the centrepiece of the toothwear examination form, conceptually reinforcing that the dentition is within an oral environment and influenced by surrounding structures that provide signs of potential imbalance. Surface-specific considerations have indicated interproximal surfaces to be least affected by toothwear. Buccal and lingual surfaces are of greater importance and the odontogram has been formulated with this in mind, focusing on the predominant surfaces affected by toothwear.

The appropriate strategy to complete the odontogram is based on *The Stages of Wear* (Table 4.3). Each of the preceding sections in this chapter has detailed one or more of these stages. Attrition (A) and erosion (B) on incisal and occlusal surfaces are often identified in

Table 4.3 Stages of wear.

Stage A	Attrition	Wear facets formed tooth-to-tooth
Stage B	Bowl-shaped erosion	On incisal edges and cusp tips
Stage C	Cervical lesion	On a tooth with occlusal attrition or erosion
Stage D	Degradation	Occlusal attrition or erosion merged with a cervical lesion
Stage E	Near exposure	Pink pulp shining through
Stage F	Frank exposure	The pulp open to the oral environment

dentitions with no cervical lesions. Cervical lesions (C) often affect the dentition at a later stage and are more commonly found on teeth also affected by occlusal or incisal toothwear. Fusion of occlusal or incisal attrition or erosion with non-carious cervical lesions (C) represents extensive loss of tooth structure, described as degradation (D). As further progression occurs, the pulpal structures may be encroached upon and areas of near-exposure (E) may be identified. Rarely will a frank exposure (F) be found. However, in rapidly progressing cases of dental erosion, the maxillary anterior teeth may be particularly susceptible. *The Stages of Wear* assessment strategy allows for identification of toothwear within a dentition and systematic charting on an odontogram. *The Stages of Wear* are not exclusive stages *per se* and instead should be considered a classification strategy to assist clinicians to decipher toothwear processes at work within a worn dentition. *The Stages of Wear* have been developed based on scanning electron microscopy assessment of type specimens (Khan et al. 1998, 1999, 2001; Teo et al. 1997; Young & Khan 2002) and utilised by the chapter authors over the past 15 years for the detailed clinical examination of 2000 documented toothwear cases referred for further diagnosis and treatment planning. The research projects have considered the surface-specific distribution of toothwear across the worn dentition. In combination with an odontogram, *The Stages of Wear* approach is applied to:

- *Chart* toothwear across the dentition
- Consider *risk status* of the patient for developing severe toothwear

- *Assess* whether affected regions are those least protected by saliva from the major salivary glands and/or most exposed to extrinsic and possible intrinsic sources of acid
- *Manage* and treatment-plan toothwear cases
- *Monitor* the severity of toothwear over time and *reassess* at intervals for changes in distribution and/or severity

When charting *The Stages of Wear*, an assessment of severity across the dentition can be made and compared to baseline at subsequent recall visits. Regions affected by toothwear can be appreciated visually on the odontogram. Generalised wear affects the majority of the dentition, whilst anterior-based wear predominantly affects the incisor and canine teeth, as is the case in patients with high-acidic-beverage-consumption habits. Frequent recoating of the anterior dentition accelerates wear in this region. The distribution of wear has implications on the restorative modalities implicated and is further discussed in Chapters 11 and 12.

Charting encompasses the chairside assistant colour-coding lesions directly onto the odontogram or alternatively marking A or B for occlusal or incisal attrition or erosion. C is charted for cervical lesions, D for degradation and, in rare cases, E or F for frank exposure. The buccal, lingual, incisal or occlusal surfaces are charted for all teeth across the dentition. Throughout the chapters of this book, interesting cases have been described. In this book, special cases in each chapter have an odontogram included alongside photo panels. Figures 4.20 and 4.21 detail four cases with completed charting of the odontograms.

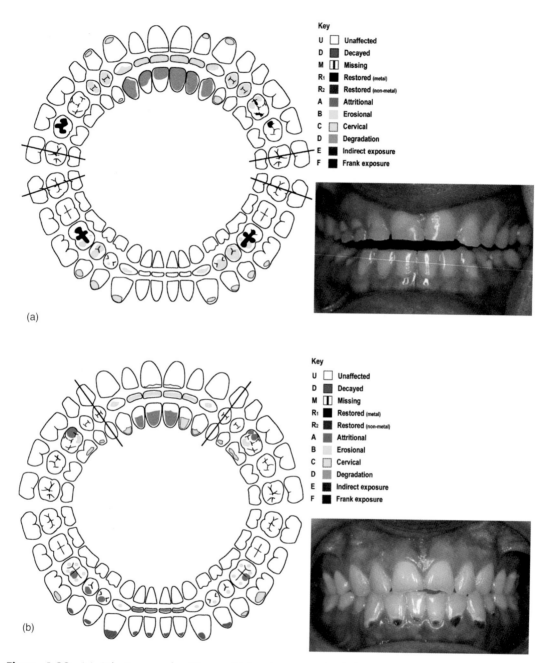

(a)

(b)

Figure 4.20 (a) Odontogram of a 28-year-old female patient. Underlying toothwear aetiology and dental erosion have continued since placement of multiple cervical restorations on the canine and premolar teeth. New cervical lesions and dental material breakdown have occurred in these regions. This case and case history are presented in detail in Chapter 6. (From Young, 2001b, with permission of Dentil Pty Ltd.) (b) Odontogram of a 19-year-old ballet dancer, who presented with significant active toothwear. Arrested dental caries was observed on the facial cervical regions of the mandibular anterior teeth. This case is further detailed in Chapter 1, Fig. 1.16. (From Young, 2001a, with permission from the *Australian Dental Journal*.)

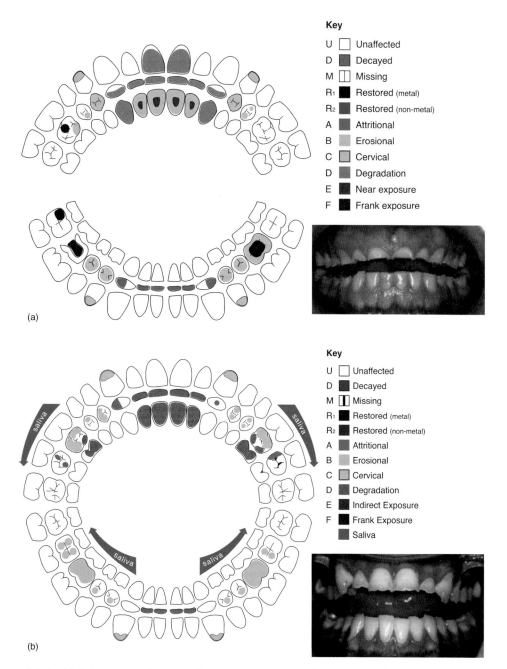

Figure 4.21 (a) Odontogram of a case of generalised severe toothwear across the dentition of a 27-year-old male patient. The case history and restorative approach for this case are detailed in Chapter 11. Extensive exposure to acids has allowed rapid loss of tooth structure to occur. Extensive loss in crown structure of all teeth, reduction in vertical dimension and near-exposures of the maxillary anterior teeth palatally was identified. (b) Odontogram of a case of a 24-year-old elite athlete, who for many years at times of sports-related dehydration rehydrated with acidic beverages. Palatal degradation on the maxillary anterior teeth extended within close proximity of pulpal structures. (From Young, 2003b, with permission of Dentil Pty Ltd.) The case history is discussed in Chapter 1, Fig. 1.8.

The application of *The Stages of Wear* classification to these and the other cases throughout this book highlight the following:

The surfaces affected by toothwear

- Between the mandibular and maxillary arch, the amount of toothwear charted is likely to be disproportionate.
- Mandibular incisor teeth commonly show incisal attrition (A).
- The opposing maxillary incisor teeth in patients who drink excessive acidic beverages or are exposed to intrinsic acids may appear disproportionately more heavily worn as dental erosion (B) accelerates and potentiates attritional tooth structure loss.
- Mandibular molar teeth are more severely affected by occlusal erosion (B) than the opposing maxillary counterparts.
- Cervical lesions (C) rarely occur on their own, whilst occlusal attrition (A) or erosion (B) commonly occur in the absence of cervical lesions and may even be severe.
- Whether or not cervical lesions (C) are associated with attrition or erosion occlusally, they commonly occur on buccal surfaces of maxillary and lower mandibular teeth and palatal surfaces of maxillary anterior and posterior teeth.
- Cervical lesions (C), associated either with occlusal attrition or erosion, occur on the surfaces of the teeth which are least protected by serous saliva, and are most subject to wear by toothbrush abrasion often secondary to erosion.
- Buccal and lingual cervical lesions (C) do not occur concurrently on the same tooth.
- The maxillary incisor, canine and premolar teeth are more prone to develop degradation, near-exposures and frank exposures (D, E and F).

The protected surfaces generally not affected by toothwear

- Mandibular anterior teeth are relatively protected as submandibular saliva affords good protection. Lingual surfaces are rarely affected by significant toothwear.
- Mandibular posterior teeth are protected on lingual surfaces and cervical lesions in these regions are very rare.
- Maxillary molar teeth adjacent to the parotid duct orifices show less occlusal erosion than mandibular counterparts. Buccally, cervical regions are also less common.
- Interproximal regions are not affected by toothwear at a clinical level.
- A collar of enamel remains along gingival margin regions, even when a tooth is affected by severe erosion (B) or degradation (D), perhaps due to the protection gingival crevicular fluid offers.

The balance of the oral environment from the time of eruption is important

- As introduced in Chapter 2, the first molar and incisor teeth are present for additional years within the oral environment, which if unbalanced at an early age, allow toothwear processes to affect these important keystones of the dentition from a young age.
- It follows that second and third molar teeth generally show much less toothwear, other than in severe cases or much older adults.
- Acidic influences are greater on the incisor, canine premolar and first molar teeth.

The explanation of a patient's multifactorial toothwear aetiology in creating such a diverse variety and spread of lesions involves aspects that extend well beyond what examination of the dentition alone can determine, and include the following:

- The role of intrinsic and extrinsic acids
- The role of attrition and abrasion
- The role of saliva protection
- The role of patient lifestyle, diet and habits
- The role of patient health and medications
- Variation of the above over time

The surface specificity observed exists as a result of interactions between protective elements, acidic insults, elements of attrition and abrasion. The worn dentition is a state created as a result of processes that develops over time. The presentation of toothwear across the adult dentition is a cumulative result of the influences of all these processes.

APPLICATION OF *THE STAGES OF WEAR* TO DIAGNOSING TOOTHWEAR

Rarely are all the teeth within one dentition affected by lesions of toothwear in one stage alone. More commonly, a dentition will have a number of teeth mildly, moderately, severely and not affected. Moreover, those affected may show attrition (A) or erosion (B) with or without cervical lesions (C) and upon fusion (D), with near- (E) or frank exposures (F) of the pulp.

Occlusal attrition across the dentition may be physiologic. More commonly, the relative loss of salivary protection is reflected in regional occurrences of occlusal attrition or erosion and abrasion. So within a dentition, teeth with stage A (attrition) or B (erosion) or stage A or B with stage C (cervical) lesions can be found. As individual teeth wear progressively to stage D (degradation), the severity of structural loss increases, so do the indications for aesthetic and functional improvements and for pulpal protection. Moreover, with loss of

occlusal surfaces, alterations take place in the patient's occlusion. These may be adaptive alterations of exaggerated wear facets, which are of no functional consequence. It follows that for any given patient, a range of restorative modalities may be appropriate to restore the different surfaces affected across their dentition. Irrespective of the restorative modality implemented, preventive approaches must continue to be reinforced to prevent those areas of mild toothwear within the dentition, not requiring restoration at this stage, from progressing.

Given the common multifactorial aetiology underlying toothwear, care must be taken in distinguishing between stage A (attrition) and stage B (erosion) as often dental erosion predisposes to attritional processes, and whilst wear facets may be identified, these may be surrounded by more subtle signs of dental erosion. Higher scanning electron microscope magnification details the transition zone, peripherally on a wear facet from the enamel to dentine and may show etching (Fig. 4.22), illustrating dental erosion potentiating further tooth structure loss via secondary attrition. Such findings must guide the preventive and management strategies, covering all the possible aetiologies involved for maximum conservation of tooth

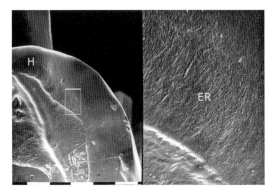

Figure 4.22 An attritional wear facet on the buccal cusp of a first premolar. The enamel is mostly flat and smooth (H). However at the amelodentinal junction, etched enamel rods (ER) can be discerned (Bar = 1 mm).

structure. The mandibular first molar, considered previously in Fig. 1.5, showed a number of cup-shaped lesions on all cusps (B) and a cup-shaped lesion with a surrounding facet (A) on the mesiobuccal cusp, again illustrating dental erosion potentiating secondary attrition. When charting toothwear, it is important to identify underlying erosion if these processes are involved, and if so, then the more severe stage B should be recorded on the odontogram.

UTILISING THE CHARTED ODONTOGRAM TO ASSESS PATIENT RISK

Toothwear risk status can in part be determined through considering the odontogram. When teeth with an advanced stage of wear are identified, the clinician should be alerted as to the high-risk status applicable to the patient (Table 4.4). Presence of degradation (D), near-exposures (E) or frank exposures (F) suggest the patient is at a high risk. Such toothwear with extensive exposure of dentine and with close proximity to pulpal structures has resulted from a combination of aetiologies that may have involved strong potentiating factors likely in combination with a lack of or reduction in protective elements. For a maxillary anterior tooth to have lost palatal tooth structure to the extent of a near-exposure (E), neighbour-

Table 4.4 Patient risk status by stage of wear identified.

Risk status	Identifying teeth with stage
High	D, degradation E, near exposure F, frank exposure
Moderate	B, erosion C, cervical lesions
Low	A, attrition No cervical lesions

Table 4.5 Patient risk status by location of lesion.

Risk status	Location of lesions
High	Areas that are normally highly protected such as lingual to the mandibular incisor teeth
Moderate	Maxillary incisors palatally and cervical regions across the dentition
Low	Occlusal surfaces only

ing teeth are likely to be similarly affected and at risk to develop the same, with further progression. Presence of cervical lesions (C) implies a moderate risk. Occurring later than occlusal or incisal toothwear, presence of cervical lesions suggests that toothwear processes have been ongoing over a substantial period of time.

Lesion location is the next risk identification variable (Table 4.5). In patients where toothwear lesions are identified in regions, which are normally protected by saliva, a higher risk category applies.

Toothwear at presentation provides historic information and is subject to ongoing change. The extent of toothwear identified may also have happened many years earlier. Health, lifestyle and diet may change again, increasing the risk of a patient developing significant toothwear. A patient reporting sensitivity in areas of non-carious cervical lesions should alert the clinician to suspect progression. Shiny wear facets suggest recent activity. A patient reporting chipping of teeth in recent times or an ongoing dry mouth sensation suggests risk of reduced salivary protection. Such clinical appreciation of risk is achieved through communication and discussion during the clinical history interview and assists the clinician in arbitrarily assigning a patient to a level of risk and therefrom decide the level of prevention and intervention applicable. Chapter 7 further details those patients at risk based on clinical history items and the appropriate preventive measures to be implemented.

SUMMARY

Toothwear is a multifactorial process. Correct identification of toothwear across a patient's dentition is important. However, consideration of toothwear within a dentition is insufficient to exclude all aetiologies involved and insufficient to base all preventive advise upon, given the diverse possibilities leading to development of a worn dentition. Work, lifestyle and health parameters of the patient may all play an important role in accelerating toothwear. In the chapters to follow, consideration is given to the role of saliva protection, the detailed clinical history interview appropriate to elucidate the above aetiological components further, how to prevent and manage toothwear and ultimately how to restore and rehabilitate *The Stages of Wear* which encompasses the worn dentition.

References

Addy, M. (2005) Tooth brushing, tooth wear and dentine hypersensitivity – are they associated. *International Dental Journal*, **55**, 261–267.

Amechi, B.T., Higham, S.M., Edgar, W.M., et al. (1999) Thickness of acquired salivary pellicle as a determinant of the sites of dental erosion. *Journal of Dental Research*, **78**, 1821–1828.

Briggs, P., Djemal, S., Harpal, C., et al. (1998) Young adult patients with established dental erosion – what should be done? *Dental Update*, **25**, 166–170.

Collins, L.M.C., Dawes, C. (1987) The surface area of the adult human mouth and thickness of the salivary film covering the teeth and oral mucosa. *Journal of Dental Research*, **66**, 1300–1302.

Daley T.J., Harbrow, D.J., Kahler, B., et al. (2009) The cervical wedge-shaped lesion in teeth: a light and electron microscopic study. *Australian Dental Journal*, **54**(3), 212–219.

Dawes, C. (2008) Salivary flow patterns and the health of hard and soft oral tissues. *Journal of the American Dental Association*, **139**, 18–24.

Greaves, W.S. (1973) The inference of jaw motion from toothwear facets. *Journal of Paelontology*, **47**, 1000–1001.

Grippo, J.O. (1991) Abfractions: a new classification of hard tissue lesions of teeth. *Journal of Esthetic Dentistry*, **3**(1), 14–19.

Kaidonis, J.A., Townsend, G.C., Richards, L.C. (1992) Brief communication: interproximal tooth wear: a new observation. *American Journal of Physical Anthropology*, **88**, 105–107.

Khan F., Young W.G., Daley, T.J. (1998) Dental erosion and bruxism. A tooth wear analysis from South East Queensland. *Australian Dental Journal*, **43**(2), 117–127.

Khan, F., Young, W.G., Law, V., et al. (2001) Cupped lesions of early onset dental erosion in young Southeast Queensland adults. *Australian Dental Journal*, **46**, 100–107.

Khan, F., Young, W.G., Shahabi, S., et al. (1999) Dental cervical lesions associated with occlusal erosion and attrition. *Australian Dental Journal*, **44**, 176–186.

Khan, F., Young, W.G., Taji, S.S. (2010) Toothwear: A Guide for Oral Health Practitioners. Copyright Publishing Pty Ltd. Brisbane, Australia.

Lussi, A., Hellwig, E., Zero, D., et al. (2009) Buonocore memorial lecture. Dental erosion. *Operative Dentistry*, **34**(3), 251–262.

Michael, J.A., Kaidonis, J.A., Townsend, G.C. (2010) Non-carious cervical lesions on permanent anterior teeth: a new morphological classification. *Australian Dental Journal*, **55**, 134–137.

Osborn, J.W. (1990) A 3-dimensional model to describe the relation between prism directions, parazones and diazones, and the Hunter-Schreger bands in human tooth enamel. *Archives of Oral Biology*, **35**(11), 869–878.

Rees, J.S. (1998) The role of cuspal flexure in the development of abfraction lesions: a finite element study. *European Journal of Oral Sciences*, **52**, 1028–1032.

Teo, C., Young, W.G., Daley, T.J., et al. (1997) Prior fluoridation in childhood affects dental caries and toothwear in a South East Queensland population. *Australian Dental Journal*, **42**(2), 92–102.

Wood, I., Jawad, Z., Paisley, C., et al. (2008) Non-carious cervical tooth surface loss: a literature review. *Journal of Dentistry*, **35**, 759–766.

Young, W.G. (1998) Anthropology, tooth wear and occlusion *ab origine. Journal of Dental Research*, **77**(11), 1860–1863.

Young, W.G. (2001a) Oral medicine of toothwear. *Australian Dental Journal*, **46**(4), 236–250.

Young, W.G. (2001b) *Oral Medicine of Toothwear CD Rom*, Dentil Pty Ltd. Queensland, Australia.

Young, W.G. (2003a) *Teeth on Edge,* Erosion Watch Pty Ltd. Queensland, Australia.

Young, W.G. (2003b) *What Colour Is Your Sports Drink CD Rom*, Dentil Pty Ltd. Queensland, Australia.

Young, W.G., Khan, F. (2002) Sites of dental erosion are saliva-dependent. *Journal of Oral Rehabilitation*, **29**, 35–43.

Young, W.G., Khan, F. (2009) *By the Skin of Our Teeth*, Erosion Watch Pty Ltd. Queensland, Australia.

Young, W.G., Messer, B. (2002) *Diet Analysis and Advice for Patients With Tooth Wear CD Rom*, Dentil Pty Ltd. Queensland, Australia.

Salivary protection against toothwear and dental caries

Colin Dawes

FACTORS CAUSING TOOTHWEAR

Toothwear may be due to abrasion, attrition, acid erosion or some combination of these processes. *Abrasion* occurs from the action of foreign bodies rubbing against the teeth. An example is the use of a hard toothbrush and an abrasive toothpaste. *Attrition* is the wear which occurs from repeated contact between opposing teeth, a process which is accentuated in patients with bruxism. *Acid erosion* is due to exposure of the teeth to extrinsic acid which is unsaturated with respect to tooth mineral. There are many different types and possible sources of such acids and they include gastro-oesophageal reflux disease (GORD, in which a weak gastro-oesophageal sphincter allows gastric juice to enter the oesophagus and then the mouth), bulimia (deliberate vomiting), acidic, soft or sports drinks, fruit juices, wine, acid fumes in the workplace, acidic medicaments, such as aspirin, and exposure to the water in an improperly chlorinated swimming pools. Of

these, the hydrochloric acid in gastric juice is probably the most potent as its concentration in it is about 0.1 mol/L. It is the plaque-free surfaces of the teeth which are attacked by these acids and they dissolve the very surface layers of the enamel (ten Cate 1979). The buccal, lingual and occlusal surfaces of the teeth are particularly affected and the approximal surfaces almost never. Loss of enamel may take a long time to be noticeable, but complete loss has been reported to occur in as little as 2 weeks after prolonged daily exposure to the water in an improperly chlorinated (low-pH) swimming pool (Dawes & Boroditsky 2008). The citric acid present mainly in fruit juices can act not only as an acid but also as a chelating agent for calcium ions, even when the pH is close to neutrality.

FACTORS CAUSING DENTAL CARIES

Dental caries is also caused by the action of acid on the teeth. However, in contrast to acid

Toothwear: The ABC of the Worn Dentition, First Edition. Edited by Farid Khan and William George Young.
© 2011 John Wiley & Sons, Ltd. Published 2011 by John Wiley & Sons, Ltd.

erosion, caries is caused by those acids, primarily lactic and acetic acids, which are produced from fermentable carbohydrates by acidogenic microorganisms in dental plaque. Thus, caries can only occur at sites on the tooth which are covered by dental plaque and will progress only when the pH of the plaque is less than the so-called critical pH (about 5.1), at which the fluid phase of plaque (plaque fluid) becomes unsaturated with respect to tooth mineral. Some investigators suggest that caries is primarily due to the metabolic activity of strongly acidogenic microorganisms, such as *Streptococcus mutans* (Tanzer 1995), and that colonisation of the mouth by mutans streptococci is the critical factor in whether caries will occur. However, many of the microbial species in plaque are acidogenic, and Hardie et al. (1977) have found caries under plaques in which the presence of *S. mutans* was not detectable. An alternative view (Marsh 2003) is the 'ecological hypothe-

sis' that frequent consumption of fermentable carbohydrate (i.e. sugars which can be converted to acid by plaque microorganisms) will favour the growth and predominance of microorganisms which are acidogenic (i.e. ones which can form acid from sugars) and aciduric (i.e. ones which can survive under acidic conditions). So if fermentable carbohydrates are consumed frequently, the proportions of acidogenic and aciduric microorganisms in undisturbed plaque will increase and caries will be more likely to progress whenever fermentable carbohydrates are consumed. Thus, the ecological hypothesis suggests that the frequency with which fermentable carbohydrates are consumed is the key factor promoting dental caries.

A critical difference between acid erosion and dental caries is that the latter begins largely as a subsurface, rather than a surface lesion (Fig. 5.1), and the lesion may extend into

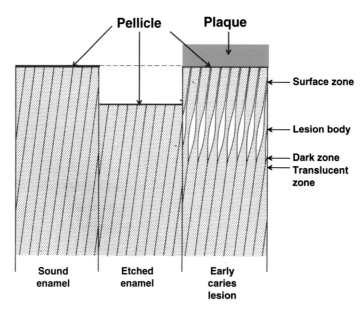

Figure 5.1   Schematic representation of the essential difference between the formation of acid-etched enamel and an early caries lesion of enamel (which is covered by dental plaque). The positions of the four zones of an early caries lesion (surface, body, dark and translucent) are shown. Pellicle is present on the surface of both intact enamel and enamel shortly after it has been acid etched. Pellicle also usually separates the enamel at the surface of an early caries lesion from the overlying dental plaque. (Modified from ten Cate, 1979, by kind permission of Prof. J.M. ten Cate.)

dentine before the relatively intact surface zone of the enamel (about 30 μm thick) breaks down to create an actual cavity.

Another difference between acid erosion and caries is that the former usually involves relatively short exposures (seconds) of the teeth to acidic fluids, whereas after consumption of fermentable carbohydrate, the plaque pH may fall below the critical pH for several hours.

WHY DOES A TOOTH DISSOLVE IN ACID?

The mineral phase of enamel and dentine is composed of an impure form of hydroxyapatite (HA) which contains many trace elements, such as carbonate, which increases its solubility, and fluoride, which decreases its solubility. The structural formula of HA is $Ca_{10}(PO_4)_6(OH)_2$, and when this is in contact with water, a small amount slowly dissolves to release calcium, phosphate and hydroxyl ions:

$$Solid \rightleftharpoons Solution$$
$$Ca_{10}(PO_4)_6(OH)_2 \rightleftharpoons 10Ca^{2+} + 6PO_4^{3-} + 2OH^-$$

The dissolution continues until the water is saturated with respect to HA, and at that point, the rate of dissolution is equal to the rate of precipitation.

The solubility of an ionic material, such as HA, is described by its solubility product (K_{sp}), which is the product of its component ions (in mol/L) raised to the appropriate power in a solution saturated with HA. This is equal to $[Ca]^{10} \cdot [PO_4]^6 \cdot [OH]^2$, where the values in square brackets represent the activities of the component ions. Since HA is relatively insoluble in water, and the ionic activities are measured in mol/L, the K_{sp} has a very low value of about 10^{-117} (Larsen & Bruun 1986). This value is a constant, but the concentrations of the three component ions may vary in different saturated

solutions, provided that their product remains at 10^{-117}.

For any given fluid such as saliva, wine or a sports drink, one can make a similar calculation from the calcium, phosphate and hydroxyl ion concentrations in these fluids to obtain a value termed the 'ion product' (I_p). This can then be compared with the K_{sp}. If $I_p = K_{sp}$, the solution is just saturated with respect to HA. If $I_p > K_{sp}$, it is supersaturated and HA will tend to precipitate out until it becomes saturated, while if $I_p < K_{sp}$, the fluid is unsaturated and HA will tend to dissolve in it until it becomes saturated.

The solubility of HA in water at pH 7 is about 30 mg/L, but since the solubility increases about tenfold for each unit fall in pH, the solubility is about 30 g/L at pH 4 (Larsen & Bruun 1986). Although the concentration of calcium in a solution is virtually independent of pH, the hydroxyl concentration changes inversely with the hydrogen ion concentration, as the product $[H^+] \cdot [OH^-]$ always equals 10^{-14} $(mol/L)^2$. Thus, in gastric juice at about pH 1, $[H^+] = 10^{-1}$ mol/L, but $[OH^-] = 10^{-13}$ mol/L. In addition, in any fluid containing inorganic phosphate, the phosphate is present in four different forms: H_3PO_4, $H_2PO_4^-$, HPO_4^{2-} and PO_4^{3-}, and the proportions change with pH, as shown in Fig. 5.2 (Dawes 2003).

It is the PO_4^{3-} form of phosphate which contributes to the I_p and K_{sp} for HA and the fraction of phosphate present as PO_4^{3-} decreases markedly as the pH falls. Thus, very acidic solutions will contain very low OH^- and PO_4^{3-} concentrations such that usually the $I_{pHA} < K_{spHA}$ and the mineral of the tooth will begin to dissolve in the acid.

The critical pH of a solution is the pH below which the solution becomes unsaturated with respect to HA. For saliva, the critical pH varies from 5.5 to 6.5 in different individuals (Ericsson 1949), the lower values being for saliva that contains higher calcium and phosphate concentrations. Since plaque fluid contains more calcium and phosphate than does saliva (Tatevossian & Gould 1976), its critical pH is

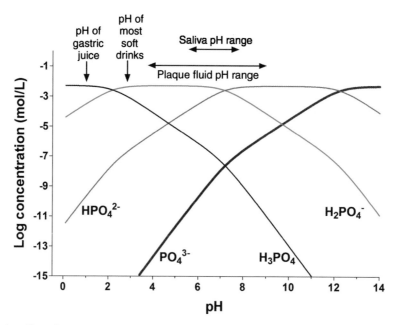

Figure 5.2 The effect of pH on the concentrations of the four different species of inorganic phosphate in saliva containing a total phosphate concentration of 5 mmol/L, as is typical of whole saliva. There is a marked decline in the PO_4^{3-} concentration (thick red line) as the pH falls. (From Dawes, 2003, by permission of the Journal of the Canadian Dental Association.)

about 5.1. During a Stephan curve, which is the fall and subsequent rise in plaque pH after exposure of plaque to a fermentable carbohydrate, caries will progress only during the period when the plaque pH is less than about 5.1.

SOURCES AND COMPONENTS OF SALIVA RELEVANT TO TOOTHWEAR AND CARIES

Sources of saliva

The fluid phase of whole saliva is a mixture of secretions from three pairs of major glands, namely the parotid, submandibular and sublingual, together with those from numerous minor mucous glands in the lips, cheeks and soft palate and secretions from the small glands in the foliate and circumvallate papillae of the

dorsum of the tongue. Table 5.1 shows the primary nature (serous or mucous) of the secretions from different salivary glands, as well as their percentage contributions to whole saliva when the flow rate is unstimulated and when it is strongly stimulated.

Figure 5.3 shows, diagrammatically, the probable net direction and volumes of saliva flow from the different glands at different locations in the mouth. The lingual and palatal surfaces of the teeth and the buccal surfaces of the molar teeth receive the greatest protection from the serous secretions of the major salivary glands.

Whole saliva also contains components of non-salivary origin, including gingival crevicular fluid (except in the edentulous), desquamated epithelial cells, microorganisms, metabolic products from the microorganisms, viruses, fungi and possibly food debris,

Table 5.1 Some characteristics of the different types of saliva.

| Glandular source of saliva | Nature of secretion | Percent contribution to whole saliva at: | | Contains bicarbonate |
		Low flow rate	High flow rate	
Parotid	Serous	25	50	Yes
Submandibular	Serous + mucous	60	35	Yes
Sublingual	Mucous	8	8	Yes
Minor mucous	Mucous	7	7	No

expectorated bronchial secretions and blood. The total volume of saliva secreted each day has been calculated to be about 600 mL (Watanabe & Dawes 1988). When whole saliva is collected into a container, it has usually been assumed that all surfaces of the mouth have been exposed to this fluid. However, the proportions of the different secretions which make up whole saliva vary considerably at different sites in the mouth (Sas & Dawes 1997), even during gum chewing, which might have been expected to cause efficient mixing of the various salivary secretions. Thus the fluid environment of the mouth shows marked site specificity.

The unstimulated salivary flow rate averages 0.3–0.4 mL/min, but with wide variability among different individuals, and the unstimulated flow rate is very low during sleep. Unstimulated flow rates <0.1 mL/min are considered objective evidence of hyposalivation, as are stimulated flow rates of <0.5 mL/min (Sreebny et al. 1992). The unstimulated flow rate is influenced by many factors, including

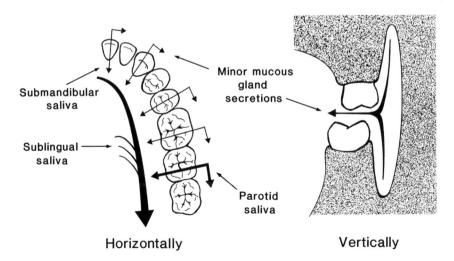

Figure 5.3 Diagrammatic representation of the anticipated directions and volumes of salivary flow in different locations in the mouth. (From Lecomte & Dawes, 1987, by permission of Sage Publications.)

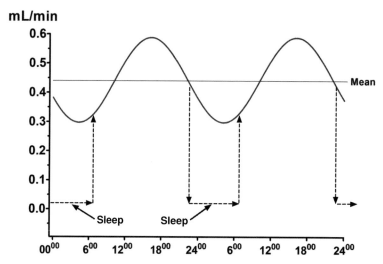

Figure 5.4 The circadian rhythm in the unstimulated salivary flow rate. The dramatic reduction in flow rate during sleep is also shown schematically.

the degree of hydration (the most important factor with respect to toothwear), body position, exposure to light, previous stimulation of the glands, smoking and circadian and circannual rhythms, as discussed in more detail elsewhere (Dawes 2004a). Figure 5.4 shows that the circadian rhythm in unstimulated salivary flow rate is of quite high amplitude, with the peak at about 5 PM being about double that at 5 AM. Figure 5.4 also illustrates that during sleep, the salivary flow rate is virtually zero.

Females tend to have smaller gland sizes and lower flow rates than males. Several hundred drugs cause hyposalivation as an unwanted side effect (Sreebny et al. 1992), and the flow rate may be virtually zero in patients with congenital absence of the major salivary glands or in patients who have been treated with radiation for head and neck cancer or have advanced Sjögren's syndrome, an autoimmune condition in which the acinar cells of the salivary glands are destroyed. Figures 5.5 and 5.6 illustrate erosion of the teeth of a man with congenital absence of the parotid and submandibular glands, who had used acidic soft

drinks to relieve his xerostomia. The lack of cervical lesions suggests mucous saliva was protective.

The salivary flow rate can be increased by the action of chewing alone, but foods also provide gustatory stimulation of taste receptors to elicit a maximum average flow rate of about 7 mL/min. Of the different gustatory stimuli (acid, salt, bitter, sweet and umami), acid is the most potent while sweet is a relatively poor stimulus of salivation.

Components of saliva

The secretions from the salivary glands consist primarily of water (99%), which is necessary for dilution and clearance of materials taken into the mouth, to be discussed in a later section. The different secretions contain a great variety of proteins and glycoproteins, electrolytes and small-molecular-mass substances which give saliva its characteristic properties. As many as 309 different proteins and glycoproteins have been identified in whole saliva by proteomic techniques (Hu et al. 2005) and over 1000 in

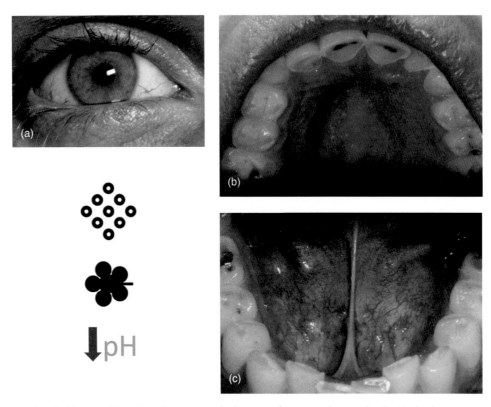

Figure 5.5 A 19-year-old male with congenital absence of major salivary glands. He had constant tearing from both eyes (epiphora) due to lack of tear ducts (a). No parotid, submandibular or sublingual glands were palpable. Degradation was present on the palatal surfaces where the exposed dentine was dull, featureless and brown reparative dentine was evident (b). Saliva came only from under his tongue and minor salivary glands were visible on the inner surface of the lip. No openings of Stenson's or Wharton's ducts were found (c). (From Young et al., 2001, by permission of Elsevier Limited.)

secretions obtained from the ducts of the parotid and submandibular glands. Helmerhorst and Oppenheim (2007) have discussed the different families of proteins in saliva and the fact that many of these are subject to rapid proteolysis and deglycosylation by enzymes secreted by oral microorganisms. Many factors influence the concentration of protein in saliva, including the rate of flow, the duration of stimulation, the degree of previous stimulation of the glands, the nature of the stimulus, and circadian rhythms, as discussed elsewhere (Dawes 2004a).

The amylase, secreted primarily by the parotid glands, may play a role in dental caries by releasing maltose from starches retained in the mouth as food debris. In addition, the antibacterial and antifungal factors in saliva may influence the composition of the oral microflora. Many salivary proteins also contribute to the formation of the acquired enamel pellicle (AEP), which is discussed in a later section.

The main electrolytes in saliva include sodium, potassium, calcium, magnesium, chloride, bicarbonate, phosphate, thiocyanate and fluoride. Their concentrations are particularly

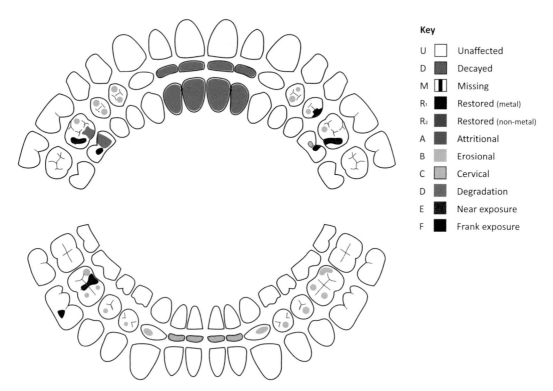

Key

U	☐	Unaffected
D	▦	Decayed
M	▯	Missing
R₁	■	Restored (metal)
R₂	■	Restored (non-metal)
A	■	Attritional
B	▨	Erosional
C	▨	Cervical
D	▦	Degradation
E	▦	Near exposure
F	■	Frank exposure

Figure 5.6 Odontogram showing erosion was evident on the incisal edges of the lower anterior teeth. Cuspal-cupped lesions were present on the premolar and first molar teeth. Remarkably only one cervical lesion was found on the palatal surface of the upper left first molar tooth, suggesting that most cervical surfaces were protected by mucous saliva despite the absence of the major glands. Degradation was present on the incisal and palatal surfaces of the upper incisor teeth and on the mesiopalatal cusp of the upper right first molar tooth.

dependent on the salivary flow rate and they also show circadian rhythms. The most important change with flow rate is an increase in the bicarbonate concentration from about 5 mmol/L in unstimulated whole saliva to about 17 mmol/L in whole saliva elicited by chewing gum and even higher values with acid as the stimulus. The pH of saliva is influenced by changes in the bicarbonate concentration, as may be calculated from the Henderson–Hasselbalch equation:

$$pH = pK + \log([HCO_3^-]/[H_2CO_3]).$$

The carbonic acid concentration is about 1.2 mmol/L, and this is constant under normal breathing conditions and is independent of the flow rate. Since the pK value of about 6.1 is almost independent of the flow rate, the pH of saliva is governed by the bicarbonate concentration. So for unstimulated whole saliva,

$$pH = 6.1 + \log(5/1.2) = 6.5$$

and for saliva elicited by chewing gum, the pH will be about 7.35.

One of the low-molecular-mass substances secreted in saliva is urea, with a concentration of about 3 mmol/L in unstimulated saliva and somewhat higher concentrations in secretions from the minor salivary glands. Urea is neutral and thus cannot protect against acid erosion. However, urea can diffuse from saliva into dental plaque, where it is broken down by bacterial ureases to form two molecules of ammonia and one of carbon dioxide. The ammonia is able to neutralise some of the acid formed in dental plaque, and it has been calculated that in the absence of urea, the plaque pH would fall an extra 0.5 units after exposure to fermentable carbohydrate (Dibdin & Dawes 1998). Thus, salivary urea provides some protection against dental caries. However, patients with renal disease and high urea levels in their saliva are much more susceptible to calculus deposition in their plaque because of the alkalinity caused by the ammonia.

Salivary clearance

Many substances pass through the mouth each day to be cleared by swallowing and these include food, beverages, microorganisms, desquamated epithelial cells and oral hygiene products. For optimum oral health, most of these materials should stay in the mouth for as short a time as possible, as the prolonged presence of sugars and acids from foods and beverages will have deleterious effects on the teeth. Thus, it is important to identify the factors which can change the rate of salivary clearance.

The Dawes model of salivary clearance (Dawes 2004b) assumes that the swallowing process can be represented as the action of an incomplete syphon. After a swallow, the mouth is not cleared completely of saliva, but a residual volume averaging 0.8 mL (range 0.4–1.4 mL) is left in the mouth. More saliva then enters and another swallow is normally initiated at a maximum average volume (V_{max}) of 1.1 mL (range 0.5–2.1 mL). Thus, the average person swallows only 0.3 mL of saliva when salivary flow is unstimulated and leaves behind 0.8 mL (Lagerlöf & Dawes 1984). If the unstimulated flow rate is 0.3 mL/min, and this saliva mixes well with the residual volume of 0.8 mL, the time for half of the material in the saliva at time zero to be cleared (the half-time) is about 2.2 min. The model applies to many materials, such as sucrose, which do not bind to

anything in the mouth, but for substances such as fluoride or chlorhexidine, which are able to bind to oral structures (termed substantivity), the clearance half-time will be longer. The clearance half-time will be longer in people with high values of the residual volume and V_{max} (who may be termed 'inefficient swallowers'), a low unstimulated salivary flow rate and a low stimulated salivary flow rate. After the last portions of food and beverages have been swallowed, gustatory stimulation will be reduced and the salivary flow rate will fall to the unstimulated level in about 1 min. The stimulated flow rate will determine how rapidly harmful substances such as sucrose and acid are diluted, and the more quickly this happens, the smaller will be the concentration gradient for sucrose to diffuse into dental plaque and the lower will be the acid concentration for causing erosion of the teeth.

Saliva as a thin film

For many years, saliva was assumed to be present in the mouth as a relatively large volume, but after the normal values for the residual volume and V_{max} had been established and the surface area of the mouth measured, it was realised that saliva must be present between any two oral surfaces as a thin film, averaging between 0.07 and 0.1 mm in thickness after and before swallowing, respectively (Collins & Dawes 1987). On individual surfaces not in contact with others, the film thickness would be about half those values. More recent studies (DiSabato-Mordarski & Kleinberg 1996) of film thicknesses on individual surfaces have shown the average thickness to vary from 70 μm on the posterior dorsum of the tongue to 10 μm on the anterior hard palate. A sense of dryness (xerostomia) is experienced when the thickness of the film on the hard palate becomes <10 μm. In patients with dry mouth and a very low unstimulated salivary flow rate, the residual volume has been found to average 71% of the normal 0.8 mL, which suggests that the sensation of xerostomia may not be due to generalised oral dryness, but due to localised areas of dryness, particularly in the hard palate region.

A critical factor influencing the rate of clearance of materials from a particular oral site is the velocity of the salivary film as it moves towards the pharynx. When salivary flow is unstimulated, the velocity has been estimated to vary from 0.8 to 8.0 mm/min in different regions of the mouth, with the lower values occurring buccal to the upper anterior teeth and buccal to all the lower teeth. The higher velocities occur on the lingual and palatal surfaces of the teeth and buccal to the upper molar teeth, where the parotid duct opens. When salivary flow is stimulated, there is only a slight increase where the unstimulated velocities are low, but a dramatic increase to >300 mm/min where the unstimulated velocities are higher.

With respect to dental caries, two types of clearance are of particular importance. The first is the clearance of ingested sugar from the salivary film overlying dental plaque. Although sugar, compared with acid, is a relatively weak stimulus for salivary flow, when a sugar-containing chewing gum is chewed, the flow rate increases initially to about 12 times the unstimulated rate before falling within about 10 min to between 2 and 3 times the unstimulated rate (Dawes 2004a). There is great site specificity in the rate of sugar clearance, the highest rate being lingual to the lower incisor teeth and the lowest rate being buccal to the upper incisor teeth (Dawes & Macpherson 1993).

The second type of clearance is that of acids produced by the microorganisms in dental plaque from the sugar that has diffused into plaque. These acids are removed from plaque either by their diffusion into the salivary film overlying the plaque or by diffusion of salivary buffers into plaque. The higher the velocity of the salivary film, the more rapidly will these acids be cleared from plaque, the greater will be the supply of salivary buffers and the shorter will be the time during which the plaque pH

is less than the critical pH. Salivary sugar and plaque acid are cleared more readily from the lingual and palatal surfaces of the teeth and from buccal to the upper molar teeth than from the other buccal surfaces, and this may be why the latter are more susceptible to smooth-surface caries (Dawes & Macpherson 1993).

The rate of clearance of acid from the mouth is also of critical importance in determining the rate at which enamel erosion occurs in people who frequently consume acidic foods and beverages. Again, because the salivary film velocity will be higher lingually and palatally and buccal to the upper molar teeth, these surfaces would be expected to show less acid erosion.

Salivary buffering

Saliva acts as a temperature buffer against hot or cold foods and beverages, but more importantly, with respect to dental caries and erosion, as a buffer against acid. The three types of salivary buffers against acid are bicarbonate, phosphate and protein. Since the protein concentration in saliva is very low in comparison with that in plasma, salivary proteins are not very effective buffers at all and will have only a minor buffering action at around pH 4, the approximate pK of free carboxyl groups.

The phosphate concentration in unstimulated whole saliva is about 5 mmol/L and this falls as the flow rate is increased. Figure 5.2 shows that at pH 6.5, the pH of unstimulated whole saliva, the majority of the phosphate is in the $H_2PO_4^-$ form and this cannot take up a hydrogen ion to form H_3PO_4 until the pH is much closer to 2.2, the pK_1 value for phosphate. At high flow rates, the pH will exceed the pK_2 value of 7.2 and the majority of the phosphate will be in the HPO_4^{2-} form, which can take up a hydrogen ion to form the $H_2PO_4^-$ species. However, the phosphate concentration falls as the flow rate increases and it may then be too low for phosphate to act as a useful buffer.

In contrast, bicarbonate, with a pK of about 6.1, is a particularly useful buffer because it reacts with hydrogen ions to form carbonic acid. The latter does not accumulate, as does the acid form of most buffers, but it breaks down to water and carbon dioxide and the latter is released into the atmosphere. The bicarbonate concentration increases with flow rate and the concentration in strongly stimulated parotid saliva may reach as high as 60 mmol/L, well above the 24 mmol/L in plasma. Most of the hydrogen ions in plaque at a low pH have been found to be bound to the surface proteins of microorganisms or other fixed buffers (Shellis & Dibdin 1988) and they are not freely mobile. Thus, a water rinse will have little effect on the pH of plaque after a meal containing fermentable carbohydrate as the bound hydrogen ions in plaque cannot diffuse out into the water. However, the bicarbonate and phosphate ions in the salivary film are able to diffuse into plaque as HCO_3^- and HPO_4^{2-} ions, bind hydrogen ions and diffuse out as $H_2CO_3^-$ and HPO_4^- ions. Bicarbonate is thus the main buffer in saliva, and an important point is that the minor mucous gland secretions contain no bicarbonate (see Table 5.1) and only about one-tenth the concentration of phosphate as that in the major salivary gland secretions (Dawes & Wood 1973). Thus, in locations in the mouth, such as buccal to the upper incisors, where minor mucous gland secretions predominate, the saliva will be very poorly buffered. In addition, because of the very high viscosity of the mucous secretions, the salivary film velocity is typically very low where minor mucous gland secretions predominate in the salivary film. These factors may contribute to the site specificity of acid erosion. When a mouthful of an acidic soft or sports drink (about 10–12 mL) is taken into the mouth, this volume greatly exceeds the residual volume of saliva (0.8 mL) and it is not surprising that a mouthful of these types of products is able to overwhelm the buffering capacity of the residual volume of saliva and cause erosion, especially if each mouthful is swished around the mouth before it is swallowed, a practice which should be avoided.

Oral hygiene procedures are particularly important before sleep, since the salivary flow rate is virtually zero during sleep (see Fig. 5.4) and the bicarbonate concentration in the saliva will be very low, so that any saliva secreted during sleep will have a very low buffer capacity.

The acquired enamel pellicle (friend or foe?)

After the teeth have erupted, the embryological integuments are worn away by frictional forces and replaced by the AEP (Dawes et al. 1963), which is about 1 µm in thickness. Pellicles formed for 1 h on bovine enamel slabs positioned at different sites in the mouth were found to vary in thickness from 0.30 to 1.06 µm, with the thicker pellicles being located lingual to the lower incisor teeth (Amaechi et al. 1999). Pellicle was originally believed to be derived entirely from salivary proteins, but it has recently been shown, by proteomic techniques, to contain 130 different proteins, 88% being of cellular origin (presumably from desquamated oral epithelial cells), 18% being from plasma (presumably mainly from gingival crevicular fluid) and only 14% being of salivary origin (Siqueira et al. 2007). However, since proteomics can identify individual proteins, but not determine their percentage contributions to the material analysed, it may be that the actual percentage of salivary proteins in the pellicle is much higher than 14%.

The most important feature of the AEP is that if it is removed from the enamel surface, it is replaced within seconds when the denuded surface contacts saliva. The AEP is partially or completely removed by the forces of abrasion and attrition, and its rapid replacement by some of the proteins in saliva gives it the property of a renewable lubricant. In the absence of the AEP, the forces of abrasion and attrition would wear the enamel much more rapidly than they normally do.

When the enamel is subject to acid erosion, the presence of the AEP has been found to give some slight protection against the acid (Amaechi et al. 1999; Hara et al. 2006). However, on plaque-free surfaces, hydrogen ions diffuse through the AEP, dissolve the underlying enamel, and may also remove the AEP. After removal of the acid and contact with saliva, a new pellicle forms and, by binding tightly to the surface enamel crystals, prevents the reformation of the enamel crystals which dissolved in the acid. Incidentally, this property of the AEP prevents the continuous enlargement of the teeth, which would tend to occur in its absence, since the enamel is bathed in saliva which is supersaturated with respect to tooth mineral.

During the acid-etch technique, usually with 37% phosphoric acid, the AEP will be removed, along with a few micrometers of surface enamel, and it is important that the clinician not allows saliva to recontact the etched surface prior to placement of composite resin, since the presence of a newly formed AEP will reduce the bond strength between the enamel and the resin.

The AEP forms the substrate to which microorganisms can attach to begin the formation of dental plaque. During the development of an early caries lesion, the hydrogen ions produced by acidogenic microorganisms in dental plaque are also able to diffuse through the AEP and create microchannels through the enamel (Haikel et al. 1983) and eventually a subsurface caries lesion.

Remineralisation

Since both saliva and plaque fluid are supersaturated with respect to HA when food has not been in the mouth for some time (i.e. when the plaque pH is above the critical pH), there is the possibility of remineralisation of the subsurface lesion of early caries. Such lesions are sterile, but once the surface zone has been broken through, oral microorganisms can penetrate to the subsurface body of the lesion where the major loss of mineral has occurred (see Fig. 5.1)

and remineralisation is no longer possible. The process of remineralisation involves the diffusion of calcium and phosphate ions through the AEP and then through the micropits in the enamel surface (Haikel et al. 1983) to create a supersaturated solution in the subsurface body of the lesion. This then allows crystal growth on the existing enamel crystals in the depth of the lesion. Such remineralisation is promoted by the presence of fluoride in the drinking water or in oral hygiene products, which facilitates the formation of fluoridated HA. Ideally, the early enamel lesion to be remineralised should be kept free of dental plaque and have good access to saliva. Stimulation of salivary flow by the use of such products as sugar-free chewing gum will be beneficial, as the higher the salivary flow rate, the greater is its degree of supersaturation with respect to HA. The use of products containing casein phosphopeptide-amorphous calcium phosphate may also help to promote remineralisation by providing an extra source of calcium and phosphate.

In contrast, as mentioned previously, remineralisation of enamel eroded by acid is not possible, because the tightly adherent enamel pellicle does not allow crystal growth of the underlying enamel crystals. Thus, an important responsibility of the dentist is to diagnose the presence of acid erosion, identify the causes and recommend changes in the lifestyle of the patient to avoid further damage to the teeth.

CONCLUSIONS

Saliva plays a critical role in protection against both dental caries and acid erosion of the teeth, and its effects are reduced in patients with hyposalivation. Patients should be advised to maintain good hydration, as the unstimulated salivary flow rate is markedly decreased during periods of dehydration, such as may occur in a hot climate and particularly while playing sports. The drinking of water rather than soft or sports drinks should be encouraged as the latter drinks are usually very acidic and may also contain fermentable carbohydrates. Between-meal snacks should be avoided to reduce the frequency of acid formation in dental plaque, thereby allowing more time between meals for remineralisation of early caries lesions to occur. The use of sugar-free chewing gum or candies can also be recommended as these stimulate salivary flow to provide a fluid of higher pH, buffer capacity and degree of supersaturation with respect to tooth mineral. Dentists have a responsibility to identify early signs of acid erosion of the teeth and recommend such lifestyle changes as may be necessary to prevent the progression of this irreversible condition.

References

Amaechi, B.T., Higham, S.M., Edgar, W.M., et al. (1999) Thickness of acquired salivary pellicle as a determinant of the sites of dental erosion. *Journal of Dental Research*, **78**, 1821–1828.

Collins, L.M.C., Dawes, C. (1987) The surface area of the adult human mouth and thickness of the salivary film covering the teeth and oral mucosa. *Journal of Dental Research*, **66**, 1300–1302.

Dawes, C. (2003) What is the critical pH and why does a tooth dissolve in acid? *Journal of the Canadian Dental Association*, **69**, 722–724.

Dawes, C. (2004a) Factors influencing salivary flow rate and composition. In: *Saliva and Oral Health* (eds M. Edgar, C. Dawes & D. O'Mullane), 3rd edn. pp. 32–49. British Dental Association, London.

Dawes, C. (2004b) Salivary clearance and its effects on oral health. In: *Saliva and Oral Health* (eds M. Edgar, C. Dawes & D. O'Mullane), 3rd edn. pp. 71–85. British Dental Association, London.

Dawes, C., Boroditsky, C.L. (2008) Rapid and severe tooth erosion from swimming in an improperly chlorinated pool: case report. *Journal of the Canadian Dental Association*, **74**, 347–349.

Dawes, C., Jenkins, G.N., Tonge, C.H. (1963) The nomenclature of the integuments of the enamel surface of teeth. *British Dental Journal*, **115**, 65–68.

Dawes, C., Macpherson, L.M.D. (1993) The distribution of saliva and sucrose around the mouth during the use of chewing gum and the implications for the site-specificity of caries and calculus deposition. *Journal of Dental Research*, **72**, 852–857.

Dawes, C., Wood, C.M. (1973) The composition of human lip mucous gland secretions. *Archives of Oral Biology*, **18**, 343–350.

Dibdin, G.H., Dawes, C. (1998) A mathematical model of the influence of salivary urea on the pH of fasted dental plaque and on the changes occurring during a cariogenic challenge. *Caries Research*, **32**, 70–74.

DiSabato-Mordarski, T., Kleinberg, I. (1996) Measurement and comparison of the residual saliva on various oral mucosal and dentition surfaces in humans. *Archives of Oral Biology*, **41**, 655–665.

Ericsson, Y. (1949) Enamel-apatite solubility. Investigations into the calcium phosphate equilibrium between enamel and saliva in its relation to dental caries. *Acta Odontologica Scandinavica*, **8**(Suppl 3), 1–139.

Haikel, Y., Frank, R.M., Voegel, J.C. (1983) Scanning electron microscopy of the human enamel surface layer of incipient carious lesions. *Caries Research*, **17**, 1–13.

Hara, A.T., Ando, M., González-Cabezas, C., et al. (2006) Protective effect of the dental pellicle against erosive challenges *in situ*. *Journal of Dental Research*, **85**, 612–616.

Hardie, J.M., Thomson, P.L., South, R.J., et al. (1977) A longitudinal epidemiological study on dental plaque and the development of dental caries – interim results after two years. *Journal of Dental Research*, **56**(Sp. no. C), C90–C98.

Helmerhorst, E.J., Oppenheim, F.G. (2007) Saliva: a dynamic proteome. *Journal of Dental Research*, **86**, 680–693.

Hu, S., Xie, Y., Ramachandran, P., et al. (2005) Large-scale identification of proteins in human salivary proteome by liquid chromatography/mass spectrometry and two-dimensional gel electrophoresis-mass spectrometry. *Proteomics*, **5**, 1714–1728.

Lagerlöf, F., Dawes, C. (1984) The volume of saliva in the mouth before and after swallowing. *Journal of Dental Research*, **63**, 618–621.

Larsen, M.J., Bruun, C. (1986) Enamel/saliva – inorganic chemical reactions. In: *Textbook of Cariology* (eds A. Thylstrup & O. Fejerskov), pp. 181–203. Munksgaard, Copenhagen.

Lecomte, P., Dawes, C. (1987) The influence of salivary flow rate on diffusion of potassium chloride from artificial plaque at different sites in the mouth. *Journal of Dental Research*, **66**, 1614–1618.

Marsh, P.D. (2003) Are dental diseases examples of ecological catastrophes? *Microbiology*, **149**, 279–294.

Sas, R., Dawes, C. (1997) The intra-oral distribution of unstimulated and chewing-gum-stimulated parotid saliva. *Archives of Oral Biology*, **42**, 469–474.

Shellis, R.P., Dibdin, G.H. (1988) Analysis of the buffering systems in dental plaque. *Journal of Dental Research*, **67**, 438–446.

Siqueira, W.L., Zhang, W., Helmerhorst, E.J., et al. (2007) Identification of protein components in *in vivo* human acquired enamel pellicle using LC-ESI-MS/MS. *Journal of Proteome Research*, **6**, 2152–2160.

Sreebny, L.M., Banoczy, J., Baum, B.J., et al. (1992) Saliva: its role in health and disease. *International Dental Journal*, **42**(Suppl 2), 291–304.

Tanzer, J.M. (1995) Dental caries is a transmissible infectious disease: the Keyes and Fitzgerald revolution. *Journal of Dental Research*, **74**, 1536–1542.

Tatevossian, A., Gould, C.T. (1976) The composition of the aqueous phase in human dental plaque. *Archives of Oral Biology*, **21**, 319–323.

ten Cate, J.M. (1979) Remineralization of enamel lesions. A study of the physicochemical mechanism. Ph.D. Thesis, Rijksuniversiteit te Groningen.

Watanabe, S., Dawes, C. (1988) The effects of different foods and concentrations of citric acid on the flow rate of whole saliva in man. *Archives of Oral Biology*, **33**, 1–5.

Young, W., Khan, F., Brandt, R., et al. (2001) Syndromes with salivary dysfunction predispose to toothwear: case reports of congenital dysfunction of major salivary glands, Prader-Willi, congenital rubella, and Sjögren's syndromes. *Oral Surgery, Oral Medicine, Oral Pathology, Oral Radiology, Endodontics*, **92**, 38–48.

Dental diagnosis and the oral medicine of toothwear

6

William G. Young and Colin Dawes

Examination of patient's facial features, oral soft tissues and teeth (see Chapters 1 and 4) yields a set of observations. Before a dental diagnosis can be made, these observations have to be explained from the patient's history and oral medicine. Four clinical cases of patients with moderate and severe toothwear are detailed in full later in this chapter to highlight their oral medicine ramifications and the importance of a detailed clinical history to better undertand all the aetiologies involved and facilitate formulation of a diagnosis. The clinical interview history is paramount in the diagnosis of toothwear given its often complex multifactorial aetiology. In no other oral condition are the history and oral medicine so important in formulating the diagnosis. This is not necessarily the case in the diagnosis of dental caries.

THE APPROACH

The dentist and the patient have to resolve five key questions:

- Why is the toothwear mild, moderate or severe?
- Is bruxism involved?
- Is abrasion involved?
- What are the sources of extrinsic or intrinsic acids?
- Why has saliva protection been lost?

MILD, MODERATE OR SEVERE TOOTHWEAR

The age of the patient helps explain why their wear is mild. In the mixed dentition phase, wear on the deciduous teeth may have been severe, yet that on the first permanent incisors and molars is mild. The patient's gender associated more severe wear with males and less wear with females of the same age (Young 2001a). However, the patient's lifestyle at that stage in their life, as a student, in an occupation or in retirement on the date of presentation determines whether their toothwear is mild, moderate or severe, more than their age.

Toothwear: The ABC of the Worn Dentition, First Edition. Edited by Farid Khan and William George Young.
© 2011 John Wiley & Sons, Ltd. Published 2011 by John Wiley & Sons, Ltd.

Severity of toothwear can be markedly affected by genetic and environmental influences on development (Khan et al. 2001). Parafunction and bruxism may affect the severity of occlusal toothwear, dental diagnosis and management of attrition (Khan et al. 1998). Historically, the severity of occlusal and approximal wear was strongly affected by abrasive particles in the diet (Young 1998). Contemporaneously, cervical wear is exaggerated by toothbrush abrasion. In the absence of saliva protection, any acidic food or drink will attack the teeth. The commonest sources are soft drinks and sports drinks containing ascorbic, citric and/or phosphoric acid as preservatives. Wines are also acidic (Young 2001a). Less commonly, gastric juice containing hydrochloric acid is regurgitated by patients with alcoholism, eating disorders and gastro-oesophageal reflux disease (GORD; Valena & Young 2002). Dry mouth (xerostomia) and enlarged major salivary glands (sialadenosis) are key symptoms and signs requiring an oral medicine explanation. Dehydration, from exertion in sports or at the workplace, is the commonest cause of lost saliva protection in healthy patients of all ages and gender with toothwear (Young 2001a). Alcohol, drugs and medications also cause dry mouth and sialadenosis (Friedlander et al. 2003).

For a variety of reasons, saliva protection is defective in the following common conditions:

- Asthma
- Depression
- Diabetes mellitus
- Hypertension
- Sjögren's syndrome

COMPLAINT/DISCOVERY

The complaint by which excessive toothwear comes to the patient's attention is rarely dramatic (Box 6.1). The teeth may be rough, chip easily or appear shorter than normal. Fill-

---

Box 6.1 Complaint/discovery questions

- When were the lesions found?
- Who noticed them and why?
- How did the lesions present: chipping, fillings falling out, roughness?
- Were the teeth sensitive to hot, cold, sweet or acid stimuli, to crisp food or to touch with the toothbrush?
- Are the pulps showing pink through the dentine? Is tertiary dentine exposed?
- Was root canal therapy indicated?

---

ings have high, sharp margins or even fall out. Worn teeth are sensitive some time after drinking soft drinks, but not after sugary foods. Episodic hypersensitivity may develop into near- and frank exposures, necessitating root canal therapy.

These signs and symptoms give a history quite different from that of dental decay. The patient needs to understand the essential differences between acid wear and dental caries for the severity of the signs and symptoms strongly influence the patient's perception of their problem and what they want done about it. The patient is reassured when their complaints result from acid wear and not dental decay. It is not an infection and can be treated by less invasive and less costly techniques if identified in its early stages.

DEVELOPMENT

There is a common misconception that patients inherit genetically 'soft teeth'. Patients need to be told that they have toothwear or dental decay and that this is not because they have inherited soft teeth. In fact, the surfaces most affected by occlusal attrition and erosion are enamel surfaces that have evolved as the strongest to resist wear throughout a lifetime. Teeth develop in the early years of life. Only rarely do they

Box 6.2 Development questions

- Does the patient have genetically soft teeth or a syndrome with abnormal salivation?
- Is the toothwear familial?
- Where did the patient live in the first 12 years of life?
- Was there fluoride in the water or were they given supplements?
- Did the patient have tetracycline in childhood?

carry the marks of adverse genetics or environmental influences from these early years. Toothwear is only marginally influenced by development, but some key considerations emerge (Box 6.2).

Teeth affected by amelogenesis and dentinogenesis imperfecta chip and wear more rapidly than normal (see Chapter 2). Hereditary absence of major salivary glands puts patients at risk of dental erosion. In Prader–Willi syndrome (PWS), a non-hereditable chromosomal abnormality, salivation is abnormal (Young et al. 2001). Down's syndrome children have excessive salivation, but drugs used to control their behaviour shut off salivary protection (Bell et al. 2002). Such syndromes are, thus, associated with increased risks of both toothwear and dental caries. Excessive toothwear in other members of a family more likely reflect socio-economic factors and dietary preferences than a genetic predisposition.

Environment during the first 12 years of life gives a helpful guide to the climatic conditions that could have established food and drink preferences. Similarly, fluoride levels in the water supply during the first 12 years can influence the resistance against dental caries and perhaps acid wear. Potentially, fluoride supplements given by parents would have similar effects. Despite this, excessive toothwear can develop in teeth even when fluoridation has been optimal (Teo et al. 1997). Tetracycline-stained teeth have a tendency to chip with age, but wear is not excessive.

ATTRITION

It is an axiom that the hardest and toughest tissues of the body, enamel and dentine, have evolved to resist wear by attrition. Attrition by tooth-to-toothwear, in the absence of abrasive particles in the diet and in the absence of oral acids, is minimal in contemporary Westernised populations (Young 1998). However, when acids etch enamel and dentine, attritional wear facets develop at an early stage (see Chapter 2). Tooth clenching and grinding habits likewise exaggerate attritional facets. Bruxism can only be diagnosed from observed parafunctional habits, muscle strain, tongue indentations and pronounced *linea alba*. The habit cannot be inferred from attritional wear facets alone.

The items provided in Box 6.3 have to be considered.

The patient may be aware of clenching or grinding their teeth when concentrating or stressed during the day. Clenching or grinding during sleep has to be confirmed by a parent or partner. Mouth breathing and snoring do not count. Muscle or joint strain or tenderness on waking may indicate bruxism.

Bruxism may have been suspected or suggested to the patient as the cause of the attrition, erosion and degradation on their teeth. Occlusal adjustments, extensive restorations and splint therapy may have been given on the basis that bruxism alone was the cause of wear (Box 6.3).

Box 6.3 Questions on attrition

- Does the patient clench or grind their teeth during the day or not?
- Does anyone they live with tell them they grind their teeth when asleep?
- Do they wake up feeling their muscles of mastication are tense or their joints ache?
- Has a dentist ever told them that their problem was caused by grinding their teeth at night (bruxism)?
- Do they wear a splint at night? Does it help?

ABRASION

Occupational tooth abrasion is largely of historical interest, being connected with work practices, habits and food preparation by archaic methods. However, this topic opens up the patient's occupation, habits, recreation and creativity in a general way (Box 6.4). Insights emerge that throw light on unusual causes of toothwear. Gemstone polishing exposes teeth to industrial abrasive dusts of silica, carborundum and diamond. Musical instruments with the reed held in the mouth may be a factor. Sewing and cutting thread, opening hairpins or holding nails cause local abrasion. Stoneground flour is abrasive because of its silica content. Bread from this flour was historically a major cause of abrasion on the teeth before steel milling was introduced.

Stains from tobacco smoking were removed with abrasive 'smoker's toothpastes'. Some tooth-whitening preparations are abrasive and the effects of bleaches on enamel hardness have yet to be evaluated. In the past, a diagnosis of 'pipe-stem abrasion' was given to regional abrasions on anterior teeth where the pipe was held habitually. The chemicals and drugs in tobacco smoke may not necessarily affect saliva protection of the teeth.

Healthy patients with excessive toothwear are not commonly smokers. However, former smokers with toothwear may have high blood pressure and be on antihypertensive medication, which reduces salivary protection.

TOOTHBRUSHING

Toothbrushing with non-abrasive toothpaste is unlikely to cause damage to the hardest and toughest biopolymers of the body – enamel and dentine. But enamel and dentine softened by acids undergo toothbrush abrasion (Box 6.5). Clinicians can be reassured that toothbrushes and toothpastes developed for plaque control and gingival health are unlikely to damage tooth surfaces, unless the teeth have been softened by oral acids in the absence of salivary protection. Eroded dentine is sensitive. So, changing methods of toothbrushing or the applications of toothpastes, densensitising gels or fluoride treatments afford only temporary relief.

As sensitivity comes and goes with episodes of acute erosion and remission, obtundent toothpastes get used sporadically and are often abandoned as ineffective. Sensitivity is the best warning to the patient of an acid attack, and a

---

Box 6.4 Abrasion questions

- Does the patient's occupation or hobbies expose them to industrial abrasives such as diamond carborundum or silica dusts?
- Do they play a musical instrument with a reed between their teeth?
- Do they break thread, hold pins or nails, or open hairpins with their teeth?
- Do they make their own bread with stoneground flour?
- Do they smoke? Have they removed tobacco stains from their teeth with bleach or abrasive toothpastes?

Box 6.5 Toothbrushing questions

- What toothbrushes do the patients use? Are the bristles soft, medium or hard?
- Ask the patients to demonstrate their method of brushing. Are they left or right handed?
- What toothpaste do they use regularly: gel or paste? Does it contain fluoride?
- How often do they brush and when in the day? How long do they usually spend?
- Have they used an obtundent toothpaste for sensitive teeth? Did it help? Obtundent toothpastes are used by patients with dentinal sensitivity.

loss of sensitivity is the best indicator of remineralisation and tooth repair by saliva.

Caution must be advised in brushing teeth soon after an incident of acid attack that has softened the enamel. Excessive brushing habits shed light on obsessive behaviour and fixation on oral hygiene, e.g. ten times a day for at least 5 min each time.

ORAL HYGIENE

Oral hygiene methods other than toothbrushing are important for the management of dentinal sensitivity and toothwear. The following insights are relevant (Box 6.6). Flossing helps sensitivity by removing impacted food and dental plaque. But excessive flossing may abrade sensitive dentine and cementum softened by acids. Chewing gum flavour stimulates salivary flow. Chewing and swallowing neutralise and clear acids from plaque and the teeth (Dawes 2004b). Patient, parental and social attitudes need to be addressed when recommending chewing gum for oral hygiene. Astringent, bactericidal mouthwashes used to combat mouth odour and dental caries precipitate protective salivary proteins. Patients complain of a ropey, whitish deposit in their mouth after using astringent toothpastes, gels and mouthwashes, which precipitate proteins from their saliva. Alcoholic and phenolic mouthwashes produce leukoedema. Excessive use of astringent may products is, therefore,

contraindicated for patients with toothwear because the protective properties of saliva are compromised. Fluoride rinses and gel applications control bacterial plaque and dentinal sensitivity. By reducing the solubility of the calcium apatites of enamel and dentine, fluoride may also be protective against intrinsic and extrinsic acids. Remineralisation of enamel and dentine by saliva is the goal of acid wear management. Therapeutic remineralising preparations are still under evaluation (Dawes 2008).

DIET EROSION

The points stated in Box 6.7 require consideration. Citrus fruits are a good source of vitamin C and excellent for stimulating saliva flow. But sucking oranges and lemon wedges or drinking undiluted lemon juice causes etching (Kunzel et al. 2000). Vitamin C (ascorbic acid) as powder, chewable tablets or added to sports and soft drinks can cause acid wear (Giunta 1983). Citric acid is commonly added to fruit drinks, soft drinks, sports drinks and cordials which, if drunk when saliva is shut off, will etch unprotected teeth. Sports gels contain citric acid and sodium citrate, and together these buffer the gels to a

---

Box 6.6 Oral hygiene

- How often does the patient floss?
- How often do they chew gum? Is it regular or sugar-free?
- Do they use a mouthwash? Which one and why?
- Have they had fluoride treatments, either as a rinse or a gel application?
- What about remineralising therapy?

Box 6.7 Questions on diet

- Is the patient fond of fresh fruit? Citrus or non-citrus? How many pieces of fresh fruit do they have per week?
- Do they take a vitamin C supplement, as powder or chewable tablet?
- What drinks do they have with meals? Water, milk, fruit juice 100%, fruit drink <30%, cordial or a soft drink?
- What soft drink do they prefer? What brand? Regular or diet? How many bottles or cans do they have per week?
- Is the patient a vegetarian? Are they slimming or on a special diet for any reason?

low pH that etches teeth. Gel sticks to teeth where saliva has been shut off by sports dehydration.

Orthophosphoric acid is a common acid in both diet and regular colas. Guarana extract is equally as acidic as orthophosphoric acid in colas. Special diets for 'health' or slimming need evaluation. Slimming pills and laxatives cause dehydration. Vegetarian diets can cause erosion from acetic acids in vinegars, used to preserve fruit and vegetables.

GASTRIC EROSION

Saliva is essential for digestive health. Swallowing it protects and heals the upper digestive tract from GORD. Accordingly, indigestion, heartburn and sour mouthfuls are common symptoms of gastric upset and GORD. Gastroscopy or radiography is used to find gastritis or ulcers. Antacid self-medication is common. Proton pump inhibitor (PPI) medications not only relieve symptoms of GORD but also reduce saliva flow rates. Gastric acid reflux brings hydrochloric acid into the mouth, so its cause and frequency are important. Bulimia nervosa exposes the teeth to hydrochloric acid. Bulimics, with enlarged salivary glands and low salivary flow, develop dental erosion (Milosevic et al. 1997).

Alcohol is the most frequent cause of heartburn and acute and chronic gastritis. Chronic nocturnal acid regurgitation is found in alcoholics with chronic gastritis. Alcohol is dehydrating. Beer is not usually acidic, but wines and spirits mixed with soft drinks are. Erosion of the lingual surfaces of the lower anterior teeth is a good indicator of chronic GORD. Erosion of the lingual surfaces of lower incisors, canines and even premolars is found in alcoholics in whom nocturnal gastric acid reflux is common. Enlargement of the major salivary glands (sialadenosis) is also found (Box 6.8).

Box 6.8 Questions on gastric problems and alcohol

- Does the patient suffer from indigestion? Bloat, heartburn or sour mouthfuls?
- Has their indigestion been investigated by tests, endoscopy or X-rays? What medication do they need?
- Have they had frequent vomiting for any reason?
- Do they know what bulimia nervosa is? Do they suffer from this?
- Do they prefer beer, wine or spirits? How many drinks per week? Have they had any problems with alcohol?

SPORTS AND SOCIAL

Sports- and work-related dehydration is the commonest risk factor for toothwear, because dehydration physiologically turns off salivary protection and increases thirst for acidic sports and soft drinks. The points given in Box 6.9 need consideration. Exertion in fitness programmes, dancing, training sessions and competitions result in frequent dehydration. Degrees of exercise-induced dehydration change from childhood to adolescence to adulthood.

Box 6.9 Sports and social questions

- Which sports does the patient play? How many training sessions, games or competitions per week?
- Is the patient at school, in a club or in a gym?
- Are they in a programme of exercise for health at their time of life?
- Is their diet altered to improve performance? Water? Sports drinks? High-carbohydrate or protein supplements?
- Does their social recreation involve alcohol, caffeine or other drugs?
- Is their occupation dehydrating? Does it involve overnight or shift work?
- What do they take to keep awake?

Sports- and work choices influence diet. Nutrition and fitness require water, minerals, carbohydrates, fats and proteins. Caffeine, alcohol and performance-enhancing drugs affect athletes and thirsty workers. Caffeine and alcohol addiction increase exposure to acids in colas, wines and spirits.

Many occupations involve dehydrating work conditions and exposure to acids. Examples include lemon and citrus farmers or battery manufacturers. Night-shift workers are at risk if they drink caffeine-containing acid soft drinks to keep themselves awake and are, thus, at risk of dental erosion, for saliva is shut off at night (Dawes 2004a).

MEDICAL

Medical conditions and treatments in which salivary protection of the teeth is lost put patients at risk of toothwear. The questions asked in Box 6.10 therefore require investigation. Systemic conditions asthma, diabetes mellitus and high blood pressure (hypertension) are common and particularly important. GORD is common in asthmatics.

There are thousands of medications that shut off saliva or are acidic. The side effects of dry mouth (xerostomia) and sialadenosis are often found to be caused by alcohol, dehydration,

---

Box 6.10 Medical questions

- Do the patients have a systemic medical condition? Asthma, diabetes or hypertension?
- What type of medication are they on? How often and what dosage?
- Do the patients suffer from a dry mouth? What causes this, when and how often in a week? Do they have dry eyes and joint problems?
- What is their height and weight? What is causing weight loss or gain?
- Are menstrual periods abnormal? Is this amenorrhea or menopause? Are they on hormone replacement therapy?

---

systemic condition or medication. Xerostomia is experienced when saliva is lacking from the anterior hard palate (Wolff & Kleinberg 1998). Many drugs diminish the production of salivary proteins (Nederfors et al. 1994; O'Connell et al. 1993). How often does dry mouth come on and how is it being managed?

Asthma medications reduce saliva flow and increase toothwear and dental decay. In type I diabetes mellitus, thirst cravings, dry mouth and acidic diet drinks may be problems. Salivary flow rates are reduced in type II diabetes. Beta-blocker antihypertensive medications produce dry mouth and sialadenosis as side effects. Dry mouth, dry eyes and joint problems are found in the systemic conditions of primary or secondary Sjögren's syndrome.

Weight loss and gain are found in many systemic conditions associated with toothwear. Exercise, exertion and slimming may be accompanied by dehydration.

Because obesity is a major risk factor for diabetes and hypertension, this cue effectively links patients' diet, lifestyle, a medical condition and medications that put them at risk. Patient's obsessions with height and weight are found in eating disorders and in the fashion and fitness industries. Weight gain from binge eating is found in bulimia nervosa, whereas excessive weight loss characterises anorexia nervosa.

Amenorrhoea in young women occurs from the excessive exercise in the competitive sports industries and fashion. It is also a symptom of the hormonal upsets that arise in anorexia nervosa. Hormonally induced sialadenosis develops in postmenopausal women on hormone replacement therapy (HRT), and is associated with dry mouth.

ADDICTIONS, FIXATIONS AND CONFIDENTIALITY

Psychological concerns of patients, children, parents and the examiner affect the diagnosis in

---

Box 6.11 Psychological questions

- What underlying concerns affect the patient's responses?
- Are the responses consistent throughout the interview?
- Do the parent and the child agree or disagree?
- Does the patient have a fixation influencing their habits or lifestyles?
- Have they had emotional stress, anxiety attacks, attention deficit and hyperactivity disorder or depression?
- Have they ever been given medication for these?
- Was there associated alcohol or drug dependency?
- How receptive is the patient to connecting their toothwear with medical and psychological concerns in lifestyle and diet?
- Are they giving informed consent?
- Did they have privacy issues within the interview?

---

the ways mentioned in Box 6.11. Inconsistent responses reveal conflicts of guilt, idiosyncrasies or parental guidance. Fixations (of the patients, parents and children) bias responses. Clinicians have their own set of biases. In some patients, there is reluctance to talk about attention deficit and hyperactivity disorder, work-related stress, anxiety attacks, anorexia nervosa or depression. Some patients believe that their medications are private matters of no concern to a dentist. Patient's receptivity to lines of questioning, suggestions and advice is influenced when they understand how their problems connect with their private concerns and that these have been respected. Informed consent is then effective.

THE CASES

The cases are natural experiments from which much can be learnt. They demonstrate that the severity and distribution of their lesions of toothwear are the result of the relative importance of saliva protection, modified by their lifestyle, medical condition or syndrome. These cases are significant learning experiences in their own right and apply the approach taken in the first section of this chapter.

Case 1. Sports dehydration

This 32-year-old male patient was seen on consultation concerning toothwear. On examination, he had no parotid or submandibular gland enlargement, no muscular tenderness on palpation or temporomandibular joint problems. Intraorally, his oral mucosa and periodontium were healthy and his occlusion was normal.

Examination of the teeth

The incisal edges of his anterior teeth showed erosion (Fig. 6.1a).

Palatal enamel loss was present on all of his maxillary incisors, canines and first premolars (Fig. 6.2b). Bilateral occlusal cuspal-cupped lesions were evident on premolars and molars in both jaws. Buccal cervical lesions were evident on his lower canines and premolars. This distribution of tooth surface loss, by stage, is shown in Fig. 6.2. No changes in stages were noted 4 years later.

Interview

He was healthy with no family history of similar tooth pathology. He had complained of sensitivity in his lower molars to hot and cold stimuli, as well as when chewing hard foods. He experienced no problems of clenching or grinding and no muscle or joint tenderness. He had no problems of gastric reflux. The patient recorded frequent consumption of citrus fruits and cola beverages when dehydrated, especially after competitive BMX cycling. He worked as a draughtsman in air-conditioned rooms and did not complain of a dry mouth.

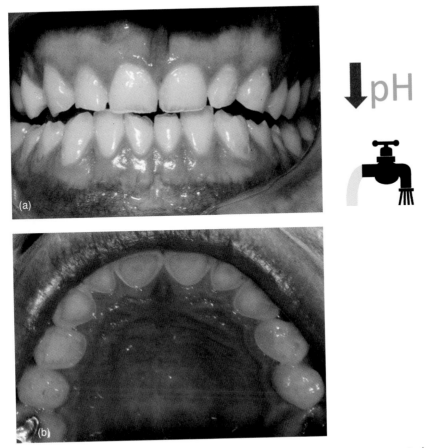

Figure 6.1 Erosion in a 32-year-old male patient with high cola beverage consumption particularly at times of dehydration from BMX bicycle competitions. The incisal edges of the maxillary anterior teeth were thinned and chipped, whilst cervical lesions affected the canines and premolars (a). (From Young & Messer, 2002, with permission of Dentil Pty Ltd.) Palatally, extensive degradation affected all anteriors and first premolars (b).

Analysis of a diary of his diet and activities kept for 6 consecutive days revealed that, as a bachelor, his evening meals regularly consisted of a 1.25 L bottle of cola beverage and a chocolate bar.

Management

This case documents a 4-year history of tooth tissue loss from dental erosion secondary to sports-related dehydration and high cola consumption. Despite counselling, diet analysis and advice, he did not reduce his cola bever-

age intake. However, a lifestyle change took place when he substituted chess for BMX cycling. This may have affected the outcome due to a reduction in sports-related dehydration.

Discussion

This case illustrates the predominant group of healthy young men with work- and/or sports-related dehydration. Dehydration reduces the salivary flow rate and the ability, with its buffering capacity, to clear acids from the mouth (see

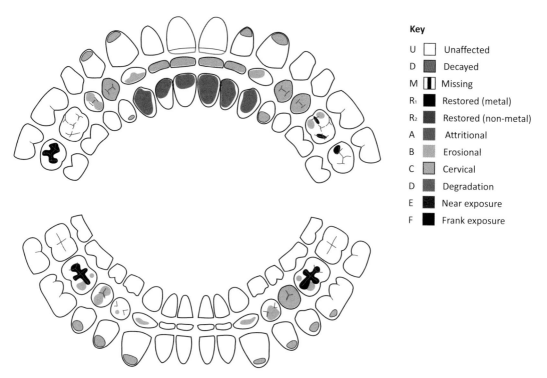

Key

U	☐	Unaffected
D	▨	Decayed
M	〖	Missing
R₁	■	Restored (metal)
R₂	▨	Restored (non-metal)
A	▨	Attritional
B	▨	Erosional
C	▨	Cervical
D	▨	Degradation
E	■	Near exposure
F	■	Frank exposure

Figure 6.2 Odontogram showing the moderately worn dentition of the patient shown in Fig. 6.1. The cuspal and incisal erosion, buccal cervical lesions and palatal degradation can be explained by loss of saliva protection from major glands in the regions of most severe toothwear.

Chapter 5). It has been demonstrated that dehydration causes a significant decrease in parotid salivary output in healthy young and older subjects (Ship & Fischer 1997). Therefore, a history of work- and/or sports-related dehydration assumes considerable importance in the diagnosis of patients with toothwear.

The distribution of lesions (see Fig. 6.2) is common in this group. Incisal and palatal lesions are found on maxillary incisors, canines and premolars. The maxillary molars are less affected than the mandibular molars, which show extensive cuspal-cupped lesions – loss of fissural dentinal hypersensitivity. The mandibular anterior teeth show attrition or erosion on incisal edges associated with shallow cervical lesions on their buccal aspects. As shown in Fig. 6.2, the dentist can read-

ily explain to the patient the relevance of salivary protection from the major glands from the pattern.

Evidence continues to mount that the dental erosion produced by soft drinks and sports drinks depends not only on their pH, but on their buffering capacity and phosphate content (Larsen & Nyvad 1999). This case also illustrates that the usual acid beverage consumed after exercise may be cola. Although the caffeine content of teas, coffees, chocolate and cola beverages varies considerably, patients whose main source of caffeine is cola put themselves at risk of dental erosion from both the citric and orthophosphoric acid content in these socially accepted, mildly addictive beverages which have additional consequences for health (Couper-Smart 1984).

Table 6.1 Prader–Willi syndrome: general and oral clinical features.

Musculoskeletal system	Slow growth/short stature Small hands and feet Lack of muscle size, strength and tone (hypotonia) Waddling gait
Endocrine system	Lack of sexual development Underdeveloped genitalia (hypogonadism) High-pitched voice Feminine appearance Lack of secondary sexual hair (lanugo)
Central nervous system	Insatiable appetite (polyphagia) Mild-to-moderate mental retardation Behavioural problems Wandering eyes (not strabismus; not myopia)
Cardiovascular system	Obesity (neck, trunk and thighs) Diabetic tendency Cardiovascular disease
Oral features	Enamel hypoplasia Dental erosion Dental caries Thick, ropey mucinous saliva

Case 2. Prader–Willi syndrome (Table 6.1)

This patient, of age 27 years, presented on referral for evaluation of severe dental erosion. His dental practitioner had performed root canal treatment on five incisors.

Soft tissue examination

His face had a juvenile feminine appearance, with a narrow frontal diameter (Fig. 6.3). His eyes showed a tendency to wander, but were not crossed as in strabismus. He had sparse moustache hair and no beard, but lanugo was present over his parotid glands. His scalp hair was normal. Some sores were present on his legs, possibly picked or scratched insect bites. His gingivae, tongue and buccal mucosae were normal. The major salivary glands were prominent, moderately enlarged and palpable, but not firm, lumpy or tender. The muscles of mastication, and temporomandibular joints, and cervical lymph nodes were normal. His saliva was frothy and mucinous (see Fig. 6.3).

Examination

Loss of tooth height and palatal enamel were evident on his anterior teeth (see Fig. 6.3). Loss of enamel and cusp height was evident in maxillary premolars and molars. Deep-cupped lesions were evident in the dentine of the occlusal surfaces of mandibular incisors, canines, premolars, first, second and third molars. One caries lesion was found in tooth 17. Teeth 11, 21, 22, 31 and 41 had been treated by root canal therapy, presumably because of exposure of their pulps by erosion of dentine. It is remarkable that despite the severity of the occlusal lesions and root canal treatments, cervical lesions were absent from all regions of his dentition (Fig. 6.4).

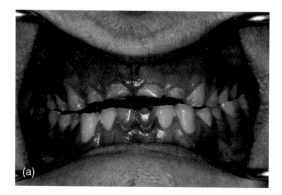
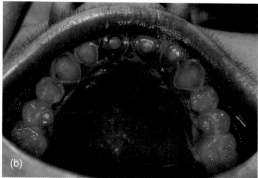
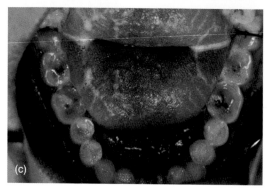

Figure 6.3 This 27-year-old male had Prader–Willi syndrome and severe toothwear (a). His occlusal lesions were severe, several teeth had near-exposures, and frank exposures had necessitated root canal therapy. Near-exposures of the pulp are seen through the degraded palatal dentine of teeth 13, 12 and 23 (b). Root canal treatment has been completed on several teeth. The saliva was perpetually mucinous (c). Sources of acid were dietary sugar-free soft drinks. (From Young et al., 2001, with permission of Elsevier Ltd.)

Interview

His speech was clear, and his use of language was good. His mother, in attendance, helped clarify or rephrase questions and verified or corrected responses. No members of his family were similarly affected. To combat the polyphagia and obesity (features of PWS), he was on a low-calorie diet. He had received dental advice to avoid oranges, grapefruits and pineapples; however, chewable vitamin C tablets were taken every day. He was allowed to buy his own choice of cordial and soft drinks. He preferred apple juice, 2–3 L/wk, and drank about 2 L/wk of reconstituted orange cordial. He had

drunk diet cola in at least the same amount until he was told to avoid this by the referring dentist.

His mother reported that his primary teeth had not been badly affected. He clenched his teeth during the day when stressed, and his mother confirmed that he used to grind his teeth at night. However, a hard plastic night guard, worn for at least 10 years before this examination, seemed to have obviated this problem. He used a fluoride-containing toothpaste, but not a fluoride mouthwash, and on occasion used an obtundent toothpaste on his dentist's recommendation. However, owing perhaps to his high pain threshold, he had not complained

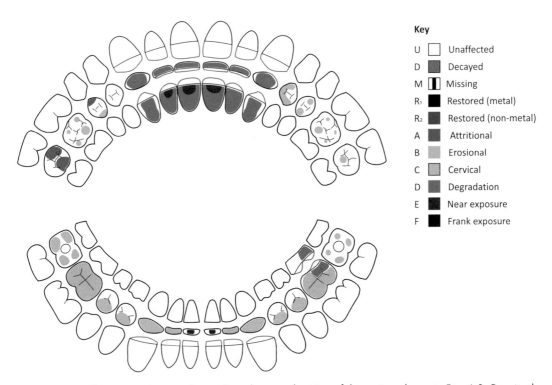

Key

U	☐	Unaffected
D	▨	Decayed
M	▯	Missing
R₁	■	Restored (metal)
R₂	▨	Restored (non-metal)
A	▨	Attritional
B	▨	Erosional
C	▨	Cervical
D	▨	Degradation
E	■	Near exposure
F	■	Frank exposure

Figure 6.4 Odontogram showing the moderately worn dentition of the patient shown in Fig. 6.3. Despite the severity of occlusal bowl-shaped lesions, degradation of the anterior teeth and near- and frank exposures, no cervical lesions were found.

much of tooth sensitivity. He used an electric toothbrush in his right hand, 3–5 min twice per day. He chewed various sugar-containing gums and bubble gums excessively. His mother said he would chew a whole ten-stick package in 1 day if allowed to do so. Perhaps as the result of hyperphagia, he had heartburn without sour mouthfuls. This had been investigated by endoscopy, but no gastritis or ulcer was found. His gall bladder had been removed after an incident of severe abdominal pain. His mother kept him at home and locked all food away from him to control his polyphagia. He was allowed to purchase certain items of food and drink in addition to his controlled low-calorie diet. His endocrinologist was generally satisfied with the state of his cardiovascular system at check-ups every 6 months. He had not

developed diabetes mellitus at this stage. The patient had only minor behavioural problems and was on no medication.

Management

The patient kept a record of his activities and diet for 6 days before he returned for dietary analysis and advice. Salivary flow was stimulated by chewing sugar-free gum, eating fresh fruit and drinking lots of water. The acid content of cordials, vitamin C tablets, fruit drinks and beverages, diet colas was explained to the patient, his mother and his dietitian. A regular fluoride mouthwash regimen in association with his night-guard wearing was instituted. The lesions were coated with a fluoride-containing adhesive resin, and his incisors

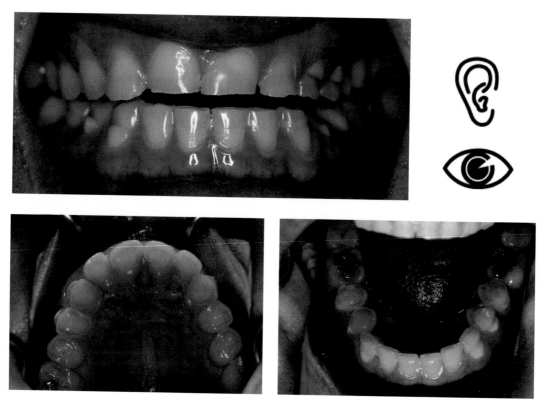

Figure 6.5 Loss of saliva protection caused by eye drops containing beta-blocker for glaucoma in this 28-year-old woman with congenital rubella syndrome produced extensive occlusal, cervical and degradative lesions. (From Young, 2001b, with permission of Dentil Pty Ltd.)

were restored with composite resin in preparation for post and core crowns. The caries lesion on tooth 17 was restored with a glass ionomer/composite material. One year later, the patient, his mother, the referring dentist and one of the authors were impressed that the teeth were shiny and hard, despite the continued frothiness of the patient's saliva. He had broken his hard plastic mouth guard, which was subsequently replaced.

Discussion

Previous reports on the oral findings in PWS have emphasised enamel hypoplasia and rampant caries as the presenting pathol-

ogy (Bazopoulou-Kyrkanidou & Papagiannoulis 1992; Salako & Ghafouri 1995). In the present case, enamel hypoplasia was absent and active caries was found in only one tooth. The pattern of occlusal lesions and palatal degradation was entirely consistent with dental erosion caused by lack of serous saliva protection (Fig. 6.5). However, despite the severity of this occlusal erosion, the absence of cervical lesions is remarkable and suggests that his mucinous saliva was protective against the acids in his sugar-free soft drinks. All studies have noted that the saliva in PWS is thick and sticky, and that the oral mucosa and lips are mildly dry (Bazopoulou-Kyrkanidou & Papagiannoulis 1992; Salako & Ghafouri 1995). Although no systematic investigations of salivary flow rate, buffering capacity or mineral content of saliva in PWS subjects have yet been reported, it is probable that salivary dysfunction is part of the syndrome and accounts for both the high prevalence of dental caries and severity of erosion. Polyphagia probably encourages snacking on candy and sweets. In addition, soft drinks, especially of the orange-flavoured types, have been used as bribes to control temper and achieve compliance with instructions. For the present patient, artificial sweeteners were part of the calorie reduction strategy of the patient's regular diet. However, he was allowed to buy his own choice of fruit and soft drinks. Unfortunately, diet colas are as acidic as regular cola beverages, and clearly these had contributed to his dental erosion. The chewable vitamin C tablets, taken daily as candy, were probably also implicated in the development of his dental erosion. In the absence of tongue indentations and linea alba, it is unlikely that bruxism contributed significantly to the severity of the incisal surface loss that resulted in the need for root canal therapy.

Case 3. Congenital rubella syndrome

History

This 28-year-old woman had severe wear on her deciduous dentition. During a recent dental examination it was noticed that wear on her permanent teeth had progressed rapidly since the last yearly check-up. She had no active caries and her restorations were intact.

Soft tissue examination

She has had bilateral deafness since birth and was wearing two hearing aids. She had no sight in one eye and had glaucoma. These are components of congenital rubella syndrome, for her mother had German measles during pregnancy. She had no overt heart damage.

Some degree of corneal opacity was noted in her eyes. Her skin, hair and lips were normal. There was bilateral *linea alba*, but no tongue indentations. Her submandibular and parotid salivary glands were firm, slightly enlarged, but not tender to palpation (sialadenosis). No muscular or temporomandibular joint tenderness was found.

Examination of the teeth

Figure 6.5 illustrates that enamel was lost from the palatal and incisal aspects of her upper anterior teeth. There were buccal cervical lesions on the canines and premolars in all quadrants, and cupping and loss of occlusal enamel, particularly on lower premolars and first molars. However, grooves had developed above these restorations. Intact amalgam occlusal restorations were present in all molar quadrants. More cervical lesions had been restored with composite materials. Lesions were absent from the lingual surfaces of all lower teeth and the buccal surface of the upper molars, consistent with protection from adjacent major salivary glands (see Figs. 4.20a and 6.5).

Interview

She did not complain of tooth sensitivity. She had lived in Brisbane, Australia, all her life – where the water was not fluoridated. Her mother had never given her fluoride tablets. There was no history of tooth abnormalities in the family. The patient said she clenched her teeth when playing with animals or small children. However, her mother confirmed that the patient did not grind her teeth at night, nor did she report muscle or joint tenderness on waking. For oral hygiene, she used a medium toothbrush and non-abrasive fluoride toothpaste with her left hand, even though she was ambidextrous. She gave no history of heartburn, gastric acid regurgitation or bulimia, or of exposure to industrial acids in her occupation as a clerk typist. However, 2 years earlier, she had left home and was drinking as much as one 2-L bottle of cola beverage daily. On return to home, she still had at least two glasses per day, in preference to any other beverage. However, in the 6-day dietary diary she subsequently kept she did not drink tea or coffee. She found her work stressful, but not dehydrating, and she exercised only moderately. For most of the patient's life, her glaucoma had been treated with twice-daily eye drops of 0.25% timolol maleate, a beta-adrenergic–blocking agent (Timoptol). Her mother was convinced that this medication was in some way connected to the patient's dry mouth and consulted the medical practitioner involved, who changed the medication to latanoprost eye drops (Xalatan), 50 µg/mL, one drop twice daily. The mother then noticed that the instructions for use of latanoprost specified that after application of the drop, the index finger was to be pressed against the inner corner of the eye against the nose for about 2 min to prevent drainage through the lacrimal duct to the nose and throat, from where it could be absorbed into other parts of the body. The patient's mother noted that she did not do this whilst using the previous medication for many years. It was probable that the beta-blocker absorbed through the nose and throat was responsible for her xerostomia. Dry mouth is recorded as a side effect of this medication. Eighteen months earlier, an antihistamine (budesonide) and antibiotics had been prescribed for a maxillary sinus infection. Within the last 3 months, the antidepressant paroxetine hydrochloride (Aropax), 10 mg daily, had been taken for work-related stress.

Management

The patient and her mother were counselled on the link between medication-induced xerostomia and loss of salivary protection against acids in the diet – in her case, cola beverage. The appropriate use of eye drops with lacrimal duct restriction was emphasised, as was the use of

chewing gum for salivary stimulation. Further diet analysis and advice were given at follow-up appointments as required.

Discussion

Congenital rubella syndrome is mostly of dental concern in cases in which congenital heart disease, the most frequent congenital rubella syndrome defect (Schluter et al. 1998) and sialadenosis or its sequelae, requires presurgical antibiotic prophylaxis against bacterial endocarditis. Increased rates of caries or dental erosion are not regularly reported in cases of this syndrome. However, her xerostomia and sialadenosis were probably direct effects of daily beta-blocker eye drops for the long-term control of glaucoma, which is a rarer ocular manifestation of the syndrome than cataracts. The concentration of the beta-blocker in the eye drops is higher than that used for the control of hypertension. Xerostomia and sialadenosis have been frequently reported as side effects of this medication (Nederfors et al. 1994; O'Connell et al. 1993).

The pattern of tooth surface loss (see Figs. 4.20 and 6.5) is entirely consistent with the concept that lesions occur in sites that are least protected by saliva when salivary flow rate is reduced by medications. The source of acid causing her dental erosion was clearly consumption of cola beverages to the exclusion of other sources of caffeine, such as tea or coffee.

Case 4. Alcoholism

This patient was a retired accountant who, at 62 years of age, recently noticed some fillings had come out. From age 50, he had a drinking problem that resulted in the breakdown of his marriage. He reformed, but was currently on antidepressant medication. The rarest form of tooth surface loss, from the lingual surfaces of his lower anterior teeth, made for important connections between alcohol and salivary gland atrophy.

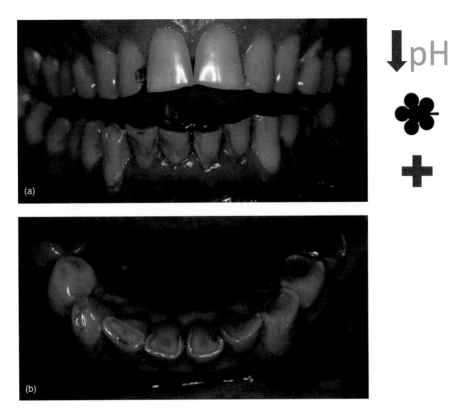

Figure 6.6 Chronic alcoholism and nocturnal gastric reflux produced an unusual pattern of toothwear in this 59-year-old man (a). (From Young & Messer, 2002, with permission of Dentil Pty Ltd.) Composite resin veneers were present on the upper central incisors. Degradation of the lingual surfaces of the lower anterior teeth is the result of gastric juice and atrophy of the submandibular and sublingual glands (b). (From Young, 2001a, with permission from the *Australian Dental Journal.*)

Soft tissue examination

He had sad, blue eyes in a ruddy, wrinkled complexion from coaching football outdoors. His hearing was normal.

No signs of temporomandibular joint dysfunction were found and he gave no history of bruxism. His tongue and buccal mucosae were normal. His gingivae and palate were also normal with the curious exception that there was supragingival calculus and stained plaque on the facial surfaces of his lower anterior teeth. The lingual surfaces of his lower anterior teeth were devoid of calculus except within the gingival crevices (Fig. 6.6). Posteriorly, his first molars met in class 1 relationship. However, he had an anterior open bite due to loss of crown height of his central incisors. His parotid glands were not palpable. In the floor of his mouth, his sublingual glands were raised and erythematous, and his submandibular glands on palpation were flabby, moderately enlarged, but not lumpy or tender.

Facial veneers were present on his upper central incisors with multiple amalgam restorations on his posterior teeth. This pattern of wear is exceptional, principally because the lingual surfaces of the lower anterior teeth are usually well protected from acid wear by submandibular and sublingual saliva (Young & Khan 2002). In contrast, the palatal surfaces of his upper teeth were not worn. These findings are

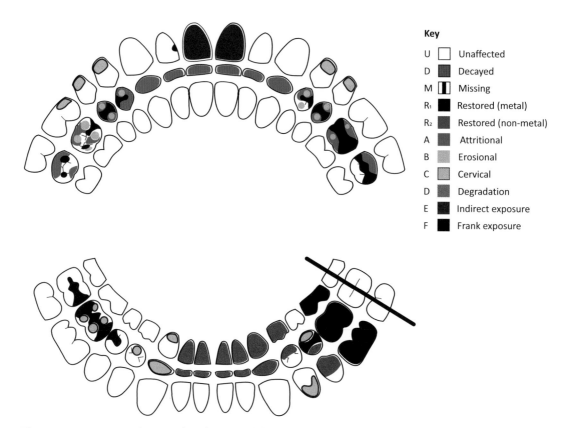

Figure 6.7 Conceptualisation of toothwear and lack of salivary protection for the patient shown in Fig. 6.6. No wear was found on the palatal surfaces of the upper anterior teeth. Incisal attrition is present on these upper anterior teeth. Buccal cervical lesions were found on upper premolars and lower canines. Degradation was found on the lingual aspects of the lower anterior teeth. (From Young, 2003, with permission of Erosion Watch Pty Ltd.)

consistent with chronic nocturnal gastric juice regurgitation and lack of protection from saliva.

The following stages of toothwear were recorded on the surfaces of his dentition (Fig. 6.7):

- No wear on the palatal surfaces of his maxillary teeth
- Attritional wear on the incisal edges of his upper anterior and posterior teeth
- Cuspal-cupped lesions on his premolars and molars
- Buccal cervical lesions on his upper premolars and lower left first premolar
- Lingual degradation on his lower anterior teeth and left first premolar

Interview

The broad dentine exposures on the lingual of lower incisors had caused him no pain or sensitivity to hot, cold or acid drinks. However, he had noticed his fillings had started to fall out. He had no history or signs of bruxism.

From age 50, as a result of marital problems, he suffered from alcoholism. This was associated with some vomiting, although this was not investigated or medicated. He gave no history of glossodynia, indigestion, rarely had heartburn and no sour mouthfuls. When he became an alcoholic, he drank beer and vodka. His cola, citrus and sports drink consumption had been negligible. His consumption of fresh fruit was mostly non-citrus, with pineapple only occasionally. He did not drink lemon juice or suck lemons, but took vitamin C chewable tablets once a day.

His general health had been good, especially in his teens and twenties when he played competitive rugby league and union, one training session and one game weekly. He continued his interest in sports, doing gym work, circuit training and sports cycling, hydrating with water and not sports drinks. He keeps physically healthy by walking, mild gym work at home and coaching football. He suffered a mental breakdown and saw a psychiatrist who prescribed PROZAC, which he took until he was 54 years old. This gave him a dry mouth, mostly on waking.

Management

This patient completed a 6-day dietary diary with close attention to detail. His diet was nutritionally very good, even with a slight excess in most food groups. Recommendations were made to keep up the good work and to follow an Erosion WATCH Plan (see Chapter 7). More generally, dentists may feel overwhelmed by the implications of a patient's drinking habits, but finding sialadenosis and excessive wear should alert them to ensure that management of patient's psychosocial and medical problems need to be addressed (Friedlander et al. 2003).

Discussion

This patient's problems were as follows:

- Rarest stage of tooth surface loss on lingual aspects of lower anterior teeth
- Salivary gland atrophy from alcoholism
- Antidepressant medication had reduced saliva protection
- Alcohol and acids in diet
- Maintaining a healthy diet

Before he developed alcoholism, he had a healthy lifestyle with frequent exercise. His dental caries was treated with amalgam and gold restorations. A taste preference for strong, sweet solutions is found in patients who develop alcoholism. This preference may be genetic (Kampov-Polevoy et al. 2001). This may account for his caries experience. However, the distribution of his erosion and the facial veneers indicate that his tooth surface loss post-dated dental caries.

Pathological toothwear is prevalent in patients with chronic alcoholism (Robb & Smith 1990) and is most likely due to nocturnal gastric acid regurgitation (Hede 1996). The parotid glands undergo changes of histology and function in patients with alcoholic cirrhosis (Dutta et al. 1989). Specifically, both stimulated and unstimulated salivary flow rates are significantly lower in patients with cirrhosis, as were concentrations of sodium, bicarbonate and total proteins.

Functional changes have histological correlates. Enlargement of acinar cells occurs from accumulated protein secretory granules. This results in the clinical appearance of parotid hypertrophy found in 30–80% of patients with cirrhosis. These changes have been ascribed to disturbances of the autonomic innervation in the glands, resulting from alcoholic neuropathy (Mandel & Hamele-Bena 1997). Conceivably, disturbance of the sympathetic neuroregulation affects protein secretion, whereas fluid and electrolyte secretion is affected by neuropathy of the parasympathetic nerves (Mandel & Hamele-Bena 1997).

Alcoholic sialadenosis is recognised initially by hypertrophy of major salivary glands and subsequently by atrophy, wherein the specialised tissues are replaced by fat and scar tissue.

In this case, the rarest form of wear, degradation of the lingual surfaces of lower anterior teeth, occurred from chronic intrinsic acid regurgitation on surfaces unprotected by saliva from the sublingual and submandibular glands. Thus, alcoholism is responsible for both.

Plaque and calculus on the facial aspects of his lower teeth indicate that mucous from the minor mucous glands in the lip is still protecting these surfaces against oral acids.

The failure of his marriage and alcohol-related problems requiring psychiatric assistance and antidepressant medication further gave him a dry mouth. Fortunately, he has been able to overcome his alcoholism and depression. His reformed lifestyle and diet reflected these changes.

As well as containing proteins, buffering bicarbonate and digestive enzymes, parotid saliva contains factors for healing. Epidermal growth factor secretion is affected by alcoholism (Dutta et al. 1992). Thus, reductions in all protective proteins in alcoholism may perpetuate and compound injuries to the oesophagus and the upper gastrointestinal tract (Christen 1983).

Medical science tends to neglect the roles of salivary glands in the health of the gastrointestinal tract. Dental science may inadvertently be ignoring the connections between toothwear and salivary protection of not only the teeth but also the oesophagus, stomach, duodenum and liver. The connections between tooth surface loss and chronic alcoholism illustrated by this case are, therefore, worthy of further investigation and consideration in patients with GORD (Bartlett et al. 2000).

SUMMARY

Considering the lessons learned from these four cases, the dental practitioner can recognise that although these conditions are rarely met in general practice, they illustrate how the patterns and severity of toothwear are markedly influenced by saliva protection or lack thereof. The reasons for loss of saliva protection vary widely from congenital absence of major salivary glands to salivary gland atrophy from al-

coholism. Yet medications that produced hyposalivation and sialadenosis were also involved. Excellent knowledge can be derived by considering these 'natural experiments', which can be applied by the dental practitioner to the commoner presentation of tooth surface loss, to explaining to the patient the importance of saliva protection of their teeth and the oral medical reasons why they have xerostomia and sialadenosis.

References

Bartlett, D.W., Evans, D.F., Anggiansah A., et al. (2000) The role of the esophagus in dental erosion. *Oral Surgery Oral Medicine Oral Pathology Oral Radiology Endodontology*, **89**, 312–315.

Bazopoulou-Kyrkanidou, E., Papagiannoulis, L. (1992) Prader-Willi syndrome: report of a case with special emphasis on oral problems. *Journal of Clinical Pediatric Dentistry*, **17**, 37–40.

Bell, E.J., Kaidonis, J., Townsend, G.C. (2002) Tooth wear in children with Down syndrome. *Australian Dental Journal*, **47**, 30–35.

Christen, A.G. (1983) Dentistry and the alcoholic patient. Dental Clinics of North America, **27**, 341–361.

Couper-Smart, J. (1984) Caffeine consumption: a review of its use, intake, clinical effects and hazards. *Food Technology in Australia*, **36**, 131–147.

Dawes, C. (2004a) Factors influencing salivary flow rate and composition. In: *Saliva and Oral Health* (eds M. Edgar, C. Dawes & D. O'Mullane), 3rd edn. pp. 32–49. British Dental Association, London.

Dawes, C. (2004b) Salivary clearance and its effects on oral health. In: *Saliva and Oral Health* (eds M. Edgar, C. Dawes & D. O'Mullane), 3rd edn. pp. 71–85. British Dental Association, London.

Dawes, C. (2008) Salivary flow patterns and the health of hard and soft oral tissues.

Journal of the American Dental Association, **139**, 18S–24S.

Dutta, S.K., Dukehart, M., Narang, A., et al. (1989) Functional and structural changes in parotid glands of alcoholic cirrhotic patients. *Gastroenterology*, **96**, 510–518.

Dutta, S.K., Moldes, O., Sheetal Vengulekur, M.S., et al. (1992) Ethanol and human saliva: effect of chronic alcoholism on flow rate, composition and epidermal growth factor. *American Journal of Gastroenterology*, **87**, 350–354.

Friedlander, A.H., Marder, S.R., Pisegna, J.R., et al. (2003) Alcohol abuse and dependence – psychopathology, medical management and dental implications. *Journal of the American Dental Association*, **134**, 731–740.

Giunta, J.L. (1983) Dental erosion resulting from chewable vitamin C tablets. *Journal of the American Dental Association*, **107**, 253–256.

Hede B. (1996) Determinants of oral health in a group of Danish alcoholics. *European Journal of Oral Sciences*, **104**, 403–408.

Kampov-Polevoy, A.B., Tsoi, M.V., Zvartau, E.E., et al. (2001) Sweet liking and family history of alcoholism in hospitalized alcoholic and non-alcoholic patients. *Alcohol & Alcoholism*, **36**, 165–170.

Khan, F., Young, W.G., Daly, T.J. (1998) Dental erosion and bruxism. A tooth wear analysis from south east Queensland. *Australian Dental Journal*, **43**, 117–127.

Khan, F., Young, W.G., Law, V., et al. (2001) Cupped lesions of early onset dental erosion in young south east Queensland adults. *Australian Dental Journal*, **46**, 100–107.

Kunzel, W., Cruz, M.S., Fischer, T. (2000) Dental erosion in Cuban children associated with excessive consumption of oranges. *European Journal of Oral Science*, **108**, 104–109.

Larsen, M.J., Nyvad, B. (1999) Enamel erosion by some soft drinks and orange juices relative to their pH, buffering effect and contents of calcium phosphate. *Caries Research*, **33**, 81–87.

Mandel, L., Hamele-Bena, D. (1997) Alcoholic parotid sialadenosis. *Journal of the American Dental Association*, **128**, 1411–1415.

Milosevic, A., Brodie, D.A., Slade, D.E. (1997) Dental erosion, oral hygiene, and eating disorders. *International Journal of Eating Disorders*, **21**, 195–199.

Nederfors, T., Ericsson, T., Twetman, S., et al. (1994) Effects of the β-adrenoceptor antagonists atenolol and propranolol on human parotid and submandibular-sublingual salivary secretion. *Journal of Dental Research*, **73**, 5–10.

O'Connell, A.C., Van Wuyckhuyse, B.C., Pearson, S.K., et al. (1993) The effect of propranolol on salivary gland function and dental caries development in young and aged rats. *Archives of Oral Biology*, **38**, 853–861.

Robb, N.D., Smith, B.G. (1990) Prevalence of pathological tooth wear in patients with chronic alcoholism. *British Dental Journal*, **169**, 367–369.

Salako, N.O., Ghafouri, H.M. (1995) Oral findings in a child with Prader-Labhart-Willi Syndrome. *Quintesscence International*, **26**, 339–341.

Schluter, W.W., Reef, S.E., Redd, S.C., et al. (1998) Changing epidemiology of congenital rubella syndrome in the United States. *Journal of Infectious Diseases*, **178**, 636–641.

Ship, J.A., Fischer, D.J. (1997) The relationship between dehydration and parotid salivary gland function in young and older healthy adults. *Journal of Gerontology Biological Science Medical Science*, **52**, M310–M319.

Teo, C., Young, W.G., Daley, T.J., et al. (1997) Prior fluoridation in childhood affects dental caries and tooth wear in a south east Queensland population. *Australian Dental Journal*, **42**, 92–102.

Valena, V., Young, W.G. (2002) Dental erosion patterns from intrinsic acid regurgitation and vomiting. *Australian Dental Journal*, **47**, 106–115.

Wolff, M., Kleinberg, I. (1998) Oral mucosal wetness in hypo- and normosalivators. *Archives of Oral Biology*, **43**, 455–462.

Young, W.G. (1998) Anthropology, occlusion and tooth wear ab origine. *Journal of Dental Research*, **77**, 1860–1863.

Young, W.G. (2001a) The oral medicine of tooth wear. *Australian Dental Journal*, **46**, 236–250.

Young, W.G. (2001b) *Oral Medicine of Tooth Wear CD Rom*, Dentil Pty Ltd. Queensland, Australia.

Young, W.G. (2003) *Teeth on Edge*, Erosion Watch Pty. Ltd. Queensland, Australia.

Young, W.G., Khan, F. (2002). Sites of dental erosion are saliva-dependent. *Journal of Oral Rehabilitation*, **29**, 35–43.

Young, W., Khan, F., Brandt, R., et al. (2001) Syndromes with salivary dysfunction predispose to tooth wear: case reports of congenital dysfunction of major salivary glands, Prader-Willi, congenital rubella, and Sjögren's syndromes. *Oral Surgery, Oral Medicine, Oral Pathology, Oral Radiology, Endodontics*, **92**, 38–48.

Young, W.G., Messer, B. (2002) *Diet Analysis and Advice for Patients With Tooth Wear CD Rom*, Dentil Pty Ltd. Queensland, Australia.

Preventive and management strategies against toothwear

Farid Khan and William G. Young

Following diagnosis and assessment, prevention and management efforts for toothwear must follow sound strategic principles to allow for, if required and desired, successful restoration and rehabilitation. Counselling patients and offering advice form an important part of the prevention and management of toothwear, and must be directed towards controlling risk factors as well as addressing any imbalances within the oral environment. The range of preventive adjuncts to supplement preventive advice is discussed later in the chapter. Toothwear and dental caries prevention principles differ significantly and cannot be utilised interchangeably (Table 7.1).

In offering preventive advice (Fig. 7.1) to patients with toothwear or at risk of its development, the approach taken must include the following:

- Discussion of risk factors in the patient's lifestyle, work and sports environment, and diet
- Consideration of the patient's health and any medications they may be taking
- The *WATCH* strategy introduced in this chapter
- Patient's education and dietary diary review (see Chapter 3)
- Provision of information sheets or brochures to reinforce recommendations

Advertising and dental health campaigns have increased awareness of the public in many parts of the world to the risks associated with frequent sugar consumption and the development of dental caries. Less awareness exists regarding dental erosion (Lussi et al. 2006) and the risks associated with high or frequent acidic food and beverage consumption. The focus of this chapter is patient-based prevention and management, and population-based measures will not be covered.

AIMING PREVENTION AT ALL AGES

Toothwear is a continuous process and a limited amount of wear continues physiologically

Toothwear: The ABC of the Worn Dentition, First Edition. Edited by Farid Khan and William George Young.
© 2011 John Wiley & Sons, Ltd. Published 2011 by John Wiley & Sons, Ltd.

Table 7.1   Preventive considerations for toothwear and dental caries.

Preventive considerations	Toothwear	Dental caries
Preventive advice	Reduce dietary acids Improve salivary protection Remineralisation products *WATCH* strategy	Reduce dietary sugars Improve oral hygiene Remineralisation products
Dietary emphasis	Reduce dietary acids Promote water rehydration Increase dairy	Decrease frequency of sugars Increase dairy
Lifestyle factors	Crucial Detailed clinical history important Advise based on clinical history	Important Sugar consumption habits
Oral hygiene advice	Limited Often have a good oral hygiene Soft toothbrush and gentle technique No brushing after acid exposure	Important Flossing Toothbrushing technique Interdental brushes
Salivary protection	Important Sugar-free chewing gum Coincide acid exposure with times of high salivary protection	Beneficial Coincide sugar consumption with times of high saliva protection at meal times
Adjunct therapies	Beneficial Sugar-free chewing gum Fluoride formulations CPP-ACP	Important Chlorhexidine products Fluoride gels, pastes, rinses CPP-ACP

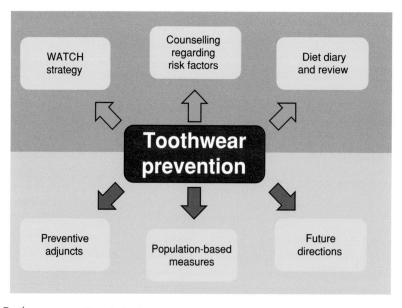

Figure 7.1   Toothwear prevention strategies.

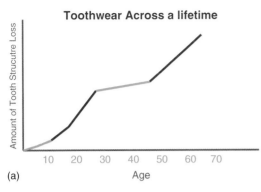

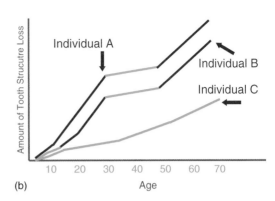

Figure 7.2 Toothwear across a lifetime involves alternating stages of toothwear progression (red) and stability (green). The arbitrary total amount of tooth structure lost over a lifetime increases with age and progresses more rapidly at certain times (a). Three different patients will, over their lifetime, experience differing amounts of toothwear (b). Individual A experienced a high rate of wear (red) in the deciduous and mixed dentition phases. The high rate of wear continued in adolescence and slowed during middle age when toothwear processes were minimal (green), increasing again at a later stage in life. Individual B experienced a slow rate of wear up until the teenage years, rapidly progressed during young adulthood and then stabilised during middle age, again accelerating in older age as health declined. Individual C went through life with relative stability and only minimal physiologic toothwear considered normal for age.

as part of the aging process. Across the patient's lifetime, alternating stages of active progression of toothwear and periods of stability occur (Fig. 7.2a). A patient may, under parental supervision, have had a good diet during childhood, whilst during teenage years and early adulthood changed lifestyle and dietary patterns with increasing consumption of acidic beverages. The same patient may in middle age have improved their diet and in later life, as health declined commenced taking medications that affected salivary protection of the dentition. This simple example details subtle variation over time that would fluctuate the rate of toothwear progression due to changes in diet. As considered in Chapter 6, the clinical history often identifies many risk variables.

Variation of toothwear progression also exists from one patient to the next. Some may experience minimal wear throughout their lifetime, whilst others more severe toothwear (Fig. 7.2b). Previously considered cases highlight such variation. The 11-year-old male patient in Fig. 1.14 had severe toothwear from a very young age. The 24–year-old male athlete shown

in Fig. 1.8 developed severe toothwear during young adulthood. When considering the appropriate preventive and management strategy for a patient, these arbitrary considerations are relevant as they identify that a patient presenting clinically may attend whilst in a period of:

• relative stability with past toothwear experiences;
• slow or rapid active progression;
• relative stability but at significant risk of developing considerable toothwear.

Preventive efforts must target all age groups, but the advice offered differs. Advice offered must be age appropriate, and variation in the preventive approaches applied for a patient must consider potential risks in the patient's lifestyle, medical history and environment, as determined by the clinical history interview. Young children and their parents must be advised of erosive potentials of foods and beverages and consumption habits to avoid. Young adults in the under-30-year age bracket, who frequently consume acidic beverages particularly during and after physical activity and as a means to rehydrate, need to be counselled accordingly. This group of patients is often of good health, and instead work- and sports-related dehydration and outgoing lifestyles need further evaluation. A third broad group are elderly patients who have developed health-related issues and are on short- and long-term medications that affect salivary protection or themselves may be acidic. The key in all three groups is to provide advice based on the imbalance identified in the oral environment.

Imbalance in the oral environment

The ultimate aim of preventively based management is to avoid all further imbalances in the oral environment in order to conserve remaining tooth structure, whilst restoration and rehabilitation aim to improve or correct problems created through past imbalances. Management must include a component reinforcing prevention. Prevention must include consideration of all external influences on the oral environment that may alter this equilibrium.

Tooth surfaces are demineralised by intrinsic and extrinsic acids and are protected by saliva. Excessive acidic influxes with or without reduced saliva protection promote dental erosion processes, which in turn potentiates further attrition and abrasion. The provision of targeted prevention and management modalities requires the complexity of underlying aetiological processes to be addressed (Fig. 7.3).

LIFESTYLE, HEALTH AND ENVIRONMENTAL RISK FACTORS

A central component for prevention of toothwear involves patient counselling regarding any potential or identified risk factors. This process should involve all members of the den-

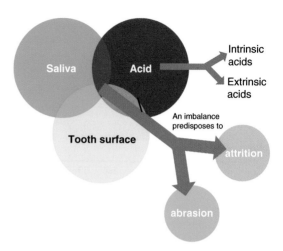

Figure 7.3 A tooth surface is protected by saliva from intrinsic and extrinsic acids. An imbalance to these components results in dental erosion that may further predispose to accelerated tooth structure loss from abrasion and attrition processes.

tal team – including dental assistants, therapists and hygienists – and not just the dentist. Preventive strategies foremost must address and reduce any risks the patient's lifestyle, health and environment may place detrimental pressures on their health and dentition. Appreciating these potential risks and identifying those that may apply to a patient allows counselling and discussion to commence to eliminate, minimise or control them. Preceding chapters have identified various health- and medication-related toothwear risks factors (Table 7.2). Patients identified with these factors should be considered at a high risk for further toothwear and managed with a strong preventive emphasis.

Whilst health ailments may create moderate and even severe toothwear in the subset of patients affected by ill health or on medications with side effects, such as salivary reduction, the predominant group of patients affected by moderate and severe toothwear are commonly healthy.

Lifestyle risk factors are most important in the majority of patients, and preventive focus must consider these risks (Table 7.3)

Table 7.2 Health and medications affecting toothwear.

Health-related considerations	Risk factors potentiating toothwear processes
Gastric reflux and conditions involving intrinsic acids	• Direct exposure of dentition to highly acidic gastric content • Secondary abrasion may occur through brushing of teeth up to 60 min subsequent to episodes
Medications	• Acidic medicines • Medicines affecting salivary protection
Chronic alcoholics	• Frequent gastric reflux or vomiting • Dehydrating effect of alcohol • Consumption of alcohol mixed with acidic beverages
Rare genetic conditions	• Affecting enamel and dentine structure and composition • Absence of salivary glands
Conditions of dietary alteration	• Bulimia nervosa • Anorexia nervosa

Table 7.3 Lifestyle-related acceleration of toothwear processes.

Lifestyle-related factors	Risk factors potentiating toothwear processes
High-frequency acidic beverage consumption	• Soft and sports drinks, juices, mixtures • Sipping and continuous reapplication of beverages • Chelation and adhesion properties of certain beverages
Sports enthusiasts	• Dehydration-induced reduction in salivary protection • Sports drink and other acidic beverage rehydration • Use of acidic slow-release supplements in gel or other formats during long-distance endurance events
Diet- and health-conscious individuals	• Lactovegetarian diets are often more acidic • Vitamin C and other supplements particularly in chewable form • Frequent juice consumption especially with artificially supplemented citric and other acids • Certain diets and slimming
Partygoers with episodes of binging	• Vomiting episodes • Dehydrating effect of alcohol and dance scene • Consumption of alcohol mixed with acidic beverages
Stress	• May promote grinding or clenching habits day or night
Patients with habits	• Swishing of acidic beverages • Sucking of lemon wedges • Biting on pencils, fishing line, sewing pins, pipe stems, seeds and nuts, foreign objects

Table 7.4 Work-related risk factors potentially accelerating toothwear processes.

Work environment	Risk factors potentiating toothwear processes
Shift workers	• Consumption of caffeine-containing beverages to remain alert • Dehydrating effect of caffeine • Caffeine-containing beverages other than coffee are often acidic • Nocturnal salivation extremely low
Outdoor workers	• Dehydrating effect particularly in warm climates • Consumption of beverages throughout the day • Acidic carbonated beverages promoted as thirst quenchers are commonly readily available
Office workers	• Sipping of beverages throughout the work day • Air-conditioned offices may have dehydrating effects • Work-related stress may influence nocturnal grinding patterns in a minority of patients
Wine tasters	• Repeated exposure to acidic wines throughout tasting periods • Swishing of wines to stimulate appreciation of taste and flavour further increases application time
Work with abrasive elements	• Dusty environments, cements and building materials • Industrial polishing abrasives
Work with industrial acids	• House cleaning with concentrated chlorine-based solutions • Battery acid factories (Petersen & Gormsen 1991)

Lifestyle changes throughout life and is never constant. Parental guidance dictates lifestyle in childhood, whilst from young adulthood onwards, the individuals choose their own leisure, sports and day-to-day activities and dietary consumption. Consumption of acidic beverages contributes significantly to the dental erosion component and toothwear in many individuals (Jarvinen et al. 1991; Lussi et al. 2004; Nunn 1996).

A great proportion of adult life is spent within the work environment. Often a regular daily routine evolves, including dietary consumption patterns. The work environment itself is important in certain circumstances and may present an environmental risk factor (Table 7.4). Whilst often not as severe a risk as health, lifestyle or dietary factors, work-related risks tend to develop slowly over many years and affect a subset of the population.

When discussing lifestyle, health and work parameters with a patient, the dental team aims to ascertain the following:

• Frequent consumption of acidic foods and beverages
• Sports- or work-related dehydration reducing salivary protection
• Acidic beverage rehydration at times of dehydration
• Health-related changes
• Medications affecting salivary protection
• Work-related exposure to acids or abrasive
• Or any combination of the above
• Any detrimental habits or dietary preferences 'Before the last line' or any combination of the above

Having identified and discussed these risks, a strategy to convey preventive advice is required.

THE *WATCH* STRATEGY

Any strategy proposed for toothwear prevention, if it is to be effective, must be straightforward, easily understood and agreed to by the patient. It needs to be in line with the best advice of dietitians, nutritionists and the medical profession.

The authors have formulated the *WATCH* strategy (Fig. 7.4), which is central to preventive counselling advice offered to any patient presenting with toothwear to allowing a tailor-made preventive approach to be communicated (Young 2005). The *WATCH* strategy is a preventive approach encouraging a lifestyle that is both healthy and dentally healthy, irrespective of whether patients present with significant toothwear or not.

For toothwear patients, this strategy can be applied either subsequent to in-depth clinical history-taking or at the review appointment at which time the diet diary is also reviewed. For all other patients presenting for routine dental examinations and treatments, the strategy can provide a succinct line of questioning and dentally relevant lifestyle advice therefrom to help reduce the risk of developing toothwear. Patients should be provided with an information sheet or brochure to reinforce key recommendations made during counselling in the clinical setting (Fig. 7.5). In training dental team members to follow the line of questioning for patients, the dentist can advise staff members to discuss the key abbreviated summary points of the *WATCH* strategy with the patient (Tables 7.5 & 7.6).

ADJUNCTIVE PRODUCTS

Adjunctive products can provide benefit in a number of ways, including the following:

- Neutralising acids
- Desensitising exposed dentine at times of acute exacerbation

- Preventing demineralisation by increasing acid resistance of the tooth surface or superficial tooth structure
- Providing a protective barrier over tooth structure
- Crystallising precipitates onto tooth structure
- Enhancing salivary protection
- Supplementing the effects of saliva
- Being added to commonly consumed acidic beverages or foods, reducing their erosive potential

The myriad of preventive adjuncts commonly available include chewing gum, topical fluoride, artificial saliva solutions, casein phosphopeptide-amorphous calcium phosphate (CPP-ACP) products and a large variety of obtundent toothpastes, to name a few. These products come in variants of gels, pastes, rinses and foam formulation.

Use of preventive adjuncts in patients with dental caries is well established and has been researched extensively. The use of fluoride and chlorhexidine formulations is well documented and supported. Research of preventive adjuncts and modalities for cases of dental erosion and toothwear is comparatively limited to date, and no doubt will be a research area of interest for the foreseeable future. A review on novel remineralising agents in the prevention or repair of dental erosion concluded that there is no formulation available at present that shows full protection (Lussi 2009). The range, availability and efficacy of preventive adjuncts will no doubt continually further evolve.

Sugar-free chewing gum

Chewing sugar-free gum is beneficial as it increases the salivary flow rate. At high flow rates, more bicarbonate is secreted from the ducts of the glands. As bicarbonate is the principal buffer in saliva, acids in the mouth are neutralised effectively by this faster flowing saliva. Saliva secretion rate falls to two to three times

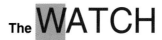 **Water**   The **WATCH**

                                                   Strategy

Do you drink enough water?
Do you play sport or go to the gym?
Do you work outdoors?
What do you drink after a sport session or whilst at work outdoors?

 Acids & Alcohol

How many cans or bottles of soft drink do you have in a week?
Do you use a straw or swish or sip your drinks?
Do you have your drink with or in-between meals?
Have you suffered from: indigestion, heartburn, reflux or frequent vomiting?

 Taste

Do you like fresh fruit?
How many pieces of fresh fruit do you eat in a week?
What fruit do you not like or are allergic to?
Is your diet healthy? Does it contain a balance of all the food groups?

 Calcium, Caffeine & Chewing gum

How many cups of tea or coffee do you drink in a day?
Do you like caffeine-containing soft drinks?
Do you avoid dairy foods (including milk) for health reasons?
Do you chew gum?

 Health

Do you have a healthy lifestyle?
What sports or exercise are you involved in?
Do you have a medical condition? Are you on medication?
Is your health affected by your diet, a medical condition or an addiction?

Figure 7.4 The *WATCH* strategy (Young 2005) for preventing toothwear.

the unstimulated flow rate in about 15 min (Dawes & MacPherson 1992). Advising patients to chew gum two or three times a day for up to 5 min at a time after meals is ideal. Patients with toothwear who suffer from heartburn or from gastro-oesophageal reflux aggravated by alcohol consumption may receive additional benefit from chewing gum. Chewing gum helps reduce postprandial acid reflux and heartburn, as the bicarbonate in saliva helps neutralise the stomach acid within the oesophagus and the healing factors reduce the oesophageal inflammation that causes heartburn (Moazzez et al. 2005).

WATCH Strategy Preventive Advice for Patients

1) Avoid dietary acids in between meals.

2) Sporting and work-related activities can be dehydrating.

3) Dehydration leads to a reduction in salivary protection of the teeth.

4) Meal times, breakfast, lunch and dinner, are the key times of salivary protection where the dentition is most capable of coping with acidic foods and beverages.

5) Chewing sugar-free gum for a few minutes after a meal is beneficial.

6) Drinking more water, particularly in between meals is ideal.

7) Dietary acids should be minimised and identified on food and beverage packaging. In particular, citric acid, ascorbic acid, sodium citrates, tartaric acid, phosphoric acid, acetic acid, lactic acid, malic acid and fumaric acid.

8) Acidic beverages should ideally be consumed quickly. Use of a straw is beneficial. Sipping or swishing of beverages is to be avoided.

9) Consumption of fruits with natural acids, in moderate quantities, stimulates salivary flow through taste and function and these are preferable sources of vitamins, as oranges are for Vitamin C.

10) Highly acidic vitamin supplements or medications should not be chewed and instead swallowed whole.

11) Avoid habits such as sucking lemon wedges, biting pens or pencils, stripping electrical wires or biting fishing lines.

12) Certain medications can dry the mouth and reduce salivary protection as a side effect. If a particular medication is drying the mouth, talk to your general practitioner to see if alternative medications are available.

13) A particular diet may be 'healthy' for the body but not so for the dentition.

14) Sensitivity indicates further loss of tooth structure in the recent period of time preceding the symptoms.

15) Absence of sensitivity indicates that the balance within the oral environment is better.

16) Toothpastes for sensitivity, whilst useful for short term use, mask the ability of the teeth to warn the patient of new periods of toothwear progression.

17) Small, soft bristle tooth brushes are ideal, utilising a circular brushing motion with bristles tilted forty-five degrees towards the gums.

18) Some whitening toothpastes may be particularly abrasive on the teeth.

19) Teeth should not be brushed for at least one hour after consuming an acidic beverage or teeth are exposed to any acids.

20) Toothwear is a condition where, in most patients, the advice offered by the clinician outweighs any treatment modality that can be offered. The acceptance of the patient to make lifestyle and dietary changes by following the *WATCH* Strategy and compliance in following the practitioner's specific advice is central to achieving long term stability and success in treating toothwear.

Figure 7.5   The *WATCH* strategy information sheet for patients detailing 20 key recommendations for preventing toothwear. (From Khan et al., 2010, with permission of Copyright Publishing Pty Ltd.)

Table 7.5 Key discussion points for the *WATCH* strategy – water, acids and alcohol, taste.

Key discussion points for water
- Patients should be encouraged to drink more water
- Two to four litres per day or eight or more standard glasses is a suitable quantity for adults
- The more water a patient consumes on a daily basis, the less the patient resorts to other drinks that would otherwise further contribute to the overall dietary intake of sugars and acids
- At times of dehydration, saliva protection is reduced, the mouth dries and the sensation of thirst is created
- Hydration with plain water to avoid dehydration is ideal
- Children dehydrate more rapidly than adults due to their body mass
- Sporting, gym and fitness enthusiasts should be encouraged to drink 1 L of water 1 h prior to the sport session

Key discussion points for acids and alcohol
- Consumption of acidic beverages contributes significantly to the dental erosion component and toothwear in many individuals
- Patients should be encouraged to restrict consumption of acidic drinks to meals times. Water is ideal in-between meals
- Both sugar-containing (regular) and sugar-free diet varieties of soft drink have similar levels of orthophosphoric acid. Hence both varieties can cause toothwear
- A high frequency of consumption and recoating of the dentition are more detrimental than a large volume consumed all at once
- Alcohol, being dehydrating, reduces salivary flow protection of the teeth. Wines and spirits with mixers are frequently highly acidic. Chronic alcoholism is associated with numerous long-term effects on the upper gastrointestinal tract and its associated glands, the liver and pancreas, and relevant to toothwear promote gastro-oesophageal reflux

Key discussion points for taste
- Taste stimulates saliva flow
- Fresh fruit and vegetables are excellent salivary stimulants
- Citric acid in oranges, grapefruit, pineapple and lemons is the best natural salivary-stimulant known (Watanabe & Dawes 1988)
- Mild erosion of the upper incisor teeth has been described in Cuban children who have a high consumption of oranges in their diet (Kunzel et al. 2000). Prolonged sucking of citrus fruit is detrimental to tooth structure due to extended contact time
- The consumption of fruit should *not* be discouraged on the basis of their acidity, as fresh fruit are still preferable to modified foods and beverages and are good sources of vitamin C

Sugar-free lozenges

Sugar-free lozenges are an alternative to gum, and have applications in cases of severe xerostomia on their own or alternatingly with chewing gum. Lozenges can be beneficial, provided no acidic flavours or additives have been incorporated. Comparatively, sucking of lozenges does not mechanically stimulate the salivary glands as well as chewing gum achieves (Dawes & MacPherson 1993).

Bicarbonate mouthrinse

Patients with intrinsic acid aetiology to their toothwear involving chronic regurgitation, vomiting episodes or bulimia nervosa can benefit from rinsing with a mix of a teaspoon of bicarbonate of soda, commonly sold as baking soda, with water. This forms a suitable alkaline mouthwash to assist in rapidly neutralising the low pH of gastric content. Patients should be discouraged from brushing their demineralised teeth for at least 1 h.

Table 7.6 Key discussion points for the *WATCH* strategy – calcium, caffeine and chewing gum and health.

Key discussion points for calcium, caffeine and chewing gum
- The diets of many children do not include the recommended dietary intake (RDI) of calcium (Moos 2005)
- Dietary calcium in milk, cheese and yogurt is to be encouraged
- Yogurts are acidic, but their high calcium content prevents them form being agents of significant dental erosion
- Coffee and tea can have a dehydrating effect
- Caffeine in larger doses can have an acute diuretic effect
- Patients should be advised to drink an extra glass of water for each cup of coffee or tea they consume
- Chewing sugar-free gum promotes saliva flow
- Short duration chewing of gum for 5 min after meals is beneficial

Key discussion points for health
- A healthy lifestyle and diet with regular exercise is ideal
- A lifestyle may be healthy for the body, but not for the dentition
- Regular exercise sessions are good for general health, but not for dental health if concluded with acidic beverage rehydration
- Frequent snacking, as recommended by nutritionists, is also healthy, but not dentally healthy
- Sports coaches may recommend consumption of supplements, vitamins and specially enhanced diets
- Vegetarians may resort to excess quantities of particular foods to supplement their nutritional intake
- Medical conditions in which patients are put at risk of toothwear (Young (2001)) include

–Asthma	–Gastro-oesophageal reflux (GORD)
–Bulimia nervosa	–Hypertension
–Chronic alcoholism	–Rare syndromes with salivary hypofunction
–Diabetes mellitus	

- The following major groups of drugs or medications may reduces salivary protection:

–Anticholinergics	–Anti-Parkinsonian medicaments
–Antidepressants	–Asthma medicaments
–Antiemetics	–Mono-oxidase inhibitors
–Antihistamines	–Neuroleptics
–Antihypertensives	–Tranquilisers

Artificial saliva

Artificial saliva and dry mouth gels are aimed at minimising the symptoms of reduced salivary flow. These products are applicable for extreme cases, especially those where the salivary glands are damaged by radiation therapy to the head and neck region. An *in vitro* erosion–abrasion cycling model study found none of the artificial salivas tested to be as effective as human saliva in protecting against dentine wear, whilst mucin-containing artificial saliva was found more effective than human saliva for enamel wear (Hara et al. 2008). Artificial saliva does not necessarily exhibit the buffering capacity of whole saliva. Such products are inappropriate for long-term use in patients with toothwear from lifestyle and dietary factors.

Water fluoridation

Water fluoridation is an important population-based dental caries prevention measure (Parnell et al. 2009). Fluoride exposure in the first 12 years of life confers improved resistance to dental caries, but its ability to reduce dental erosion and toothwear is limited (Teo et al. 1997). Another study in the North West of England

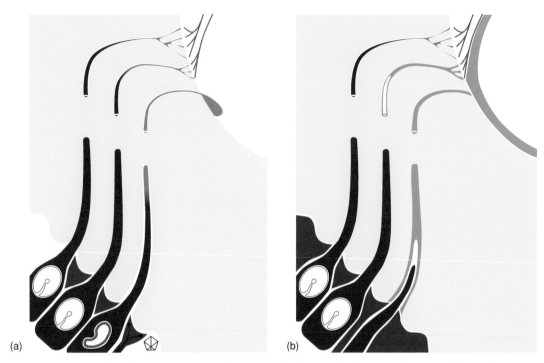

(a)

(b)

Figure 7.6   (a) Odontoblasts within patent dentinal tubules branch finely beneath the amelodentinal junction. The tubules increase in diameter the nearer they are to the pulp. Patent tubules leak dentine fluid on surfaces denuded of enamel. This activates dentinal sensitivity by hydrodynamic stimulation of nerve endings in the pulp. (b) Odontoblasts deposit intratubular dentine in response to nocuous stimuli. By narrowing tubule diameters, the hydrodynamic mechanisms of dentinal sensitivity are disrupted. Tracks of tubules filled with intratubular dentine are sclerotic and insensitive. Reparative dentine seals sclerotic dentine on the pulpal wall (brown). (From Young & Khan, 2009, with permission from Erosion Watch Pty Ltd.)

found a decrease in the risk of smooth-surface toothwear by a factor of one and a half times (Bardsley et al. 2004).

Demineralisation/ remineralisation

Remineralisation requires a lattice for crystal regrowth. Etching destroys the enamel crystals and matrix at the enamel surface (Dawes 2003). In contrast, cariogenic plaque fluid demineralises the subsurface enamel, leaving the matrix intact. Hence, there is no crystalline lattice on etched enamel surfaces to allow remineralisation, whereas the porous enamel of the white spot lesion of enamel caries preserves a lattice on which repair crystals can form. Understand-

ing this demineralisation/remineralisation dichotomy between toothwear and dental caries is essential to evaluating the further adjunct therapies discussed. Unfortunately, salivary pellicle is not a matrix that can itself become mineralised. Hence, etched surfaces covered by pellicle do not regrow surface enamel. The salivary pellicle prevents teeth from 'enlarging' in the supersaturated saliva (Dawes 2008).

However, there may also be softening of enamel in the initial stage that with a persistent attack is eventually etched away (Lussi et al. 2006). Much of the research to date has focused on remineralising abilities of adjuncts on this acid-softened layer of enamel, which may easily be removed by secondary attrition and would conceptually be of an extremely minimal thickness. It is possible that toothbrushing could wear away parts of the demineralised enamel layer, hence not allowing time for remineralisation of this layer when high-fluoride dentifrices are used (Hara et al. 2009). Importantly, research is also focusing on hardening of dental surfaces to decrease the risk of dissolution by acids of dental erosion by increasing surface resistance to acidic dissolution in the first instance.

Topical fluoride

Topical fluoride gels, rinses, toothpastes, high-concentration formulations and in-office products have been utilised for many years and continue to be used widely in high-risk patients to protect against dental caries. Fluoride application trays are custom-fitted for at-home use. Such trays, filled with strong fluoride-gel formulation, may be used on a weekly basis. This technique has its greatest application in caries management. Mouthrinses are often recommended to be used on a daily basis.

However, high-concentration fluoride gels can be used for patients presenting with toothwear-related acute-sensitivity flare-ups. Lower concentrations can be used on a daily basis for patients with toothwear, but the extent of the benefit achieved is uncertain. Lussi et al. (2006) noted that whilst most toothpastes globally contain fluoride, dental erosion appears to be on the increase, and the low levels of fluoride that standard formulations contain are ineffective. As considered earlier, water fluoridation may confer some resistance, but is also insufficient to protect against dental erosion and toothwear. A recent review of the literature (Bartlett 2009) on dental erosion noted the following:

1. Most evidence on fluoride's protective effect has been based on laboratory studies.
2. Fluoride ions appear to increase the micro-hardness of enamel and thus improve its re-

sistance to dissolution, although no clinical intervention research has been carried out to date.
3. Use of a daily fluoride rinse may be beneficial, but no research is available to support such application.

Thus, there is general support of beneficial effects of fluoride for toothwear, but also clear limitations to the current knowledge of the nature and extent of any benefit achieved. Recent *in situ* studies of fluoride dentifrices have found benefits in use of higher fluoride formulations (Ganss et al. 2004, 2007; Hara et al. 2009). Hara et al. (2009) concluded fluoridated dentifrices were able to enhance the remineralisation of eroded enamel and, importantly, reduce its susceptibility to new erosive attacks.

Casein phosphopeptide-amorphous calcium phosphate

Preparations containing CPP-ACP are available commercially in a variety of formulations, including a topical cream, tooth mousse (GC Asia Pty Ltd, Japan) and chewing gum (Recaldent™). Various other manufacturers also offer calcium-based formulations. As some of the calcium and phosphate ions in saliva are normally attached to carrier proteins, it has been proposed that the carrier protein, casein phosphopeptide, with amorphous calcium phosphate may be an adjunct therapy to augment the action of similar phosphopeptides naturally present in saliva. By maintaining a state of supersaturation on tooth surfaces or in plaque fluid, enamel demineralisation may be prevented and remineralisation may be enhanced. This range of products has been shown to have the ability of remineralising subsurface porosity beneath classic white spot lesions of caries (Reynolds et al. 2003, 2008). Particularly in newer formulations that also incorporate fluoride. Reynolds et al. (2008) have reported additive anticariogenic effects through production of novel nanoclusters of calcium, fluoride and phosphate to remineralise subsurface enamel lesions with fluoroapetite. Further detailed reviews in support of (Reynolds 2009) and questioning the usefulness and application (Zero 2009) of these products have recently been compiled subsequent to the International Conference on Novel Anti-caries and Remineralising Agents in 2008. Further research to clarify their effectiveness in cases of toothwear is required.

Obtundent toothpastes

Obtundent toothpastes are commonly available in supermarkets. Toothpastes containing potassium nitrate, potassium chloride and potassium citrate have been commercially available for many years and are thought to diffuse along dentinal tubules and decrease the excitability of intradental nerves by altering their membrane potential, although dental research on the topic is still inconclusive (Orchardson 2006). Alternatively to brushing, patients may apply such products topically, instead allowing a longer application time. Obtundent toothpastes are useful in short-term applications at times of acute hypersensitivity. However, alternative adjunctive products that offer higher levels of benefit are preferable for longer term use in cases of toothwear.

Varnishes and dentine-bonding agents

Varnishes containing fluoride and dentine-bonding agents have been marketed to act as densensitising agents. While dentine-bonding agents are primarily used in adhesive dentistry, they also have applications in a short-term topical desensitising role. Temporarily occluding open tubules allow time for the formation of sclerotic dentine. Most of these products are light cured, allowing quick application and subsequent curing on command. Their ease of use makes them a suitable choice also on shallow or grooved cervical lesions

to reduce tissue loss from abrasion. Clear dentine-bonding agents allow the area to be visualised after placement. In a review of dentine hypersensitivity, Orchardson (2006) remarked that the trials on adhesive topical desensitising materials to date have tended to be pragmatic and further research into this area is required.

Future directions

Further research into presently available products will help clarify their efficacy. One of the limitations with many available adjuncts at present is that their intended effect after application quickly reduces with repeated acidic insults of a low pH. An office worker may sip at an acidic beverage numerous times over throughout a work session of many hours, recoating the dentition with acids time and time again. The protective effect of a fluoride rinse early in the morning will have much-reduced effect when followed by such repeated insults. To receive significant protection, a higher level of protection must be offered. Alternatively, a strategy for ongoing release of such an adjunct or frequent reapplication would be required.

Alternatives to traditional fluoride formulations are being considered. Schlüter et al. (2009a, b) considered various fluoride-containing compounds and found formulations with tin to show promising results in surface hardening to prevent erosion by diffusing deeper into the enamel surface, increasing its resistance to dissolution, compared to traditional fluorides precipitating as CaF_2, which as previously discussed readily dissolve at low pH. In a recent *in situ* study, gels containing matrix metalloproteinase inhibitors were shown to impart superior dental erosion preventive effects compared to fluoride (Kato et al. 2010). Dentine-bonding agents, with longer periods of resistance, are being further developed.

Research is ongoing to add adjuncts to foods and beverages in order to decrease their acidic potential. Some manufacturers have added fluoride and calcium to beverages, such as orange or other juices, and limited ranges are available commercially, particularly in Europe. Early efforts by Sovari et al. (1986) considered the addition of fluoride and magnesium into sports drinks and their subsequent effects on molar teeth in rats. Attin et al. (2003) modified citric acid solutions with low concentrations of calcium, phosphate and fluoride, and noted a reduction in the erosive potential, but noted that enamel dissolution could not be completely prevented. Ramalingam et al. (2005) have added CPP-ACP to sports drinks, finding significant reduction in the erosive potential of the beverage without affecting taste. Hara and Zero (2008) analysed ten acidic beverages, of which five were commercially available with calcium already supplemented, and found these to have a reduced capacity to demineralise enamel when compared to five standard beverages. Further research into such applications appears warranted, given this would form a major step towards prevention on a population level, reducing the erosive potential in foods and beverages. However, it is chemically impossible to modify all erosive foods and beverages and their taste may be affected (Lussi 2009).

Other avenues being considered include increasing acid resistance of the enamel, preventively utilising laser techniques in combination with fluoride treatments. Moslemi et al. (2009) utilised laser irradiation with acidulated phosphate fluoride gel; finding this provided higher enamel resistance to acid dissolution. Steiner-Oliveira et al. (2010) considered pulse CO_2 laser treatment of enamel and dentine, with and without fluoride gel. This laser alone was not able to prevent enamel or dentine loss from dental erosion, whilst fluoride gel did show some protection. This study concluded the effect was likely due to fluoride as opposed to a synergistic effect. Vlacic et al. (2007) utilised a range of lasers *in vitro* to activate neutral sodium fluoride and concluded that under such experimental conditions, laser-activated fluoride showed protection against dental erosion in enamel. Equipment cost may be a considera-

tion as it would hinder widespread application, particularly if other more cost-effective preventive adjuncts are commonly available, unless the chosen equipment shows a notably superior and longer term protection against dental erosion and toothwear.

Recommendations

In addition to recommending the *WATCH* strategy, providing dietary advice through review of the patient's diet diary and provision of patient information brochures or sheets, that discuss oral health and incorporate selective recommendations for the use of preventive adjuncts, is appropriate. Particularly in patients in whom unfavourable oral environmental states persist, or at the extreme cannot be controlled for health, lifestyle or compliance reasons, preventive adjuncts play an important role. Given the limitations of presently available adjuncts and deficiency inconclusive research and clinically based results on the topic, for patients presenting with significant toothwear and those with a moderate or high risk of developing toothwear, a combination of preventive adjuncts should be recommended to offer supplemental preventive and protective effects (Table 7.7).

The risk of toothwear on oral health should not be considered in isolation and neither should its prevention. Instead, in recommending the use of preventive adjuncts, if deemed necessary, the clinician should do so whilst also keeping caries and periodontal disease prevention in mind. Toothwear and dental caries have previously been discussed as independent processes that may, however, occur at different stages in a patient's life through dietary and other changes (see Fig. 1.16). A patient with severe toothwear, who has the oral environment stabilised and reduces intake of dietary acids, after composite resin or prosthodontic rehabilitation of their dentition will then have numerous restorative margins on many teeth. Each marginal region is susceptible to marginal leakage and dental caries over time in an

Table 7.7 Key recommendations for the use of preventive adjuncts.

- Adjuncts need to be used regularly and the patient should form a routine
- Daily rinsing with a fluoride rinse can be supplemented with topical application of calcium phosphate formulations at a different time in the day
- Patients should avoid rinsing their mouth with water immediately after applications of adjuncts to allow longer contact time
- Sugar-free chewing gum for short periods of time, two or three times a day after meal times, is highly beneficial
- Daily applications of low-fluoride formulations are likely to confer greater levels of anticaries protection than against toothwear
- High-strength fluoride toothpaste formulations and calcium-containing pastes should be recommended to patients where the underlying toothwear aetiology cannot be further controlled, such as in a case of bulimia nervosa
- Patients experiencing intrinsic acids within the oral environment should be advised not to brush their teeth within 1 h of the episode. Use of a bicarbonate of soda rinse is beneficial to rapidly neutralise acids
- Sugar-free chewing gum with calcium phosphate supplementation has become available
- Patients experiencing acute dental sensitivity can benefit from short-term applications of calcium phosphate, fluoride or desensitising gels, pastes and other formulations
- Care must be taken in advising parents and children. Recommended formulations must be age appropriate. Many high-strength fluoride pastes are appropriate for adults, but not for children. Calcium phosphate–based formulation may be more appropriate
- In the phase leading to restoration, daily use of fluoride or calcium phosphate products may assist in improving tooth surface characteristics to enhance bond strengths of conventional restorative materials to the surface

oral environment that was previously free of caries. The use of a fluoride mouthrinse or stronger toothpaste formulation in such cases is important.

DIET DIARIES AND REVIEW

The diet diary is an important component of counselling as it offers a means of communicating a patient's diet, identifying healthy, beneficial, detrimental or unhealthy dietary consumption trends. The diet diary should also consider lifestyle and activities in between the meals and the environment where they took place. Some patients complete the diary truthfully and others write what they feel the dentist would like them to write. Working through the diet diary, identifying the frequency of consumption of dietary acids is more important

than the total quantity consumed. A can of soft drink, consumed all at once, using a straw, with a meal is far less damaging to the dentition as opposed to an office worker sipping on a can of drink slowly at intervals between lunch and the conclusion of the work day. In either case, the diet diary may indicate that one can of soft drink was consumed. In formulating strong preventive dietary advice, consumption variables require consideration (Table 7.8). Diet diary approaches are further discussed in Chapter 3.

PATIENT'S REPORTING SENSITIVITY

Dentinal sensitivity is a common presenting complaint in many patients. Dentine hypersensitivity is associated with dentine exposures

Table 7.8 Acidic food and beverage consumption variables.

- Quantity consumed
- Frequency of consumption
- Method of consumption – drinking from a bottle, cup or straw.
- The latter is more favourable
- pH and more importantly buffering capacity of the beverage
- Chelation properties
- Consumption habits – sipping or swishing drinks, sucking of lemon wedges

resulting from loss of enamel or gingival recession and subsequent loss of cementum (Zero & Lussi 2005). Rapid movements of fluid within the dentinal tubules are sensed as pain by nerve endings in the pulp (see Fig. 7.6a). The hydrodynamic theory holds that the outward flow of dentinal fluid occurs when tubules are opened (Brännström 1986), and stimulated mechanoreceptors give rise to dentine sensitivity. Sensitive teeth have been found to have many more (×8) and wider (×2) open dentinal tubules on buccal cervical surfaces than are found on non-sensitive teeth (Absi et al. 1987). Absence of tooth sensitivity may be used to indicate effective control of the erosive process (Wickens 1999). As such it is an indicator of a stable oral environment in the recent time frame. Use of obtundent toothpastes and preventive products can provide short-term relief of sensitivity. Concurrently, their use also deactivates a useful dental warning signal to inform a patient of the imbalance within the oral environment that existed in days preceding the symptoms. Presence of sensitivity is a good indicator of progression, further loss of tooth structure and open dentinal tubules. However, sensitivity is highly subjective, and what one patient considers sensitivity, another considers as pain. Without treatment, sensitivity can fluctuate on weekly basis.

When enamel is removed through, the underlying dentinal tubules become filled in with an amorphous calcified tissue, called intratubular dentine, which is secreted by the odontoblasts (see Fig. 7.6a). Initially, the diameters of the tubules are narrowed by the build-up of this material within their walls. Subsequently, the odontoblastic processes retract, leaving behind tubules completely occluded by intratubular dentine. Dentine so modified is called sclerotic dentine. Sclerotic dentine can extend within the tooth crowns from the amelodentinal junction to the pulp. Reparative dentine seals the pulpal ends of sclerotic tubules. Slow-progressing toothwear, such as a shallow wear facet exposing dentin, allows reparative dentine to form pulpally (see Fig. 7.6b). Hence, such areas are commonly not sensitive and fewer older patients present with toothwear-related sensitivity as sclerotic dentine is laid down physiologically with age. Therefore, elderly patients will be less able to use reduction of dentine sensitivity as a measure of success in their therapy.

Cervical lesions are the most frequent sites of sensitivity. Toothwear does not involve dental plaque, and patients with active erosion often have maintained plaque- and caries-free mouths. Oral hygiene methods may even have been overzealous. Often shallow and wedge-shaped cervical lesions have an underlying erosion component potentiating abrasive elements. Advice should include specifying soft-bristled brushes and to ideally go for a lower abrasive gel toothpaste. Various whitening products and toothpastes can have a high abrasive content. Some patients experience sensitivity with use of such products. Wedge-shaped cervical lesions often occur in older individuals and are generally symptom free because intratubular dentine is formed on the ceiling and floor of the lesion and reparative dentine on the pulpal wall. Preventive management advice and adjuncts available for managing acute dental sensitivity are outlined in Table 7.9.

A slow progression of toothwear allows for further reparative dentine to be laid down defending the pulp as the zone of surface wear

Table 7.9   Home advice for managing sensitivity.

Where applicable:

- Dietary changes and reducing frequency and quantity of acidic intake
- Changing consumption patterns of 'acids' to avoid intake at times of dehydration
- Implementing the *WATCH* strategy
- Oral hygiene instruction
  - Soft toothbrush
  - Circular brushing motion, bristles 45° to the gingival margin
  - Avoid abrasive toothpaste
  - Avoid brushing for 1 h after acid exposure
  - Avoid brushing just prior to an acid exposure to maintain the salivary pellicle
- Adjunct therapies
  - Sugar-free chewing gum
  - Bicarbonate rinses for cases with intrinsic acid influx
  - Topical high-fluoride rinses, gels and toothpastes (neutral pH formulations)
  - Casein phosphopeptide-amorphous calcium phosphate (CPP-ACP)
  - Short-term repeated topical application of obtundent toothpaste

approaches. Hence the pulpal tissues recede in advance of the slow-progressing erosion and related toothwear processes and often present minimal symptoms to the patient. However, in acute exacerbations and rapidly progressing forms of toothwear, these lesions may proceed faster than the pulpal tissues can retreat, in such cases creating a more severe symptomatic response, and application of adjunctive products can be beneficial and restorative intervention for pulpal protection may be warranted. Dental adjuncts should particularly be considered for short-term relief of sensitivity, but should not be exclusively relied upon over the long term. Exclusive reliance on dental adjuncts without the provision of lifestyle and dietary advice cannot be recommended and is unlikely to negate the detrimental effect of underlying processes.

TREATMENT PLANNING

Conceptually, the ideal management approach incorporates a treatment plan which includes the following:

- Analytically diagnosing toothwear aetiology
- Preventively orientating advice and treatment, aiming to conserve tooth structure
- Restoration or rehabilitation to rebuild the worn dentition if required
- Monitoring and frequent reviewing to ensure stabilisation and improvement over time

Examination of the face and soft tissues (see Chapter 1), examination of the dentition and charting *The Stages of Wear* (see Chapter 4), completion of a comprehensive clinical history (see Chapter 6), taking a set of impressions for study models to measure the progression of toothwear over time (see Chapter 8) and clinical photographs all form essential components of the analytically diagnostic process. These steps should ideally be completed over two appointments. The second appointment commences with a review of the completed diet diary the patient brings to the appointment. At this time, discussion of the *WATCH* strategy and provision of information brochures form an appropriate baseline preventive approach, which may be supplemented with selective use of preventive adjuncts.

Management of the worn dentition does not necessarily imply restoration. Instead, restoration and rehabilitation are procedures the clinician and the patient may agree to embark on in order to improve aesthetics, function and protection of the dentition when balance within the oral environment is reestablished. Cases with mild-to-moderate toothwear may, based on agreement between the dentist and the patient, be preventively managed with the *WATCH* strategy, dietary advice and selective use of preventive adjuncts.

The ideal treatment plan is presented in Table 7.10 and incorporates management ideals. Irrespective of whether a treatment plan involves a restorative phase or not, frequent review, monitoring and comparison to baselines study models is indicated. Restoration and rehabilitation of the worn dentition is detailed in Chapters 11 and 12.

THE REVIEW APPOINTMENT

A review appointment should be scheduled no sooner than a week from presentation and ideally a longer period of time. At the review appointment, the clinician should consider what changes the patient reports they have made to their diet and lifestyle, their level of reported compliance and change in the level of sensitivity experienced.

Restoration of the worn dentition upon first presentation is far from ideal. Toothwear processes have gradually worn the dentition, and whilst a patient may be keen to commence restorative treatments, this approach is not recommended. For cases in which multiple restorations or rehabilitation is planned, treatment should not commence until sensitivity has reduced. Indicators to defer or commence restorative treatment phases are detailed in Table 7.11.

Toothwear takes years to develop. When a patient initially presents, the dentition is often expressing dentinal sensitivity. The patient may

Table 7.10 The ideal treatment plan.

- Patient completes general details and medical history questionnaire
- Basic patient history and reason for attendance
- Review medical history
- Clinical examination
  - Assessment of extraoral features
  - Assessment of intraoral soft tissues
  - Charting of DMFT and periodontal assessment
  - Charting of toothwear stages A–F
- Discuss patient demands and aspirations
- Treatment and stabilisation of acute condition
  - Sensitivity, toothache, pain
  - Provision of products that may help alleviate acute symptoms
- Detailed clinical history
- Information gathering
  - Clinical photography
  - Diagnostic models
  - Bite registration and articulation if required
- Elucidate aetiology and formulate diagnosis or consider referral
- Patient completes a 6-day dietary diary
- Review dietary diary. Offer advice on diet and lifestyle
- Review sensitivity
- Evaluate success or failure of lifestyle and dietary changes
- Evaluate patient compliance
- Formulate treatment plan(s)
- Discuss restorative options, risk and limitations. Obtain informed consent
- Commence rehabilitation
  - With provisional restorative phase if substantially increasing vertical dimension
  - Stage treatment pending complexity
  - Or alternatively embark on direct restorative approach
- Clinical photographs of completed case
- Frequent review

express aesthetic concerns and desire an immediate start to restorative treatment. The crucial consideration before commencing in haste is whether the oral environment is ready or not for restoration. Is the balance within the oral environment favourable?

Table 7.11 Criteria for deferring and initiating rehabilitation.

	Criteria for deferring rehabilitation	Criteria for initiating rehabilitation
Signs	• Chalky, etched enamel • Clean, matt-finished dentine • Enlarged salivary glands	• Shiny, translucent enamel • Stained, sclerotic and reparative dentine • Supragingival calculus
Symptoms	• Dentinal sensitivity • Dry mouth	• No dentinal sensitivity • No dry mouth
History	• Dehydrating lifestyle • Patient is not compliant in changing diet and lifestyle • Frequent acid drink consumption • Medication or medical condition	• Low-risk lifestyle • Dietary improvements and good patient compliance • Patient is accepting recommendation • No medications or current medical condition

Management strategies whilst ideal for some may not be ideal for others. Chronic and slow-progressing toothwear may be monitored, particularly when the clinician is confident the aetiology has been elucidated and the dentition is reported to be asymptomatic. Patients presenting with active and rapidly progressing wear should still be approached with a maximum of preventive and conservative efforts, education and advice. In a subset of this group of patients, the underlying processes of erosion, attrition and abrasion, with or without salivary protection compromises, cannot be controlled. Restorative efforts in such patients are undertaken to offer protection, having informed the patient of the compromised dentition and associated reduced prognosis of rehabilitation that is anticipated.

Adjuncts can selectively be recommended, including sugar-free chewing gum, topical fluoride gels and rinses, artificial saliva solutions, CPP-ACP as mousse and chewing gum, and a large variety of toothpastes. These have an important role in conservation of tooth structure when the patient's health and lifestyle impose limits on the success of the *WATCH* strategy alone. The range of commercially available adjuncts is rapidly expanding. Some patients mentally thrive on a gel, cream or rinse, which gives them immediate help. If use of adjuncts encourages patients to be more compliant and conscious about their dental health, then this too can be a positive benefit. Basing prevention and management of toothwear on adjuncts exclusively is an approach that is difficult to justify.

SUMMARY

Toothwear in an individual can be prevented by identifying and eliminating intrinsic and extrinsic acids, identifying times of low salivary protection and using adjuncts where appropriate. If the *WATCH* strategy is successfully implemented by the patient and if done so early enough in the toothwear process, this constitutes ideal prevention and management (Fig. 7.7). Prevention is far simpler than restoration, but relies heavily upon the patient's compliance to follow the preventive regimes and make lifestyle and dietary changes, which are paramount to long-term success. The balance of the oral environment not only has implications on the presentation of toothwear in adults and toothwear lesions across the dentition, but also has prevention and management modalities instigated. Selective application of preventive adjuncts supplements the benefits

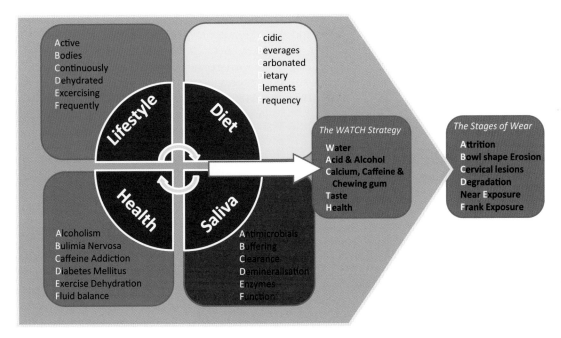

Figure 7.7 The ABCs of the *Worn Dentition*. Prevention and management must address diet, lifestyle, health and saliva. The *WATCH* strategy offers the dental team the means to provide relevant counselling advice. The level of balance between these components reflects in *The Stages of Wear* within the dentition.

achieved from lifestyle and dietary changes the patient instigates. From the literature to date, it would appear that whilst adjuncts may have role in preventing toothwear by hardening the dental hard tissues, their remineralisation potentials require further investigation. Lussi (2009), in a review of remineralisation products for the prevention or repair of dental erosion, discussed research on formation of a protective layer which is a promising focus for future research, but concluded at this standpoint that there is no formulation available showing full protection. During management of acute phases, adjuncts have beneficial short-term applications. Moreover, these products are highly applicable where compliance failures with preventive strategies are identified or handicaps or physical dexterity are present.

The diagnostic, assessment and preventive management process should at the minimum be completed over two appointments and ide-

ally over a longer period, during which proper assessment of compliance and improvement in resolution of symptoms can be monitored. Correct implementation of the *WATCH* strategy by the patient is essential, has far-reaching effects, and when applied in conjunction with selective preventive adjuncts forms the current gold-standard approach to preventive management of *The Worn Dentition*.

References

Absi, E.G., Addy, M., Adams, D. (1987) Dentine hypersensitivity: a study of the patency of dentinal tubules in sensitive and nonsensitive cervical dentine. *Journal of Clinical Periodontology*, **14**, 280–284.

Attin, T., Meyer, K., Hellwig, E., et al. (2003) Effect of mineral supplements to citric acid on enamel erosion. *Archives of Oral Biology*, **48**, 753–759.

Bardsley, P.F., Taylor, S., Milosevic, A. (2004) Epidemiological studies of tooth wear and dental erosion in 14-year-old children in North West England. Part 1: the relationship with water fluoridation and social deprivation. *British Dental Journal*, **197**, 413–416.

Bartlett, D. (2009) Etiology and prevention of acid erosion. *Compendium*, **30**(9), 616–620.

Brännström, M. (1986) Hydrodynamic theory of dentinal pain: sensation in preparations, caries, and the dentinal crack syndrome. *Journal of Endodontology*, **12**(10), 453–457.

Dawes, C. (2003) What is the critical pH and why does a tooth dissolve in acid? *Journal of the Canadian Dental Association*, **69**(11), 722–724.

Dawes, C. (2008) Salivary flow patterns and the health of hard and soft oral tissues. *Journal of the American Dental Association*, **139**, s18–s24.

Dawes, C., MacPherson, L.M. (1992) Effects of nine different chewing-gums and lozenges on salivary flow rate and pH. *Caries Research*, **26**(3), 176–182.

Dawes, C., MacPherson, L.M.D. (1993) The distribution of saliva and sucrose around the mouth during the use of chewing gum and the implications for the site-specificity of caries and calculus deposition. *Journal of Dental Research*, **72**, 852–857.

Ganss, C., Klimek, J., Brune, V., et al. (2004) Effects of two fluoridation measures on erosion progression in human enamel and dentine in situ. *Caries Research*, **38**, 561–566.

Ganss, C., Schlueter, N., Friedrich, D., et al. (2007) Efficacy of waiting periods and topical fluoride treatment on toothbrush abrasion of eroded enamel in situ. *Caries Research*, **41**, 146–151.

Hara, A.T., Ando, M., González-Cabezas, C., et al. (2009) Influence of fluoride availability of dentifrices on eroded enamel remineralization in situ. *Caries Research*, **43**, 57–63.

Hara, A.T., González-Cabezas, C., Creeth, J., et al. (2008) The effect of human saliva substitutes in an erosion-abrasion cycling model. *European Journal of Oral Sciences*, **116**, 552–556.

Hara, A.T., Zero, D.T. (2008) Analysis of the erosive potential of calcium-containing acidic beverages. *European Journal of Oral Sciences*, **116**(1), 60–65.

Jarvinen, V.K., Rytoomaa, I.I., Heinonen, O.P. (1991) Risk factors in dental erosion. *Journal of Dental Research*, **70**, 942–947.

Kato, M.T., Leitel, A.L., Hannas, A.R., et al. (2010) Gels containing MMP inhibitors prevent dental erosion in situ. *Journal of Dental Research*, **89**(5), 468–472.

Khan F., Young W.G., Taji S.S. (2010) *Toothwear: A Guide for Oral Health Practitioners*. Copyright Publishing Pty. Ltd. Brisbane, Australia.

Kunzel, W., Cruz, M.S., Fischer, T. (2000) Dental erosion in Cuban children associated with excessive consumption of oranges. *European Journal of Oral Sciences*, **108**, 104–109.

Lussi, A. (2009) Dental erosion – novel remineralizing agents in prevention or repair. *Advances in Dental Research*, **21**, 13–16.

Lussi, A., Hellwig, E., Zero, D., et al. (2006) Erosive tooth wear: diagnosis, risk factors and prevention. *American Journal of Dentistry*, **19**, 319–325.

Lussi, A., Jaeggi, T., Zero, D. (2004) The role of diet in the aetiology of dental erosion. *Caries Research*, **38**(1), 34–44.

Moazzez, R., Bartlett, D., Anggiansah, A. (2005) The effect of chewing sugar-free chewing gum on gastro-oesophageal reflux. *Journal of Dental Research*, **84**, 1062–1065.

Moos, M.K. (2005) Have your teenagers had their calcium today? *Preventive Chronicals*, **9**(4), 324–326.

Moslemi, M., Fekrazad, R., Tadyon, N., et al. (2009) Effect of Er,Cr:YSGG laser irradiation and fluoride treatment on acid resistance of the enamel. *Paediatric Dentistry*, **31**, 409–413.

Nunn, J.H. (1996) Prevalence of dental erosion and the implications for oral health. *European Journal of Oral Science*, **104**, 156–161.

Orchardson, R. (2006) Managing dentin hyper-sensitivity. *Journal of the American Dental Association*, **137**, 990–998.

Parnell, C., Whelton, H., O'Mullane, D. (2009) Water fluoridation. *European Archives of Paeditric Dentistry*, **10**(3), 141–148.

Petersen, P., Gormsen, C. (1991) Oral conditions among German battery factory workers. *Community and Dentistry and Oral Epidemiology*, **19**, 104–106.

Ramalingam, L., Messer, L.B., Reynolds, E.C. (2005) Adding casein phosphopeptide-amorphous calcium phosphate to sports drinks to eliminate in vitro erosion. *Pediatric Dentistry*, **27**, 61–67.

Reynolds, E.C. (2009) Caseine phosphopeptide-amorphous calcium phosphate: the scientific evidence. *Advances in Dental Research*, **21**, 25–29.

Reynolds, E.C., Cai, F., Cochrane, N.J., et al. (2008) Fluoride and casein phosphopeptide-amorphous calcium phosphate. *Journal of Dental Research*, **87**, 344–348.

Reynolds, E.C., Cai, F., Shen, P., et al. (2003) Retention in plaque and remineralization of enamel lesions by various forms of calcium in a mouthrinse or sugar-free chewing gum. *Journal of Dental Research*, **82**, 206–211.

Schlüter, N., Duran, A., Klimek, J., et al. (2009a) Investigation of the effect of various fluoride compounds and preparations thereof on erosive tissue lose in enamel in vitro. *Caries Research*, **43**, 10–16.

Schlüter, N., Hardt, M., Lussi, A., et al. (2009b) Tin containing fluoride solutions as anti-erosive agents in enamel: an in vitro tin-uptake, tissue-loss, and scanning electron micrograph study. *European Journal of Oral Sciences*, **117**, 427–434.

Sovari, R., Koskinen-Kainulainen, M., Sorvari, T., et al. (1986) Effect of a sport drink mixture with and without addition of fluoride and magnesium on plaque formation, dental caries and general health of rats. *Scandinavia Journal of Dental Research*, **94**, 483–490.

Steiner-Oliveira, C., Nobre-dos-Santos, M., Zero, D.T., et al. (2010) Effect of a pulsed CO_2 laser and fluoride on the prevention of enamel and dentine erosion. *Archives of Oral Biology*, **55**, 127–133.

Teo, C., Young, W.G., Daley, T.J., et al. (1997) Prior fluoridation in childhood affects dental caries and tooth wear in a Southeast Queensland population. *Australian Dental Journal*, **42**, 92–102.

Vlacic, J., Meyers, I.A., Walsh, L.J. (2007) Laser-activated fluoride treatment of enamel as prevention against erosion. *Australian Dental Journal*, **52**(3), 175–180.

Watanabe, S., Dawes, C. (1998) The effects of different foods and concentrations of citric acid on the flow rate of whole saliva in man. *Archives of Oral Biology*, **33**, 1–5.

Wickens, J.L. (1999) Tooth surface loss. 6. Prevention and maintenance. *British Dental Journal*, **186**(8), 371–376.

Young, W.G. (2001) The oral medicine of tooth wear. *Australian Dental Journal*, **46**(4), 236–250.

Young, W.G. (2005) Tooth wear: diet analysis and advice. *International Dental Journal*, **55**, 68-72.

Young, W.G., Khan, F. (2002) Sites of dental erosion are saliva-dependent. *Journal of Oral Rehabilitation*, **29**, 35–43.

Young, W.G., Khan, F. (2009) *By the Skin of our Teeth*, Erosion Watch Pty Ltd. Queensland, Australia.

Zero, D., Lussi, A. (2005) Erosion. Chemical and biological factors of importance to the dental practitioner. *International Dental Journal*, **555**, 285–290.

Zero, D.T. (2009) Recaldent TM evidence for clinical activity. *Advances in Dental Research*, **21**, 30–34.

Measurement of severity and progression of toothwear

William H. Douglas and William G. Young

Toothwear belongs to the general classification of loss of dental hard tissues from the mouth. The Pindborg (1970) general classification of attrition (tooth-to-tooth contact), abrasion (third-body contact wear, e.g. toothbrush), erosion (chemical loss of surface contour, due to mineral acids) and dental caries (subsurface loss of hard tissue), which is perhaps the only true direct pathological process, still remains useful. These factors are very likely to overlap (see Chapter 1). Toothwear in all of its manifestations gives rise to changes on the surface anatomy of the tooth. Measurement of these changes is critical for assessment of the lesion severity and progress and for the effectiveness of any treatment or preventive regimes. To measure progression of dental erosion and attrition over time, profilometry offers a gold standard for the measurement and monitoring of toothwear. Two clinical cases where profilometry techniques were applied are presented later in this chapter.

NON-PARAMETRIC OR SEMI-PARAMETRIC APPROACHES

The first serious approach to measurement of loss of dental contour was made by Ryge and Snyder (1973), and adopted by the US Public Health Service (USPHS). This was a pure ranking or non-parametric approach based on A (alpha), B (beta), C (charlie), etc., with anatomical landmarks to guide the clinician when (say) A became B and B became C. It had much to commend it: it was fast, inexpensive and easily learnt by assessors. There are many variations of the Ryge chairside measurement system designed to meet special needs such as the studies in pure erosion. A very useful review of these kinds of indexes with appropriate anatomical landmarks is given by Bardesley (2008).

Leinfelder et al. (1986) and his colleagues took the Ryge system one step further by the

Toothwear: The ABC of the Worn Dentition, First Edition. Edited by Farid Khan and William George Young.
© 2011 John Wiley & Sons, Ltd. Published 2011 by John Wiley & Sons, Ltd.

creation of calibrated stone models with increasing toothwear in 100-μm steps. Real clinical models could then be compared to these models with a better level of accuracy than the Ryge system. This was effectively a semiparametric system of measurement.

PARAMETRIC MEASUREMENT OF TOOTHWEAR

Xhonga et al. (1972) used profile tracings from sectioned study models to estimate an average daily rate of erosion in cervical lesions. Despite treatment with sodium fluoride paste, approximately 7 μm/d was recorded over 5 months from treated and untreated lesions.

The real problem of measurement of toothwear by profilometry is that volumetric loss of tissue has a complex shape which defies assessment by simple geometric calibration, such as a 'ruler' might give. The location and shape of this volume of loss are important for diagnosis and treatment. The answer to the problem of course lies in the capture of the entire anatomical tooth surfaces of the before and after time interval. These two images must now be fixed in space in the correct relation to each other, a processing known as 'fitting'. Then the surfaces can be inspected (interrogated) for differences that occurred over the time interval from the point of view of extent of wear and location. This requires a digital technique with software facilities for computer image rendering, fitting and measurement.

Contact stylus technique

There are a number of displacement contact stylus techniques which are applicable to *in vitro* simulations of wear or clinical tooth contact roughness (Lambrecht et al. 1989). These are usually displacement styli, which are very accurate, but over a short range. One that is applicable to clinical wear is the null point stylus (Delong et al. 1985; Fig. 8.1).

Here, the stylus is fixed in space and the clinical model of the tooth moves underneath the stylus, with the digital scan mapped out in the computer. A large number of scans can be covered with a grayscale rendition and the image of the tooth appears – a kind of clinical interface (Fig. 8.2).

Fitting the computer models together

The fitting procedure of computer models is a key step and is in part a matter of clinical judgement. Necessarily, the worn model (after) will fit inside the original model (before). The clinician must identify the surfaces with no change or at least minimal change and initiate a least-squared-difference fit, which is then performed automatically by the software, as shown in Fig. 8.2 for profile 46. The renditions of the teeth show the differences due to tooth loss, which can now be displayed in many useful ways. The goodness of least-squared fit of the two models in part determines the accuracy of the measurement. With this accuracy, much more information of the wear process can be obtained than from chairside observation.

Optical techniques

Optical techniques, including laser (Kramer et al. 2006) and white light (Delong et al. 2003), have advantages over a contact stylus in that they do not require as much attention to how the tooth model is mounted. However, as they are reflective techniques, they are very sensitive to the condition of the model or tooth surface. One such optical technique is shown in Fig. 8.3.

The triangulation method by which the profiler determines the anatomical location of the wear area is illustrated in Fig. 8.4. One hoped-for advance in this field is the emergence of hand-held digitisers, which are accompaniments to computerised restorative dentistry. These obviate the need for a stone model of the

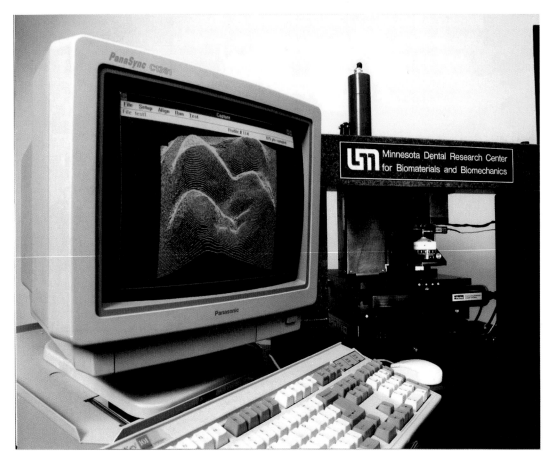

Figure 8.1 Null point stylus fixed in space and the model of the tooth which moves underneath the stylus. Note with the digital scans rendered on the computer, giving the appearance of the tooth.

teeth, but do not yet have quite the accuracy of fixed extraoral digitisers. More importantly, it is very difficult to recover the files in a usable format for current wear measurement software. No doubt in future, hand-held devices will succeed fixed digitisers in this field.

Microcomputer tomography scanning method

All of the methods described so far, including straightforward chairside assessment, use line-of-sight observation. However, interproximal areas and areas of undercut cannot be as-

sessed by line-of-sight methodologies. Using micro-computer tomography (micro-CT) scanning methods with good models this problem can be addressed. The micro-CT scanning method establishes the centre of gravity of the sample and then from a series of X-ray scans, calculates the X-ray absorption of every point within the sample. The result is a series of 'slices' presented as JPEG images, which are then finally assembled as a 3D model of the tooth. Micro-CT 3D models are extremely large files, and large computer facilities are required to manage them. The assembled dental models can be used to address a number of

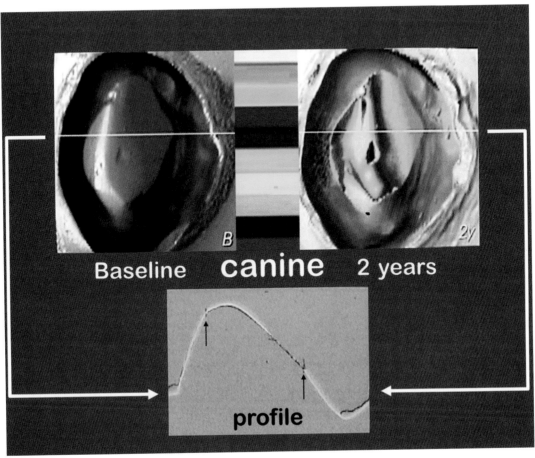

Figure 8.2 Wear on the incisal edge of a canine. The grayscaling shows the anatomical detail before (B), and wear is superimposed as a colour reference 2 years after baseline (2Y).

problems, including prototyping (Magne 2010) and quantitative dental anatomy (Pintado et al. 2007). Most usefully for wear measurement, the exterior contour of this model can be 'fitted' exactly as described for the line-of-sight models above, provided software is in a compatible language. The advantages of micro-CT profiling are shown in Fig. 8.5, where the undercut areas of a cervical abrasion are now included in the complete rendition of the lesion. Complete numeric dimensions can also be provided for the lesion and chosen slices can be highlighted for special attention (Fig. 8.5).

REPORTING TOOTHWEAR

Volume reporting

Reporting toothwear as a volume loss (mm^3) is the most complete description of the process. Volume loss is a material property of the substrate only, such as that of composite, enamel or dentine. Further, there is a direct correspondence between volume loss and the cause of the wear, such as chemical, abrasive or their combinations, and there is usually reasonable linearity between cause and effect with respect to

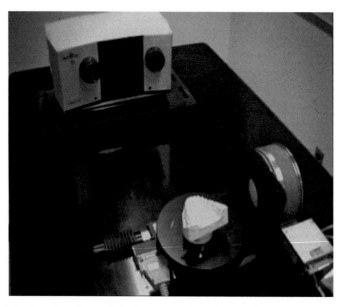

Figure 8.3   White-light digital profiler, with light being emitted from one port and detected by a CCD camera in the other. The reflective properties of the model are very important.

volume loss due to toothwear. To report volume loss, some digital method is necessary. Typical values for an occlusal composite are $0.05 \, mm^3/y$ and for a severe cervical abrasion, $0.85 \, mm^3/y$ over 26 years.

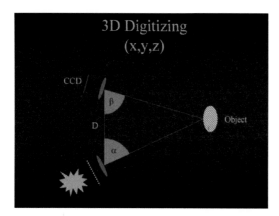

Figure 8.4   Diagram of digital profiler, showing the three-point triangulation necessary to determine the anatomical location of the wear area.

Other reporting methods

Toothwear can also be reported as a depth loss or as an increase in area of contact, especially in areas of occlusal contact. In nominal terms, depth × area = volume. Reporting depth loss is much favoured by clinicians because it affects the clinical height of the tooth, and if the whole occlusal surface is involved then the facial height may be reduced. The approximate relationships between the different methods of reporting rate of wear are shown in Fig. 8.6.

Conservation of facial height

It might be thought that a discussion of different methods of wear reporting is for those with an absorbing interest in mathematics – nothing could be further from the truth, for the following reasons. The young occlusion is characterised by well-formed cusps, with a cusp to fossa relationship under conditions of normal occlusion (Fig. 8.7). Especially in high-wearing surfaces there is a steady loss of hard tissue,

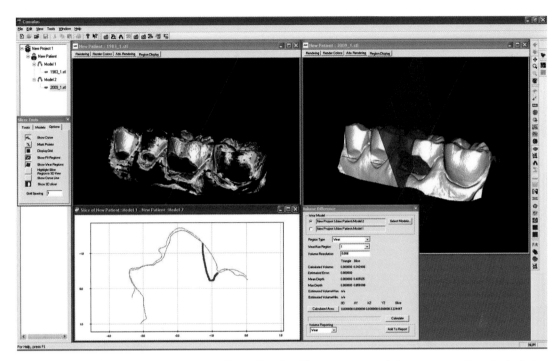

Figure 8.5 Micro-computer tomography–derived model of long-term cervical abrasive wear. Note the inclusion of undercut in the total profile of the lesion.

which can be expressed as volume. However, there are increasing areas of occlusal contact and dentine exposure. This must mean that the rate of loss of depth lags behind the same wear expressed as rate of volume loss (see Fig. 8.6). But as has been pointed out, depth loss affects the clinical crown height and facial height where many tooth are involved. Loss of occlusal surfaces or lower permanent first molars and of palatal surfaces of upper permanent incisors occurs in children from the initial establishment of the occlusion in the mixed dentition (see Chapter 10).

Canines and premolars later lose cuspal form under these conditions, and with increasing patient age, the process advances to group function. This process is easily seen in Fig. 8.8, where the loss of buccal cusp morphology is demonstrated over an 8- and 11-year period. Well-formed cusps provide ample surfaces for increasing area of contact due to wear so that even with high volume loss corresponding loss due to depth is much less. This was demonstrated by Pintado et al. (1997) in a 2-year wear study in young adults. Facial height is conserved in young patients with high wear rates by passive eruption of the worn teeth. This position is reversed in older patients, with loss of cuspal morphology and a flat occlusal table. By this stage, the area of contact is fixed, hard tissue volume loss is fully reflected in a corresponding loss in depth, and facial height is no longer conserved.

Study models

Whilst study models have limited application for patients with dental caries, unless major rehabilitation in cases of rampant caries is planned, for patients with toothwear, diagnostic study casts are crucial. Impressions for study models make quick and reliable records

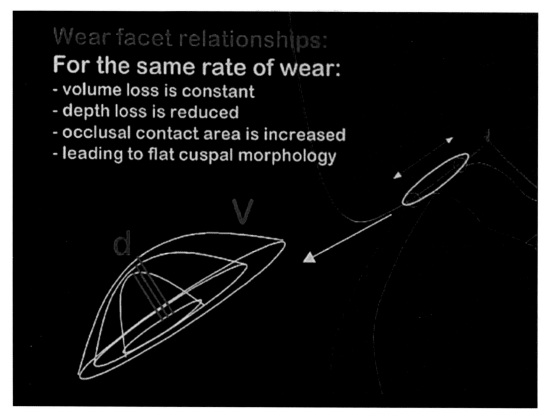

Figure 8.6 Approximate relationships between the different methods – volume, depth and contact area – of reporting wear. These observations refer to rates of change not to absolute values of wear. (Diagram courtesy of Dr. P. Magne.)

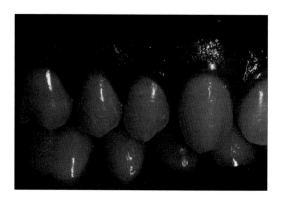

Figure 8.7 The occlusion of a young adult characterised by well-formed cusps, with a cusp to fossa and marginal ridge relationships.

of *The Stages of Wear*, distribution of toothwear across occlusal and cervical surfaces, surface susceptibility and the occlusion (Table 8.1). The clinician can either use these baseline models to confirm the clinical severity of the lesions and plan the treatment or provide the patient with the models for follow-up studies. Before and after models over time can confirm the success of therapy or whether the toothwear has progressed. Polyvinylsiloxane materials, when light and heavy body formulations are utilised in tandem, offer an excellent record of tooth surface detail across the dentition. However, basic alginate materials offer adequate surface detail replication for clinical diagnostic purposes. Impressions should be taken at the time

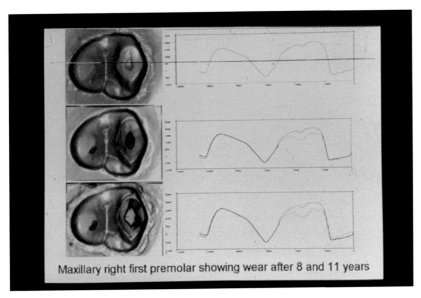

Maxillary right first premolar showing wear after 8 and 11 years

Figure 8.8 Loss of buccal cusp morphology over an 8- and 11-year period. This is due to attrition from cuspal guidance. Note the breached enamel and the progressive dentinal surface involvement. Wear due to mastication of food is minimal and represented by the small blue area on the buccal incline of the palatal cusp.

of presentation and stored for comparison at time intervals. New impressions should ideally be taken every 2 years. Often study models offer better visualisation of toothwear on occlusal and cervical surfaces than direct visualisation of the dentition clinically, given lighting, moisture and access variables. Matching facets are also often more easily discernible on articu-

Table 8.1 What can before and after models show?

- Teeth with occlusal attrition (stage A) also develop cuspal-cupped lesions (stage B).
- Cupped lesions enlarge to bowl-shaped lesions, extending over marginal ridges and fissures.
- Teeth with occlusal attrition or erosion develop, in addition, cervical lesions (stage C).
- Incisal edges and cusps degrade with merger of occlusal and cervical lesions (stage D).
- Glass ionomer restorations (GIC) dissolve.
- Metal restorations develop high margins, or are even lost.
- Changes in occlusal vertical dimension.

lated models than intraorally. Study models at intervals allow comparisons to be made of the surfaces affected. Development of new cup or cervical lesions or dentine exposure may be discernible. Whilst it is possible to section an impression of a diagnostic cast taken at a recall visit in a buccolingual direction, refitting this sectioned portion of the impression over the baseline cast and assessing for visible change has limited clinical applications. Profilometry, further discussed in the following sections, describes the gold-standard technique applicable to discerning subtle volumetric changes on the various tooth surfaces to further describe how toothwear progresses on differing tooth surfaces.

Laboratory studies

Study models made from epoxy resin or die stone are essential for laboratory studies, which measures severity and monitors progression reliably. Measurements on replicas by profilometry provide the gold standard against which

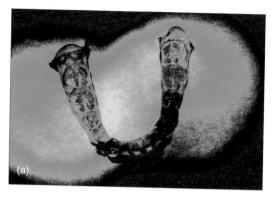
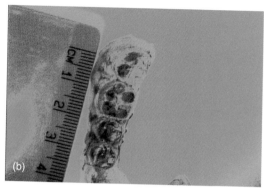

Figure 8.9   Epoxy resin models of a lower arch. The cuspal-cupped lesions contain dye to enhance the images captured by video camera (a). One-millimetre icons in use to measure the internal diameter of each lesion (b). (From Khan et al., 2001, with permission from the *Australian Dental Journal*.)

the validity of stages, grades and toothwear indices can be established. When many models are to be evaluated in cross-sectional or longitudinal studies of patients with toothwear, data can be compiled directly from the models (Bartlett 2003; Khan et al. 2001). In the former cross-sectional study of occlusal erosion, a stereoscopic light microscope was used at low magnification (×40) to capture the images of cuspal-cupped and bowl-shaped lesions filled with dyes. The images were then subjected to computerised data analysis (Khan et al. 2001). Software interpretation of the images allowed the conversion of light intensity to be converted into optically discernible colour wavelengths. Three circular icons were selected of 0.5, 1.0 and 2.0 mm diameters to measure the maximum internal diameter of each lesion (Fig. 8.9a).

Cuspal-cupped lesions were then categorised as small, medium or large with internal diameters between 0.5–1.0, 1–2 and greater than 2 mm. Fissural erosion was recorded when dye accumulated over exposed dentine greater than 0.5 mm at its widest buccolingual extent in dentine exposed across oblique or marginal ridges and in occlusal fissures. Study models of 119 patients yielded 2380 molars and premolars on which 10 472 occlusal lesions were recorded. The data from the permanent molars of 59 younger (13–27 years) and 57 older (28–70 years) patients are reported here (Table 8.2).

Small, medium and large occlusal erosions

In the maxilla, on the upper first and second molars, the numbers of small lesions was greater in younger than in older subjects, whereas on the upper third molar, fewer small lesions were found in the younger group than in the older group (Table 8.2). These significant differences indicate that occlusal erosions increase in size with age, influenced by the number of years each tooth has been in the mouth.

In the mandible, the numbers of small lesions found diminished in the sequence – first, second and then third molar – again indicating the number of years of exposure to the oral environment. However, the numbers of lesions of all sizes on lower first molars were greater in the younger group than in the older group (see Table 8.2). Thus, although the numbers of lesions increase on all three molars with age, in the older group, the lesions were not necessarily larger. Hence cuspal-cupped lesions on lower molars did not appear to increase in size in the older patients of this population.

Table 8.2 Comparisons of the numbers of cuspal-cupped lesions of three sizes, and of unaffected sites, on maxillary and mandibular permanent molars of 59 younger (13–27 years) versus 57 older (28–70 years) subjects. Degrees of significance from chi-square analysis are given where NS, not significant; *$p < 0.01$; **$p < 0.005$ between age groups.

	Tooth	Lesion size	Young SS	Old SS	Significance
Maxilla	First molar	Small	210	161	**
		Medium	66	74	
		Large	14	30	
		Unaffected	130	118	
		Total	420	383	
	Second molar	Small	109	85	**
		Medium	24	23	
		Large	1	14	
		Unaffected	169	121	
		Total	303	243	
	Third molar	Small	6	21	*
		Medium	0	11	
		Large	0	5	
		Unaffected	31	68	
		Total	37	105	
Mandible	First molar	Small	169	114	**
		Medium	174	101	
		Large	82	80	
		Unaffected	76	102	
		Total	501	397	
	Second molar	Small	140	117	NS
		Medium	48	52	
		Large	36	27	
		Unaffected	110	96	
		Total	334	292	
	Third molar	Small	8	13	NS
		Medium	3	11	
		Large	10	2	
		Unaffected	34	53	
		Total	55	79	

It is clinically important that these lesions are more frequently found and are, in general, larger in the mandible than in the maxilla. It is significant that whereas wear facets (stage A: *attrition*) normally occur in equal numbers between the jaws, bowl-shaped lesions (stage B: *erosion*) are more numerous and larger in the mandible than in the maxilla. This difference has now been confirmed by profilometry.

Buccal and lingual cusps

The numbers of small (0.5–1.0 mm), medium (1–2 mm) and large (>2 mm) lesions on the cusps of first permanent molars are compared in Fig. 8.10. Buccal cusps of lower first molars have more larger cupped lesions than the buccal cusps of the uppers. Thus, lower buccal cusps are most frequently and severely affected

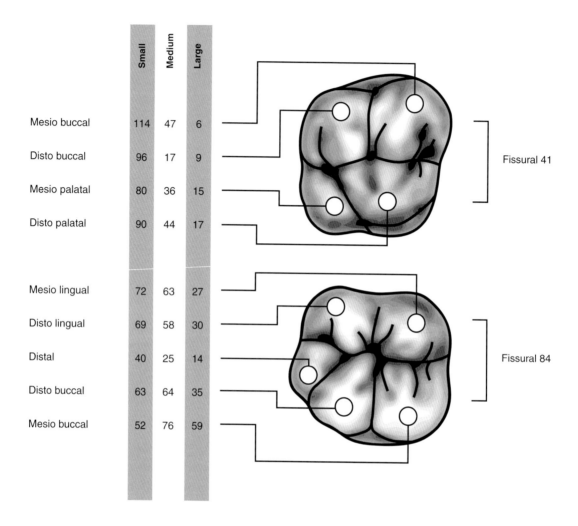

	Small	Medium	Large	
Mesio buccal	114	47	6	
Disto buccal	96	17	9	Fissural 41
Mesio palatal	80	36	15	
Disto palatal	90	44	17	
Mesio lingual	72	63	27	
Disto lingual	69	58	30	
Distal	40	25	14	Fissural 84
Disto buccal	63	64	35	
Mesio buccal	52	76	59	

Figure 8.10 The distribution of small diameter (0.5–1.0 mm), medium (1–2 mm) and large (>2 mm) cupped lesions found on buccal, palatal or lingual cusps, and of fissural lesions (>0.5 mm) on 229 maxillary and 224 mandibular first, permanent molars. (From Khan et al., 2001, with permission from the *Australian Dental Journal*.)

by occlusal erosion. Lingual cusps of lower first molars also have more larger cupped lesions than palatal cusps of the uppers. The mesiopalatal cusp of the upper first molar, arguably the largest cusp of the dentition, has more large lesions than the other cusps on this tooth. Mesiobuccal cusps of upper first molars, which normally occlude over the central buccal

fissure of lower first molars, have fewer large and more small lesions than mesiopalatal cusps. Twice the numbers of fissural erosions were found on the lower than on the upper first molars. Thus, the loss of enamel from fissures and by merger of bowl-shaped erosions across marginal ridges in the mandible is the commoner clinical problem.

This cross-sectional study on molars raises the possibility that these cupped lesions evolve rapidly as the teeth erupt sequentially in young adults (Khan et al. 2001) and implies that dental erosion is not a slow, linear process in our patients but occurs rapidly in young susceptible individuals. Clinically, spoon excavators are a suitable 'measuring' device for rapid lesion size approximation whilst charting cup lesions on occlusal surfaces of molars and premolars. Periodontal probes also offer a suitable measurement device. As further discussed later, diagnostic models form an important record or baseline to compare to at-recall visits.

Tooth tissue lost from all lower cusps and fissures allows the large upper mesiopalatal cusp to overerupt into a large bowl-shaped lesion. Erosion of upper mesiopalatal cusps further exaggerates this alteration in occlusal relationships found in severely worn dentitions. As loss of occlusal vertical dimension between first molars is frequently associated with degradation of the palatal surfaces of upper anterior teeth, the less worn lower anterior teeth overerupt, causing a deepening of the overbite. These concurrent alterations in the occlusal plane pose problems for the clinician seeking space to restore on the occlusal surfaces of lower first molars and the palatal surfaces of upper anterior teeth damaged by erosion (see Chapter 10).

Measuring toothwear in three dimensions

Laboratory methods for measuring and monitoring toothwear in three dimensions by profilometry and computer imagery are currently expensive research tools. Such research is time consuming and technically exacting, but it produces a wealth of detail on individual teeth and their cusps, fissures and cervical worn areas.

From the clinical perspective, profilometry can establish whether attrition or erosion is the more rapid progression. Occlusally, both attri-

Table 8.3 Objectives of toothwear measurement by profilometry.

- Is occlusal attrition or erosion the more rapid process?
- Does the rate of erosion differ on different molars?
- Does the rate of erosion differ on different cusps on the same tooth?
- Is the rate of erosion affected by preventive therapy?
- Is the rate of attrition affected by splint therapy?
- Does the rate of cervical tissue loss relate to occlusal loss?

tional and erosive lesions are found commonly on teeth of subjects with bruxism (Khan et al. 1998). Evidence of erosion must therefore be sought in all cases of presumed dental attrition (Lewis & Smith 1973; Meurman & ten Cate 1996). However, the management of patients depends on whether attrition or erosion is the faster process. Some clinical objectives that can be answered by profilometry are given in Table 8.3.

THE CASES

Measuring rates of tooth surface loss over time are essential to monitor preventive and management strategies against bruxism, attrition, abrasion or erosion. This next section reports the results of measurements by profilometry on a patient case. Lesions on permanent posterior teeth were measured, at first presentation and at later periods, by digitised profilometry. This enabled the nature of the lesions and volume of tooth tissue lost per year to be evaluated and objectives to be addressed (Table 8.3). The results show that in the absence of preventive advice or interceptive therapy, dental erosion causes severe, measurable loss of tooth surfaces. However, in the cases that accepted preventive advice and interceptive therapy, the loss of tooth tissue was not serious. The case highlights the importance of comprehensive diagnosis in patients with dental erosion and bruxism and suggests that interceptive strategies against erosion can effect measurable reductions in tooth tissue lost. Occlusal attrition is less rapid than erosion on the same tooth.

Profilometry methods

Measurement of the volume of tooth tissue lost with time has been achieved by surface profilometry and computer graphics (Delong et al. 1985). This technique has enabled the loss of tooth tissue in young adults with parafunctional habits to be estimated (Pintado et al. 1997). Patients had impressions taken of their dentitions at their initial presentation and at various intervals of months and years thereafter. Impressions were taken in disposable plastic trays with polyvinylsiloxane putty and light body impression material by the two-stage technique. Study models were replicated in epoxy resin. Individual tooth crowns of premolars, first and second molars were sectioned from the models. Before and after replicas of individual teeth were aligned in registration mounts for profilometry.

Using a servohydraulic-controlled stylus, profiles at 100-μm intervals were recorded by Ansur NT software (Regents, University of Minnesota, Minneapolis, MN). The software generated grayscale images of the before and after models and calculated the loss of tooth tissue in cubic millimetres per tooth (mm^3) and maximum and mean depths of lesions in micrometres. Contour maps on the after images registered regions of wear on a colour scale corresponding to intervals of 0–900 μm in depth.

Case 1

The 22-year-old individual described in Figs. 4.1, 4.2 and 8.11 reported having had fruit drinks daily and cola beverages frequently. After tennis and exercise, he drank a sports drink. When he lived in the United States of America at 17–18 years of age, he got into the habit of drinking cola beverages daily. As a teenager at school he played football, soccer, tennis and cricket. At university he continued to play tennis and squash twice a week, and after exercise, he would take a can of sports drink. His new 'exercise' became rave dancing at nightclubs

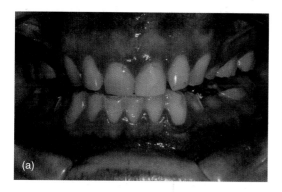
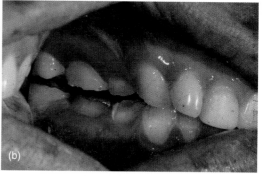

Figure 8.11 This case of a 22-year-old male was described in Figs. 4.1 and 4.2. Gold onlays placed in this 22-year-old man's lower first molars, to prevent tooth tissue loss from bruxism, had become undermined by cervical erosion. Lower canine premolars were also degraded on their buccal aspects. The patient was lost to follow-up for 85 months, enabling comparison of toothwear progression from his models (Fig. 8.10) and of his molars by profilometry (Fig. 8.11 & Table 8.4). (From Young, 2003, with permission of Erosion Watch Pty Ltd.)

where he drank white wine or cola and experimented with recreational drugs. He smoked five cigarettes a day and occasionally marijuana. He had not been on any medication for stress, anxiety or depression, but vomited frequently subsequent to rave parties.

At the time of first presentation, he was 19 years of age. He had lateral indentations of his tongue and bilateral *linea alba*, indicative of parafunctional habits. His major salivary glands were normal to palpation. In profile, his mandible was not prognathic; however, his vertical rami were broad and markedly perpendicular to the lower border. Consequently, the areas of attachment of his masseters were large, denoting masseteric hypertrophy, which gave prominence to both sides of his face.

Examination of the teeth

His teeth showed the following severity at 19 years of age. Stage A: all of his toothwear had progressed beyond the stage of exaggerated wear facets. Stage B: incisal edge erosion was evident on his lower anterior teeth. Cuspal-cupped lesions were present on his premolars except where the occlusal surfaces had been restored. Stage C: palatal cervical lesions were present on his upper premolars buccally on his lower premolars and beneath the restorations on 36 and 46. Stage D: the palatal surfaces of his upper anterior teeth were degraded. Facial veneers were present on his upper incisors, gold onlays on 36 and 46, and Ketac™ silver restorations occlusally on 16 and 46. All first premolars had been removed for orthodontia and the gaps had closed. Caries and periodontal disease were absent. These stages are charted in Fig. 8.12a.

Study models of both arches were taken for analysis at the time of first presentation. However, the patient attended irregularly, failed to keep subsequent appointments and was lost to follow-up. Clinical photos were taken at age 22. Upon returning a few years later, new models were taken 7 years from the time of initial presentation and his toothwear had increased in severity (Fig. 8.12b). Specifically, the palatal cusps of his upper premolars and first molars and the buccal cusps of his lower premolars were degraded. The occlusal surfaces of his lower second molars were almost completely eroded. *The Stages of Wear* severity recorded in Fig. 8.12b were as follows: Stage A: no new exaggerated wear facets; Stage B: erosion on teeth 37 and 47 advanced from cuspal-cupped lesions to total loss of the entire occlusal surfaces; Stage C: cervical lesions on the premolars progressed to degradation of their palatal and buccal cusps; and Stage D: the facial surfaces of the lower canines and the palatal surface of the upper left first molar were degraded. The facial veneers on his upper incisors were still intact. However, the gold onlays were so substantially undermined that one came loose and had to be replaced.

Toothwear measurements by profilometry

Replicas of all of the patient's molars were prepared for profilometry, and the statistics of wear were calculated by Ansur™ computer software. Full-coverage gold onlays were present on his lower first permanent molars and minimal changes were recorded on the gold surfaces. Tooth tissue loss from his lower left second molar was so excessive that fitting of the profiles was not possible due to loss of landmarks on the second set of models. Table 8.4 records the volumes of tooth tissue lost from his upper molars and lower right second molar.

Over the 85-month period, 80 mm^3 were lost from his unrestored maxillary left first molar (see Table 8.4), whereas 13 mm^3 were lost from his maxillary right first molar, on which a Ketac™ silver restoration had been placed, whereas 2 mm^3 were lost from his upper left second molar. Thus, the losses were greater from the upper first than from the upper second molar for a restoration had reduced the volume lost. Tooth surface loss from erosion on

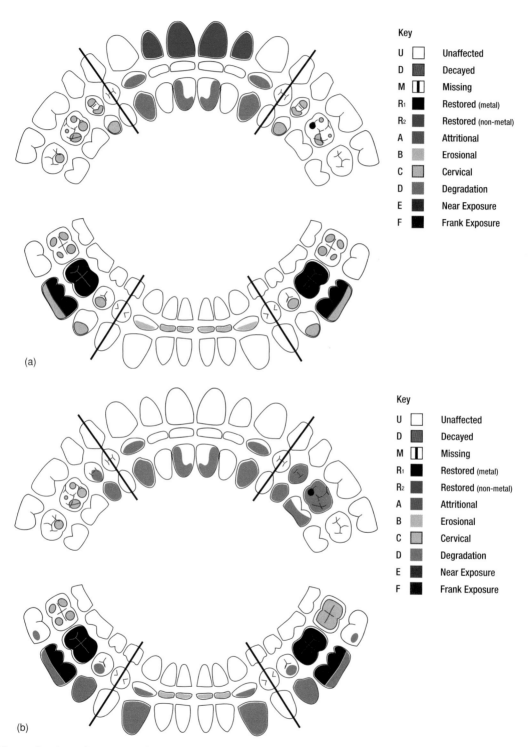

Figure 8.12 Odontograms of the case depicted in Fig. 8.10 at initial presentation (a) and 85 months apart (b). Comparatively, bowl-shaped lesions on 16, 37 and 47 have extended. A buccal cervical lesion has developed on tooth 47. Degradation of palatal cusps has occurred on 15, 13, 23, 25 and 26 and on buccal cusps of 35, 33, 43 and 47.

Table 8.4 Occlusal volumes loss per tooth (mm³) over an 85-month period and estimated volumes lost per year (mm³/y) for eight molar – case 1.

17	16*	26	27
5.39 mm³	13.42 mm³	80.15 mm³	2.29 mm³
0.76 mm³/y	1.90 mm³/y	11.31 mm³/y	0.32 mm³/y
47	46**	36**	37
35.67 mm³	0.77 mm³	0.18 mm³	***
5.03 mm³/y	—	—	—

*Ketac™ silver restoration.
**Gold onlays.
***Excess wear.

lower molars was greater than that on the upper. The lower first molars covered by onlays lost considerable volumes of tissue from subadjacent cervical lesions which were not measured. The changes in volume reflected changes in their surfaces (see Table 8.4). The lower right second molar lost 35.67 mm³ from its occlusal surface within the 85-month period. The lower left second molar (37) was so badly damaged that the before and after images could not be fitted to obtain data.

Estimated volume loss per year

The volume loss from the upper right first molar was 13.42 mm³ in 85 months, which equated to 1.9 mm³/y. In comparison, tooth 26 lost 80.15 mm³, which equated to 11.31 mm³/y. Volume losses on the upper second molars were 5.39 and 2.29 mm³ respectively. These equated to losses of 0.76 and 0.32 mm³/y (Table 8.4). Before and after profilometry over the 85 month period shows this volumetric loss on a lower first molar tooth (Fig. 8.13).

Case summary

Comparing the clinical changes in *Stages of Toothwear* severity in this case from models, the odontograms clearly identified the extent of damage sustained over a 7-year period. Profiliometry of the molars confirmed that rates

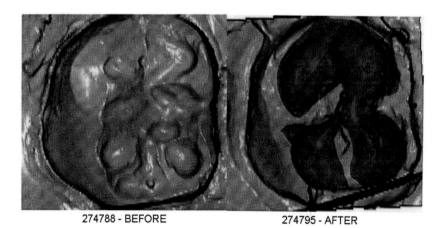

274788 - BEFORE   274795 - AFTER

Figure 8.13 Before and after grayscale images 7 years apart. Occlusal erosion (red) and a cervical lesion (blue) were measured with profilometry. (From Young & Khan, 2009, with permission of Erosion Watch Pty Ltd.)

of wear were greater in lower than on upper molars and first molars. First molars wore at faster rates than second molars. Restorations with gold and Ketac™ silver modified the rate of occlusal erosion by virtue of reducing the surface area of dentine exposed to the oral environment. However, buccal cervical lesions progressed and new ones appeared, thus emphasising the need to prevent erosion before restoration of the teeth to ensure a better long-term outcome.

Case 2

This second case, presented in brief, is of a male adult who was under the age of 30 at the start of the study. His non-carious cervical lesions were observed over 14 years. He grew up in a Minnesota community with fluoridated water. His periodontal health and oral hygiene were excellent and he used no abrasive toothpaste. He brushed primarily with electric toothbrushes. No unusual dietary habits were recorded. He was restoration free, and had minor orthodontic treatment to correct the alignment of his anterior teeth. He stated that he bruxed and clenched, but he did not report any pain or discomfort in his muscles of mastication or temporomandibular joints. Full maxillary and mandibular arch die stone models from the subject were used as the 1983 baseline and subsequently additional models were prepared in 1991, 1994 and 1997.

Examination of the teeth

Articulation of the casts revealed a class III malocclusion (group function) on the right and a class I canine-guided occlusion on the left. All replicas were digitised with a series of profiles. Each profile was separated by 100 μm, and within each profile, the surface was digitised in 50-μm steps (Pintado et al. 2010).

Profilometry

The three teeth studied had buccal cervical lesions that differed in their morphology (Pintado et al. 2010). The premolar cervical lesions first appeared as saucer-shaped depressions, i.e. shallow cervical lesions, which became more angular with time. The lesion on the second premolar became almost box-like (Fig. 8.5), but on the first molar, a wedge-shaped lesion was found that maintained its shape throughout the study period.

Profilometry results are shown in Table 8.5 for the occlusal surface changes and Table 8.6 for the cervical surface changes (Pintado et al. 2010). Although occlusal wear commences before cervical wear, it proceeds more slowly. Presumably, this is because initial losses are from the enamel of wear facets (stage A: *attrition*), whereas the more rapid rates from buccal cervical surfaces are from both enamel and dentine. These findings accord with the contention that cervical lesions (stage C) develop later than

Table 8.5 Occlusal volume losses (mm³) per year and mean depths on premolars and molars – case 2.

Occlusal	1991 (8 y)			1994 (11 y)			1997 (14 y)		
Tooth	Volume loss (mm³)	Per year	Mean depth (μm)	Volume loss (mm³)	Per year	Mean depth (μm)	Volume loss (mm³)	Per year	Mean depth (μm)
First premolar	0.40	0.05	72	0.68	0.06	99	1.18	0.08	146
Second premolar	0.94	0.12	79	1.77	1.16	137	1.89	0.14	123
First molar	3.69	0.46	115	4.98	0.45	184	7.79	0.56	231

Table 8.6 Cervical volume losses (mm³) per year and mean depths on premolars and molars – case 2.

Cervical	1991 (8 y)			1994 (11 y)			1997 (14 y)		
Tooth	Volume loss (mm³)	Per year	Mean depth (μm)	Volume loss (mm³)	Per year	Mean depth (μm)	Volume loss (mm³)	Per year	Mean depth (μm)
First premolar	0.90	0.11	252	0.96	0.09	266	1.64	0.12	330
Second premolar	1.39	0.17	287	1.63	0.15	303	2.72	0.19	415
First molar	4.62	0.58	390	8.18	0.74	557	11.50	0.82	772

stage A on a tooth and become more severe because greater volumes are lost as larger surface areas of cervical dentine become exposed.

Summary

Profilometry offers a gold-standard approach to assessing volumetric loss from toothwear processes over time. Clinically, diagnostic models offer a cost-effective record of the toothwear across a patient's dentition at time of initial presentation and at recall intervals. New diagnostic casts should ideally be taken every 2 years for patients considered at risk or presenting with significant established toothwear. Monitoring toothwear and its progression over time forms an important part of patient management both prior to and after restorative intervention.

References

Bardesley, P.F. (2008) The evolution of tooth wear indices. *Clinical Oral Investigations*, **12**(1), S15–S19.

Bartlett, D.W. (2003) Retrospective long term monitoring of tooth wear using study models. *British Dental Journal*, **194**(4), 211–213.

DeLong, R., Heinzen, M., Hodges, J.S., et al. (2003) Accuracy of a system for creating 3D computer models of dental arches. *Journal of Dental Research*, **82**, 438–442.

DeLong, R., Pintado, M.R., Douglas, W.H. (1985) Measurement of change in surface contour by computer graphics. *Dental Materials*, **1**(1), 27–30.

Khan, F., Young, W.G., Law, V., et al. (2001) Cupped lesions of early onset dental erosion in young southeast Queensland adults. *Australian Dental Journal*, **46**, 100–107.

Khan, F., Young, W.G., Daley, T.J. (1998) Dental erosion and bruxism. A tooth wear analysis from South East Queensland. *Australian Dental Journal*, **43**(2), 117–127.

Kramer, N., Kunzelmann, K.-H., Taschner, M., et al. (2006) Antagonist enamel wears more than ceramic inlays. *Journal of Dental Research*, **85**(12), 1097–1100.

Lambrecht, P., Braem, M., Vuylsteke-Wauters, M., et al. (1989) Quantitative *in vivo* wear of human enamel. *Journal of Dental Research*, **68**, 1752–1754.

Leinfelder, K.F., Taylor, D.F. Barkmeier, W.W., et al. (1986) Quantitative wear measurement of posterior composite resins. *Dental Materials*, **2**(5), 198–201.

Lewis, K.J. & Smith, B.G.M. (1973) The relationship of erosion and attriton in extensive tooth-tissue loss. *British Dental Journal*, **135**, 400–404.

Magne, P. (2010) Virtual prototyping of adhesively restored, endodontically treated molars. *Journal of Prosthetic Dentistry*, **103**(6), 343–351.

Meurman, J.H. & ten Cate, J.M. (1996) Pathogenesis and modifying factors of dental erosion. *European Journal of Oral Sciences*, **104**, 199–206.

Pindborg, J.J. (1970) *Pathology of the Dental Hard Tissues*. WB Saunders, Philadelphia, PA, pp. 294–300.

Pintado, M.R., Anderson, G.C., DeLong, R., et al. (1997) Variation in tooth wear in young adults over a two-year period. *Journal of Prosthetic Dentistry*, **77**(3), 313–320.

Pintado, M.R., Chapeau, B., Larson, M., et al. (2007) A Self-directed method of learning dental anatomy. *Journal of Dental Education*, **71**(1), 102–103.

Pintado, M.R., DeLong, R., Ching-Chang, K., et al. (2000) Correlation of noncarious cervical lesion size and occlusal wear in a single adult over a 14-year time span. *Journal of Prosthetic Dentistry*, **84**(4), 436–443.

Pintado, M.R., Delong, R., Douglas, W.H., et al. (2010) Volumetric hard tissue loss in abfractions calculated from micro-CT data. *Journal Dental Research*, Abstract 1509.

Ryge, G., Snyder, M. (1973) Evaluating the clinical quality of restorations. *Journal of the American Dental Association*, **87**, 369–377.

Xhonga, F.A., Wolcott, R.B, Sognnaes, V. (1972) Dental erosion II. Clinical measurements of dental erosion progress. *Journal of the American Dental Association*, **84**, 577–582.

Young, W.G. (2003) *Teeth on Edge*, Erosion Watch Pty Ltd. Queensland, Australia.

Young, W.G., Khan, F. (2009) *By the Skin of Our Teeth*, Erosion Watch Pty Ltd. Queensland, Australia.

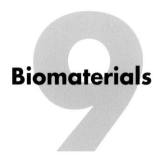

Biomaterials

Stephen C. Bayne

INTRODUCTION

Definitions and terminology

In dentistry, most clinical wear events are categorized on the basis of visual inferences of the principal causes of the events. As such, we end up with the main categories introduced in Chapter 1 of attrition, erosion, and abrasion. At the microscopic level, many more things may actually be happening than can be described by these simple terms. In materials science and engineering, wear is classified on the basis of microscopic mechanisms occurring at the surface of interest. While there are strong similarities between the dental and engineering classifications, there are also some exceptions that need to be recognized (Fig. 9.1 & Table 9.1). Attrition is associated predominantly with physical properties of a material (e.g. friction and adhesion). Erosion, in materials engineering parlance, is associated mainly with a collection of chemical properties that include solubility/disintegration, chemical corrosion, electro-chemical corrosion, and etching, but do not always involve acids. Abrasion is heavily aligned with the mechanical response of a substrate in response to an opponent solid or a solid particle.

Other areas of this text emphasize that all intraoral events are multifactorial processes. A method to consider all of these combinations is to plot the degree of involvement of each corner process (see the triangle in the middle of Fig. 9.1). Any event that is primarily erosion would be plotted inside the triangular zone closest to the erosion corner. Something representing an equal combination of erosion and attrition would be plotted half-way along the line connecting those two corners. Something deemed an equal combination of all three processes would be plotted exactly in the middle of the triangle.

Wear events also may be grouped as physiologic, pathologic, prophylactic, and surfacing ones (Table 9.2). Physiologic are ones associated with intraoral functions. Pathologic ones result from disease or dysfunctional patterns.

Toothwear: The ABC of the Worn Dentition, First Edition. Edited by Farid Khan and William George Young.
© 2011 John Wiley & Sons, Ltd. Published 2011 by John Wiley & Sons, Ltd.

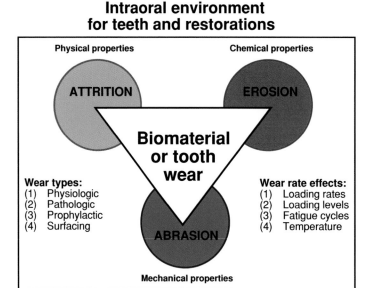

Figure 9.1 Superposition of dental and engineering wear events to include material properties likely to be involved, intraoral wear situations, and environmental factors influencing wear rates.

Prophylactic ones occur because of patient or dental professional efforts at health maintenance. They intentionally may result in wear that eliminates excess material. Surfacing ones involve intentional abrading, finishing, and polishing during restorative procedures. Abrading is intentional reduction in surface height or volume, generally to flatten it. Finishing is an effort to smoothen a surface and often reduces surface irregularities to approximately 1 μm sizes. Polishing is the removal of unwanted surface debris and/or further surface smoothening to reduce irregularities to the range of 0.1–1.0 μm (Bayne et al. 2006; Bayne & Thompson 2006).

In addition to wear categories and types, there are secondary effects from other things. The rate of loading (fast vs. slow) affects the material response (and apparent hardness). The loading level influences the number of fatigue cycles that the process may take to induce failure. The temperature alters the materials properties. The small range of intraoral temperature

changes (5–60°C) may affect polymer phases, but will not affect metal or ceramic phases much at all.

The goals of this chapter are to use these definitions and terminology to assess biomaterials' resistance to wear, consider the principles and concepts that govern wear rates, and determine the risk management necessary for successful use of biomaterials in different intraoral situations. Risk factors should allow any clinical situation to be judged as involving opportunities for short-term (0–5 years), medium-term (5–10 years), or long-term (10–20 years) success.

Properties versus structure

Any textbook (Bayne et al. 2004) on biomaterials science quickly points out that no material has a single value for each of its properties. Properties are determined by the structure of a material and that can vary for any composition. A quick review is the following: properties depend on the (a) arrangement (extent

Table 9.1 Comparison of wear definitions from dentistry and engineering.[a]

Dentistry (Chapter 1)	Engineering (quoted in part from ASM 1992, pp. 1–20)
Wear: Loss of tooth substance or restorative material as a function of normal or abnormal intraoral events	**Wear:** Damage to a solid surface, generally involving progressive loss of materials, which is due to relative motions between that surface and a contacting substance or substances
Attrition: Attrition involves two-surface wear, tooth to tooth related	**Attrition:** Removal of small fragments of surface material during a sliding contact
Erosion: Erosion, less commonly referred to as corrosion, results from acidic dissolution of mineralised tooth structure	**Erosion** (erosive wear): (1) Loss of material from a solid surface due to the relative motion in contact with a fluid that contains solid particles (abrasive erosion = parallel; impingement erosion or impact erosion). (2) Progressive loss of original material from a solid surface due to mechanical interaction between that surface and a fluid, a multicomponent fluid, and impinging liquid or solid particles
	Erosion–corrosion: A conjoint action involving corrosion and erosion in the presence of a corrosive substance
Abrasion: Abrasion on a surface comprises wear from externally applied particles or objects	**Abrasion:** A process in which hard particles or protuberances are forced against and moving along a solid surface. *Note:* Sometimes this term is used to refer to abrasive wear. See also 'abrasive erosion'
	Abrasive erosion: Erosive wear caused by the relative motion of solid particles which are entrained in a fluid, moving nearly parallel to the solid surface. See also 'erosion'
	Abrasive wear: Wear by the displacement of materials caused by hard particles or hard protuberances. Wear due to hard particles or hard protuberances forced against and moving along a solid surface

[a]Note that dental erosion presumes that acid is present and the engineering definition just assumes that liquid is present.

of crystallinity), (b) bonding patterns (types of primary and secondary bonding that might exist), (c) composition (number of phases, distribution of the phases, and sizes of the crystals), and (d) defects (point, line, area, and volume types). A change in the degree of crystallinity changes the properties. A change in crystallisation pattern changes the properties. A change in the concentration or distribution of line defects changes the properties. A change in the porosity present changes the properties. The last case is extremely important for dental materials. Manipulation that increases the porosity content by as little as 10% could effectively reduce the mechanical strength by as much as 40–50%. Most materials are strongly defect limited. Dental personnel have a major effect on

defects present in final materials and thus on their properties. Therefore, the final wear resistance of any materials must be seen as operator dependent.

Principles and concepts for biomaterials wear

What follows in this chapter is an explanation of how different wear events are controlled by different intraoral circumstances. At first, however, consider the following overall principles and concepts:

- *Operators:* Operators are more important than materials. Significant variability exists among even good operators. Materials

Table 9.2 Physiologic, pathologic, and prophylactic wear situations in dentistry.

Intraoral wear event	Type of wear	Substrate	Opponent	Lubricant	Abrasive slurry or other substance
Physiologic causes of wear					
Noncontact wear	Three-body	Tooth/restoration	...	Saliva	Silica in food
Direct-contact wear	Two-body	Tooth/restoration	Tooth/restoration	Saliva	...
Sliding-contact wear	Two-body	Tooth/restoration	Tooth/restoration	Saliva	...
Pathologic causes of wear					
Bruxism	Two-body	Tooth/restoration	Tooth/restoration	Saliva	...
Xerostomia	Two-body	Tooth/restoration	Tooth/restoration	...	...
Erosion	...	Tooth/restoration	...	Saliva	...
Anorexia	...	Tooth/restoration	...	...	HCl
Unusual habits	Two-body	Tooth/restoration	Foreign body	Saliva	...
Prophylactic causes of wear					
Toothbrushing with dentifrice	Three-body	Tooth/restoration	Toothbrush	Water	Dentifrice abrasive
Prophylactic pastes	Three-body	Tooth/restoration	Polishing cup	Water	Pumice
Scaling/cleaning instruments	Two-body	Tooth/restoration	Instrument	Saliva	...
Surfacing operations (cutting, finishing, and polishing)					
Cutting burs/diamonds	Two-body	Tooth/restoration	Bur/diamond	Water	...
Finishing burs/diamonds	Two-body	Tooth/restoration	Bur/diamond	Water	...
Polishing pastes	Three-body	Tooth/restoration	Polishing cup	Water	Abrasives in slurry

Source: (After Powers & Bayne 1992).

properties are defect limited (i.e. operator limited).

- *Environmental factors:* Failure/success of a biomaterial depends on environmental forces (physiologic, pathologic, prophylactic, and surfacing), extent of those cycles, intensity of those cycles, and time.
- *Tooth locations:* Intraoral tooth sites and intra-tooth surface locations determine the relative susceptibility to wear.
- *Wear mechanisms:* Different mechanisms at different tooth surface locations are affected differently by attrition, erosion, and abrasion.

On the basis of the above, one can already assess some biomaterials' chances of survival. Is a good-to-great clinical operator involved? If so, almost anything will fare reasonably well. What is the risk status of the patient for caries? If the patient is one of the 20% considered high risk, all restorative materials outcomes will be limited in success. Does the patient display abnormal physiologic behaviors (e.g. bulimia and clenching)? Then both tooth structure and biomaterials will be significantly challenged. If the wear mechanism is countervailed by the material's compositional design, then the material may wear very slowly over long time periods. Now, let us look at more details about each of these.

OVERVIEW OF BIOMATERIALS WEAR

Wear couples (wear assemblies)

Understanding any local wear situation in dentistry requires identification of all the parts of the teeth/materials assembly (called the 'wear couple'). Any assembly includes (a) a solid substrate surface (involving tooth structure [enamel, dentin, and cementum] and/or restorative materials [amalgam, composite, bonding agent, glass ionomer restorations, all-

ceramic, porcelain fused to metal (PFM), gold alloys, stainless steel, prosthetic teeth, sealants, and/or atraumatic restorative technique (ART) materials]), (b) a solid opponent surface, (c) a lubricant (typically saliva), and/or (d) an interposed fluid phase (food, dentifrice, and polishing paste). This is schematically summarised in Fig. 9.2. This assembly is affected by the local temperature, pH, and intraoral functions. Wear is not a continuous event. It is cyclical depending on chewing cycles (loading cycles), pH cycles, or other physiologic rhythms. When the two surfaces are in direct contact with each other (even if a lubricant is present), the assembly is involved with two-body wear. If there is an interposed phase, then wear is called three-body wear.

Once one knows the wear couple, it is possible to ask crucial questions about the wear event itself. What is the relative 'potential' for wear (high, medium, or low)? What is the typical 'wear rate' (i.e. kinetics or rate of the process [material loss/time])? What are the 'microscopic events' (i.e. wear mechanism)? How long will wear continue (i.e. extent of damage)? Each is dealt with in the following paragraphs.

Wear potential

A plethora of mechanical properties are associated with wear processes, but the key one is a material's 'hardness'. Material surfaces display elastic and plastic deformation in response to wear stresses. The hardness is the resistance to the onset of plastic deformation. Under a standard set of conditions, it is possible to rank comparative hardness using a variety of scales. Moh's hardness scale is one of those scales and is simply the resistance to being scratched by comparison to a reference set of materials. A softer material gets scratched by a harder one. The reference materials are reported in Table 9.3 along with a range of dental materials examples.

As noted earlier, properties for a single composition can be quite variable, depending

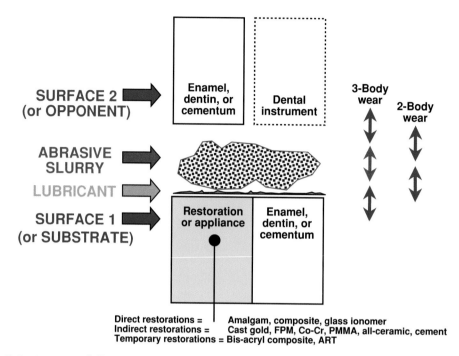

Figure 9.2 Summary of all possible wear couples for teeth and restorations. The major components of substrate, opponent, lubricant, and abrasive slurry are shown. Two- and three-body wear are contrasted. The range of restorative materials is listed.

on the arrangement, bonding, compositional phases, and defects. Consider a couple of quick examples.

SiO_2 (silica or silicon dioxide) can exist in four allotropic forms (silica glass, cristobalite, tridymite, and quartz). Silica glass is the least hard. Quartz is the most hard. Composite formulations generally choose modified silica glasses (silicates) for fillers so that the compositions can be more easily abraded, finished, and polished. Finishing and polishing agents employ abrasives that are harder than composite filler particles.

Unmodified glass ionomers are predominantly hydrogels. Their properties depend very much on the presence of an equilibrium concentration of water in the matrix. Excessive drying of the surfaces during prophylaxis procedures or in geriatric patients' mouths with reduced saliva flow will locally deplete the surface con-

centrations of water and weaken the surface layers, lowering the surface hardness.

Wear rates of materials involve either contact with an opponent and/or contact with a fluid slurry (e.g. food and dentifrices) that contains abrasive particles. Under each circumstance, the potential for wear can be easily estimated by comparing the relative hardness of the contacting material to the substrate of interest (Fig. 9.3). If the ratio is high (>1.2), there is a high tendency toward wear. If the ratio of hardness is low (<1.0), there is very little tendency toward wear. Prophylaxis pastes use abrasives of low hardness that are still capable of dislodging *material alba* and biofilms, but which are not capable of scratching enamel or restorative materials.

Estimating wear based on hardness was originally formalized by Archard (1953) as Archard's law ($W = kWS/3H$). The volume (V)

Table 9.3 Moh's hardness values for reference materials and typical dental materials.[a]

Reference material	Moh's hardness value (1–10)	Dental material
Diamond, C	10	Cutting diamonds (10) Yttria-stabilized zirconia (9–10)
Corundum, Al_2O_3	9	Alumina (99)
Topaz, $Al_2SiO_4(OH-,F-)_2$	8	Cobalt–chromium alloys (7–8)
Quartz, SiO_2	7	Quartz polishing particles (7) CAD-CAM ceramics (6–7) Dental porcelain (6–7)
Feldspar (orthoclase), $KAlSi_3O_8$	6	Composite (5–7) Glass ionomer (5–7) Glass fillers (5–6) Dental enamel (5–6)
Apatite, $Ca_5(PO_4)_3(OH-,Cl-,F-)$	5	Dental amalgam (4–5)
Fluorite, CaF_2	4	Hard gold alloys (3–4) Dentine (3–4)
Calcite, $CaCO_3$	3	Pure gold (2–3) Denture acrylic (2–3) Cementum (2–3)
Gypsum, $CaSO_4 \cdot 2H_2O$	2	Diatomaceous earth (1.0–1.5) Nylon toothbrush bristles (1–2)
Talc, $Mg_3Si_4O_{10}(OH)_2$	1	

[a]By comparing different dental values it is possible assess the relative potential for wear of the substrate.

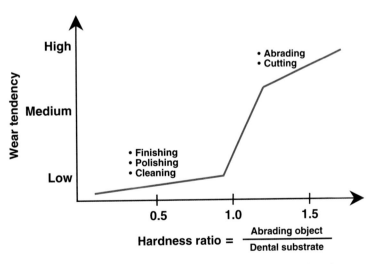

Figure 9.3 Wear tendencies (low, medium, and high) versus hardness ratios of the key wear assembly parts. (After ASM 1992, p. 188.)

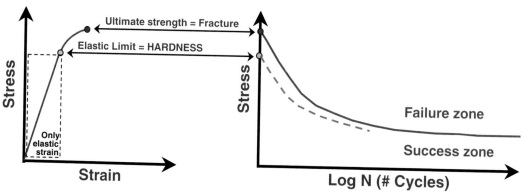

Figure 9.4 Stress–strain curve (left) for single loading cycle relationship to fatigue curve (right) for multiple cycling. Hardness is the resistance to the onset of plastic deformation and equivalent to the elastic limit.

of wear is proportional to some constant involving the abrading material (k), times the pressure or load (W) of the contacting material, times the total sliding distance (S), and divided by the hardness of the substrate (H). As the substrate hardness increases, the wear decreases.

Recall the standard descriptions of mechanical properties for dental materials and review the two parts of Fig. 9.4. Consider a uniaxial loading or wearing situation. When a load per unit area (stress) is applied to a material, the resulting deformation per unit length (strain) tends to be elastic at first (and linear in response) and then plastic at more extreme deformations. The onset of plastic deformation is defined as the elastic limit (the proportional limit) or the 'hardness' and reported in units of stress (MPa). Beyond that point, increasing stress produces more and more plastic deformation that is coupled to less and less further elastic deformation. Ultimately fracture occurs. This diagram is very useful for single-cycle loading descriptions. However, most real situations involve cyclic loading. If one monitors the point of failure for different extents of cycling at different loads, a fatigue curve can be generated (shown to the right in Fig. 9.4). All points above the curve represent failure and ones below the curve represent success.

The fatigue curve shows the cycles to failure for every cycling load. Everyone finds it curious that a material could fail below the level predicted by the single-cycle curve. The reason is as follows: In a single cycle of load up to the elastic limit, one presumes that only elastic behavior occurs. That is almost true. There is actually a very small amount of plastic strain involved (e.g., <0.1%) that is imperceptible in that single loading cycle. However, over thousands of cycles, these small amounts accumulate to significant amounts and contribute to major plastic deformation and failure.

In the fatigue curve shown to the right in Fig. 9.4, one can imagine that the actual hardness values after many loading cycles are represented as a collection of points along and below the failure curve. The hardness value of the material after 10 000 000 cycles is quite different than what it might have started out to be. In a single year, the typical number of loading cycles from mastication is about 1 000 000 cycles. Most materials are engineered to survive ~10 000 000 cycles under average conditions.

Wear rates

Wear rates can be approximated from two-body and three-body hardness differences, but they also depend on a couple of additional variables. Pressure (or load) and particle size (for three-body wear) are also important. During normal food mastication, quite a bit of pressure (load or force) can be generated to press food onto tooth surfaces. After some wear occurs, the occluding surfaces do not come quite as closely together, and this pressure tends to locally decrease. Larger particles tend to create more local stress during abrasion, but may not necessarily produce wear depending on the wear mechanism involved.

Accumulated wear

How much wear accumulates over time? Accumulated wear is a balance between losses (the wear rate vs. time) and gains (repairs or remineralisation). Loss of tooth substance or biomaterial increases in proportion to the hardness differences, pressures, and time. Yet wear does not continue forever, and it generally does not lead to a major failure. With increasing material loss, the pressure drops and wear slows down or even stops.

Intraoral processes may counteract wear and replace lost volume of teeth or restorative materials. Teeth remineralise under favorable conditions using the calcium and phosphate ions present in saliva. This is a natural and continual process. Restorative materials may also replace some of their lost surface volume. Dental amalgam is the best example of this. Amalgam continues to slowly expand for many years. As it does, it extrudes itself toward the unrestrained sides of the tooth preparation. This new volume appears to replace lost material. Along actively wearing surfaces, there can be equilibrium between lost and gained material. In clinical locations undergoing relatively little wear, the expansion actually extrudes the amalgam out of the tooth preparation. It is quite common to see a dental amalgam sticking out above the enamel margins for a class 5 restoration.

CLINICAL WEAR PERFORMANCE OF BIOMATERIALS

Clinical outcome factors

Predictions for biomaterials clinical performance are often attempted from average values of laboratory properties. Yet, despite the desire to predict clinical performance this way, it is almost impossible to do so. Clearly, there are other mitigating factors that are more important than just materials properties (Bayne et al. 1993; Jokstad et al. 2003). A simplistic aggregation of clinical outcome factors (or risk assessments) includes (a) clinical operator factors, (b) design factors, (c) materials properties, (d) intraoral location factors, and (e) patient factors (see Table 9.4).

Clinical operator factors include the technical skill of the operator, the impacts of aging on psychomotor skills and eyesight, and fine motor control. Design factors include choices for outline form, retention form (undercuts, grooves, and ferules), margin design, remaining dentin thickness, and thickness of restorative materials. Materials factors include the physical, chemical, mechanical, and biological properties of the assembly of restorative materials. Intraoral location factors consider differences between maxillary and mandibular arches, anterior versus posterior locations, and premolar versus molar locations. Patient factors include patient dental IQ, fluoride history, and intraoral personal hygiene success (flossing, choice of toothbrushes, dentifrices, psychomotor skills to use personal hygiene equipment, diet, and compliance). There are strong indications that the greatest risk factor among the group involves the clinical operator. A good operator using less-than-ideal materials can produce clinical success and generally longer term success. It has been estimated that operators constitute 50% of the risk factors involved in clinical outcomes.

Table 9.4 Clinical outcome factors.

Clinical outcome factors	Associated variables
Operator factors	• Eyesight (and use of magnification) • Age • Technical ability • Experience
Design factors	• Outline form • Resistance form (and use of ferrules for extensive preparations) • Occlusal margin choices (e.g., butt joint for composite) • Other margin choices • Internal retention (undercuts, grooves, retention points) • Smear layer
Material factors	• Choice of amalgam, composite, glass ionomer, gold alloys, PFM alloys, all-ceramic • Choice of liners and bases • Choice of bonding systems • Product age • Variables at the time of use (temperature, relative humidity, ambient light)
Intraoral location factors	• Intraoral position (anterior, posterior) • Intraoral arch (maxillary, mandibular) • Intratooth location (occlusal, proximal, lingual-labial)
Patient factors	• Oral hygiene IQ • Psychomotor skills for daily prophylaxis • Caries risk factors • Fluoride history • Diet (abrasiveness of food) • Mouth vs. nose breather

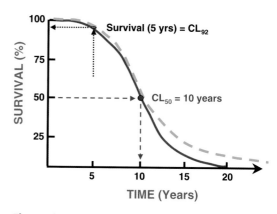

Figure 9.5 Longevity curve. (This shows the typical reverse s-shaped behavior for a group of restorations expressed as percentage succeeding or failing as a function of time.)

Clinical longevity curves

Because many factors are involved in success, there may be quite a wide distribution of overall outcomes. Clinical longevity curves track success (or failure) for a population of treatments in practice or in a clinical trial. The result is a reverse s-shaped response (see Fig. 9.5). Imagine a pool of 100 treatments. Generally, there are few if any early failures. A few failures may occur in the first few years. After a few years, the rate of failure may accelerate for a time. Some treatments may continue to be successful for moderately long time. A few may appear to last forever. This failure curve is shifted right or left depending on comparatively better or worse clinical skills of operators. The curve is shifted right or left depending on the intraoral environmental challenges being fewer or greater, respectively.

The midpoint of the curve is a point at which 50% or half of the restorations have failed and is called the CL_{50} or clinical longevity for 50%. The red curve in the figure is the idealised curve. The green dashed curve is an example of a typical behavior for a real distribution of restorations. Note that the final few restorations appear to succeed forever. Because the full curve is not known for most materials, it is typical to report a CL value for the longest recorded information (e.g. $CL_{92} = 5$ years). This is stated as clinical longevity for 92% of the population at 5 years. This is often deceptive because the future failure rate will be much greater.

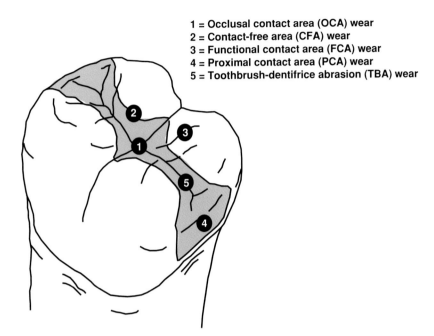

1 = Occlusal contact area (OCA) wear
2 = Contact-free area (CFA) wear
3 = Functional contact area (FCA) wear
4 = Proximal contact area (PCA) wear
5 = Toothbrush-dentifrice abrasion (TBA) wear

Figure 9.6 Intrarestoration wear variations.

Intrarestoration variations in wear couples

Restoration surfaces may involve at least five types of wear couples: (a) contact area wear, (b) contact-free area wear, (c) functional contact area wear, (d) proximal contact area wear, and (e) dentifrice-toothbrush wear (Bayne 2006) (see Fig. 9.6). These may not all function all of the time. At restoration placement, restoration contact areas will exist, but may wear out of occlusion. Other contacts on enamel surfaces will maintain the occlusion and prevent further direct contact area wear. In the absence of excessive toothwear, contact area wear will stop. Noncontact area wear is primarily caused by small abrasive silica particles in food acting along the surfaces of the restoration.

From early clinical wear studies (Kusy & Leinfelder 1977), it was clear that food abrasion (CFA wear) seemed to quickly dominate and produce extensive occlusal abrasion (Fig. 9.7). Microscopic surface examination showed no evidence of wear of filler particles, but did show apparent matrix phase loss.

Protection hypothesis

Bayne and colleagues (1992) explained non-contact area wear of composites in terms of a

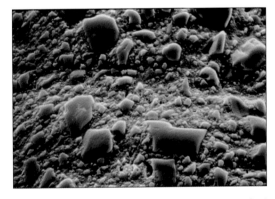

Figure 9.7 Worn composite restoration. Magnified view showing protruding and unworn filler particles on a traditional composite surface.

'protection hypothesis'. At a microscopic level, the hypothesis recognises that composite fillers are much harder than the resin matrix. During food mastication, small abrasive particles of silica in the food are forced into contact with the composite surface. If the particles are smaller than the local interparticle spacing of filler particles, then they can tear or abrade the composite resin and eliminate the matrix support for the filler. This continually removes the composite surface as filler particles are plucked or fall out. If the filler particles are closer together than the width of the abrasive particles, they locally protect (microprotection) or shelter the resin matrix. Enamel is much more resistant to wear than the composite. As surface of the composite is gradually lost, an enamel margin is exposed. It becomes progressively harder to force the food against the composite surface with high pressures and the abrasive action slows down. This is called 'macroprotection' or sheltering of the surface.

Wear occurs in a linear fashion at first for both traditional (black curve in Fig. 9.8) and newer composites (green curve). Traditional

composite wear rates are high (50–100 μm/y), but begin to slow down considerably after 100–200 μm of wear to a very low wear rate. The initial wear rate is a function of the degree of 'microprotection' (or sheltering) of the low-hardness resin matrix by the much harder filler particles from ~0.1 μm diameter silica abrasive particles dispersed in most foods. Loss of composite surface decreases contact pressures with the food (called 'macroprotection') and wear is dramatically reduced. In these situations, wear does not wear through composites and expose dentine or base. Long-term clinical trial results (Sturdevant et al., 1988; Wilder et al., 1999) are well-explained by the protection hypothesis (Bayne et al., 1992).

The last two decades of composite design have focused on developing higher loading levels of fillers, better packing of fillers, and reduced interparticle spacing. A large number of approaches have demonstrated success. As indicated in Fig. 9.9, the typical wear rate for contemporary composites is much lower, but still not zero. The reason for some continuing wear is the heterogeneity of composite

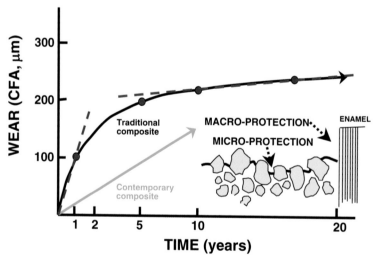

Figure 9.8 Composite wear curves (from food, contact-free area wear) for occlusal posterior restorations versus time from long-term clinical trials (Wilder et al. 1999).

Heterogeneous interparticle spacing along surface

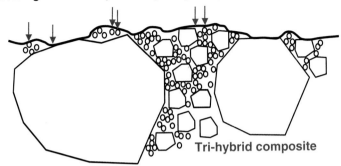

Tri-hybrid composite

Figure 9.9 Schematic view of the worn surface of a contemporary trihybrid dental composite indicating a range of interparticle spacing that determines the relative microprotection.

microstructures that allows some larger interparticle spacing to continue to exist on composite surfaces (see Fig. 9.9).

Protection appears to be a valid explanation for a large variety of dental materials wear behaviors, which involve two phases (continued resin matrix phase and dispersed filler particle phase) and have large differences in hardness of the dispersed versus continuous phases (ratio ≥1.0). Consider the situations schematically portrayed in Fig. 9.10 that compare glass ionomer, dental porcelain, and dental amalgam to composite. One would expect similar mechanisms of wear for glass ionomers because of the hardness ratios of the phases. The effect would be smaller in dental porcelains and

dental amalgams because of more similar hardness of phases.

COMMENTS ON SPECIAL WEAR SITUATIONS

There is no evidence that bonding agents contribute to increased wear resistance of restorations per se. One might intuitively anticipate that more well-bonded margins would discourage wear, but that does not seem to be detectable in long-term clinical trials. Likewise, the presence or absence of various liners and bases does not seem to affect the overall wear resistance of the superimposed restoration.

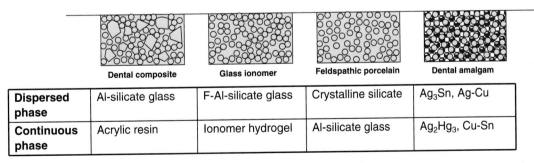

	Dental composite	Glass ionomer	Feldspathic porcelain	Dental amalgam
Dispersed phase	Al-silicate glass	F-Al-silicate glass	Crystalline silicate	Ag_3Sn, Ag-Cu
Continuous phase	Acrylic resin	Ionomer hydrogel	Al-silicate glass	Ag_2Hg_3, Cu-Sn

Figure 9.10 Schematic comparison of microstructures for several restorative materials: dental composite, glass ionomer, dental amalgam, and two-phase feldspathic dental porcelain. In each case, the dispersed phase is harder. In the first two cases, the dispersed phase is much harder. In the last two cases, it is only slightly harder.

Wear resistance seems to be confined to the surface properties of the biomaterial. There are, however, arguments that tooth structure at risk may be protected by the application of superficial bonding agent films (Azzopardi et al. 2004).

Most biomaterials are selected on the basis of having either good corrosion resistance (inactive) or protective surface films (passive) that prevent destructive corrosion. In the latter case, wear could continually remove the protective oxide films to the point that the necessary elements in the alloy substrate would become depleted and active corrosion would begin.

The presence of biofilms may have competing effects on wear. Biofilms could contribute to the chemical erosion of the underlying substrate if there is an active plaque. However, the biofilm might actually protect the underlying surfaces from intraoral events such as food abrasion. These events have not been actively studied.

Tooth structure and dental materials both are susceptible to dissolution below pH $\sim$3.5 values when challenged by certain acidic beverages (e.g. colas and beer), foods high in acids (e.g. fruit sucking), or chronic regurgitation (e.g. gastroesophageal reflux disease, eating disorders, and alcoholism; Verrett 2001). However, if acid challenges are short lived and infrequent, and saliva stays in place and to protect surfaces, then erosion does not occur. There is very little documented evidence of the destruction of dental materials from these erosive wear situations. Most reports indicate that tooth structure is more rapidly dissolved than restorative materials (Yu et al. 2009). One might speculate that restoration destruction may be accelerated by the loss of tooth structure support.

Despite the hard microstructural components of teeth, they can and do flex. Individual teeth are described to flex like a bow during intercuspation and produce tension along the facial surfaces and compression at the lingual surfaces (Heymann & Bayne 1993). Tooth flexure

has been quite a controversial subject during the last two decades because of the hypothesis that it explains the presence and progression of most cervical lesions, and it could explain other classic events (Grippo et al. 2004). What is important for the present discussion is recognising that the presence of local mechanical stresses not only contributes to mechanical fatigue but also accelerates processes such as corrosion and erosion.

Patients and dental professionals fall into the pattern of reporting toothbrush abrasion when in fact the real wear mechanism involves the abrasive particles in the dentifrice (Wiegand et al., 2008). Toothbrush bristles are commonly made of nylon which has a very low hardness value (Moh's, 1–2). Bristles generally are 150 μm in diameter, may be tufted, and do not produce wear along tooth or restorative materials surfaces. Powered toothbrushes have vibrating, oscillating, or sonicated bristle motions that are more efficient at keeping the abrasive particles suspended in the dentifrice slurry with water while agitating the slurry against tooth surfaces to produce cleaning.

Tooth cleaning can be accomplished by blasting tooth surfaces with air- or water-abrasive slurries from a nozzle. The effectiveness of the cleaning action depends on the kinetic energy of the particles impacting the surface. The imparted surface energy is related to the density of the particles, abrasive particle sizes and shapes, distance of the tip, and angle of the stream from the tip to the surface. There is rapid energy loss with increasing distance away from the surface. There is also rapid loss of effectiveness if the rebounding particles interfere with the incoming stream. The danger for cleaning or abrading devices in this manner is that close proximity of the tip or use for longer than normal times can produce rapid surface destruction of enamel and restorative materials. Even instruments designed for prophylaxis could potentially drill holes in enamel or restorative materials if misused.

References

Archard, J.F. (1953) Contact and rubbing of flat surfaces. *Journal of Applied Physics*, **24**, 981–988.

ASM (1992) Glossary of terms. In: *ASM Handbook, Volume 18, Friction, Lubrication, and Wear Technology*. ASM International, Materials Park, OH, pp. 1–21.

Azzopardi, A., Bartlett, D.W., Watson, T.F., et al. (2004) The surface effects of erosion and abrasion on dentine with and without a protective layer. *British Dental Journal*, **196**, 351–354.

Bayne, S.C., Heymann, H.O., Sturdevant, J.R., et al. (1991) Contributing co-variables in clinical trials. *American Journal of Dentistry*, **4**, 247–250.

Bayne, S.C., Powers, J.M., Swift, Jr, E.J., et al. (2006) Chapter 13: Biomaterials. In: *Mosby's Comprehensive Review of Dental Hygiene* (ed M.L. Darby), 6th edn. pp. 516–555. Mosby Elsevier, St. Louis.

Bayne, S.C., Taylor, D.F., Heymann, H.O. (1992) Protection hypothesis for composite wear. *Dental Materials*, **8**, 305–309.

Bayne S.C., Thompson, J.Y. (2005) *Biomaterials Science*. Brightstar Publishing, Chapel Hill, NC (Online only). Available at: http://www-personal.umich.edu/~sbayne/BS-book/B00-TOC/bs-toc.htm.

Bayne, S.C., Thompson, J.Y. (2006) Biomaterials. In: *Sturdevant's Art and Science of Operative Dentistry* (ed T.M. Roberson), 5th edn. pp. 135–242. Mosby, St. Louis.

Grippo, J.O., Simring, M., Schreiner, S. (2004) Attrition, abrasion, corrosion, and abfraction revisited: a new perspective on tooth surface lesions. *Journal of the American Dental Association*, **135**, 1109–1118.

Heymann, H.O., Bayne, S.C. (1993) Current concepts in dentin bonding. *Journal of the American Dental Association*, **124**, 26–36.

Jokstad, A., Bayne, S., Blunck, U., et al. (2001) Quality of dental restorations – FDI Commission Project 2-95. *International Dental Journal*, **53**, 117–158.

Kusy, R.P., Leinfelder, K.L. (1977) Pattern of wear in posterior composite restorations. *Journal of Dental Research*, **56**, 544.

Powers, J.M., Bayne, S.C. (1992) Friction and wear of dental materials. In: *ASM Handbook, Volume 18, Friction, Lubrication, and Wear Technology*. ASM International, pp. 665–681. Materials Park, OH. Available at: http://products.asminternational.org/hbk/index.jsp and http://www.asminternational.org/portal/site/www/contact-us/.

Sturdevant, J.R., Lundeen, T.F., Sluder, Jr, T.B., et al. (1988) Five-year study of two light-cured posterior composite resins. *Dental Materials*, **4**, 105–110.

Verrett, R.G. (2001) Analyzing the etiology of an extremely worn dentition. *Journal of Prosthodontics*, **10**, 224–233.

Wiegand, A., Schwerzmann, M., Sender, B., et al. (2008) Impact of toothpaste slurry abrasivity and toothbrush filament stiffness on abrasion of eroded enamel – an in vitro study. *Acta Odontologica Scandinavica*, **66**, 231–235.

Wilder, A.D., May, K.N., Bayne, S.C., et al. (1999) Seventeen-year clinical study of ultraviolet-cured posterior composite Class I and II restorations. *Journal of Esthetic Dentistry*, **11**, 135–142.

Yu, H., Wegehaupt, F.J., Wiegand, A., et al. (2009) Erosion and abrasion of tooth-colored restorative materials and human enamel. *Journal of Dentistry*, **37**, 913–922.

The role of toothwear in occlusion

Anders Johansson and Gunnar E. Carlsson

This chapter discusses various aspects of occlusion in relation to toothwear based on an evaluation of the available literature. As background information, some relevant historical perspectives on the subject are provided.

Extensive toothwear seems to have been the norm in ancient societies, with factors such as dietary habits, food composition and its preparation, and age being among its main contributory factors (Johansson et al. 2008). The consequences went beyond extensive deterioration of occlusal morphology to include notable changes in dentoalveolar and craniofacial morphology over a lifetime. These changes are considered to have maintained an efficient masticatory system, which was vital for survival (Hylander 1977). The effects on craniofacial morphology of excessive function, quite apart from occlusal and proximal toothwear, are primarily passive tooth eruption, lingual tilting of the anterior teeth and an anterior rotation of the mandible, resulting in a more 'edge-to-edge' anterior relationship (Begg & Kesling 1977; Hylander 1977; Johansson 1992; Fig. 10.1).

The frequency of malocclusions in primitive man is lower than in his modern counterpart, and it has been speculated that this resulted from attrition-caused alterations in the dentofacial morphology. Low frequencies of crowding, impacted molars, rotations, amongst others, in primitive populations can be attributed to the substantial gain of space in the dental arch following proximal attrition, thus preventing space-related malocclusions (Begg & Kesling 1977). As wear progresses, different opinions have been expressed as to whether facial height is reduced or whether it is unaffected. It is likely that this depends on the rate at which toothwear is occurring: if the rate is slow, compensatory dentoalveolar growth mechanisms will compensate for the decrease of facial height caused by the shortening of teeth, while if there is a rapid toothwear, these mechanisms may not be able to fully compensate and the occlusal vertical dimension (OVD) may be reduced. Begg and Kesling (1977) speculated that the facial height of modern Western man increases during life because of a lack of attrition. That

Toothwear: The ABC of the Worn Dentition, First Edition. Edited by Farid Khan and William George Young.
© 2011 John Wiley & Sons, Ltd. Published 2011 by John Wiley & Sons, Ltd.

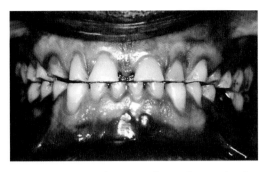

Figure 10.1 Development of an edge-to-edge bite in a contemporary 50-year-old Saudi man. (With permission from Johansson & Carlsson 2006.)

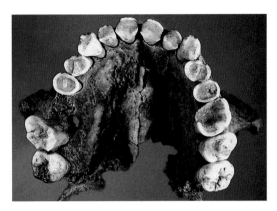

Figure 10.3 Extensive toothwear of maxillary teeth in a medieval man estimated to be 35–45 years old. The loss of the first right molar was most certainly caused by wear penetrating into the pulp, subsequently leading to an inflammatory process in the periapical jawbone. (By courtesy of Dr. M. Wretemark, editor of *S:t Per i Skara*, a book on excavations of a medieval graveyard in the Swedish town Skara, published in Swedish 2010; photograph taken by L.G. Olsson.)

facial height increase in adulthood has indeed been confirmed in several studies (Kollias & Krogstad 1999). However, whether the sole cause for this is an absence of attrition is not clear. Changes of craniofacial morphology similar to those observed in ancient materials have also been found in modern high-wear subjects (Fig. 10.2; Kiliaridis et al. 1995). The anthropological observations described provide some insight into causation, progression and features of severe toothwear. The similarities they show with today's patients with severe toothwear are remarkable and may to an extent contextualize the outcomes seen both before and after attempts at managing such conditions in today's patients. In addition, the continuing alteration

of craniofacial morphology is also of significance to explain the infraposition sometimes seen in implant-supported crowns (Thilander 2009).

In historical skull materials, toothwear was a more common cause of tooth damage and tooth loss than either dental caries or periodontal disease (Fig. 10.3). In Egyptian mummies, almost all abscesses in the jaws were ascribed to toothwear and only a fraction to caries. Even though toothwear in modern man is usually far less extensive, its impact on patients' satisfaction with their dentition can be severe and affect their quality of life (Al-Omiri et al. 2006).

In the anthropological literature, it has been assumed that toothwear had a linear progression, so that it could be used for age determination in historical skull materials (Fig. 10.4; Wedel et al. 1998).

The linearity of its progression is evident also in contemporary populations before they adopted Western lifestyles, e.g. in the Australian aborigines some 50 years ago, as described by Beyron (1964; Fig. 10.5).

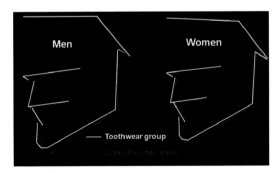

Figure 10.2 Mean facial diagrams of men and women in occlusal wear samples and cephalometric norm values. (With permission from Kiliaridis et al. 1995.)

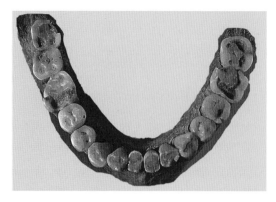

Figure 10.4 Mandibular teeth from a medieval person with estimated age 25–35 years. Some crowding in the premolar regions and extensive toothwear on the first molars, but no caries. (With permission from Wedel et al. 1998.)

In contrast to linear progression, modern man more likely experiences 'bursts' of wear, coinciding with the presence of certain causative factors, which can explain part of the

widely differing severities and patterns of wear found in people today, and even amongst those of the same age (Johansson 2002). Today, dental erosion is widely considered to be a major cause of toothwear (Bartlett 2005), yet the morphological features of the wear seen show a remarkable similarity with those seen in our ancestors (Figs. 10.6a & b).

DEVELOPMENT OF OCCLUSION

Comparative anatomy demonstrates wide differences among species in tooth morphology and occlusion, jaw architecture, muscles and temporomandibular joints (TMJ). The differences can be related to, and indeed reflect, variations in functional activities, and in turn, have evolved over millions of years in response to needed adaptations to type of diet and the role of feeding (Creanor & Noble 1994). In

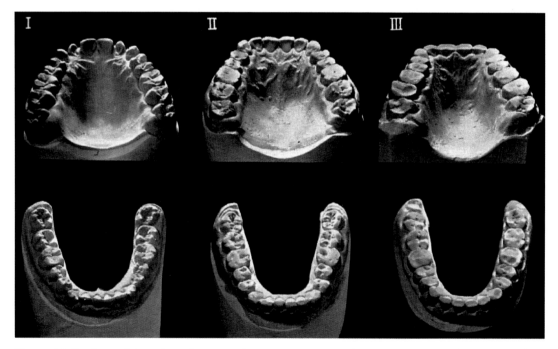

Figure 10.5 Casts of Australian aborigines showing increasing toothwear with age. (With permission from Beyron 1964.)

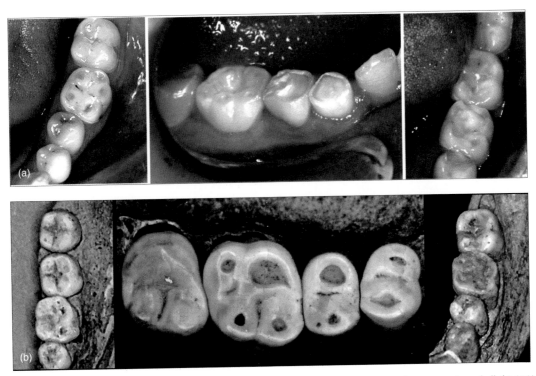

Figure 10.6   Severe toothwear with 'cuppings' in a contemporary patient (a) and in an ancient skull (b) (18). Note how closely the patterns and distributions of wear resemble each other. (With permission from Johansson & Carlsson 2006.)

comparison, modern humans (*Homo sapiens*) have a relatively short history (30 000–40 000 years) but have roots that reach back much earlier. Among the differences between modern man and early hominids is the relative proportion of cranium to jaws due to both an increase in cranium size and a decrease in jaw size in *H. sapiens*. A change in feeding habits, in addition to, and also coupled with the 'mechanisation' brought about by the use of hand-held tools has been suggested to be the major factor in the reduction in tooth size as well as the modification of the lower part of the face during evolution.

The deciduous and mixed dentitions

At the age of about 8 months, the first deciduous teeth erupt, generally beginning with the mandibular central incisors. Then follow the other maxillary and mandibular incisors, and at about 16 months of age, the deciduous first molars erupt. By the time that the first molars intercuspate, dental occlusion is established for the first time. The eruption of the deciduous dentition and occlusion are usually complete around 2.5 years of age (Ingervall 1988). There is considerable growth of the jaws and alveolar processes during the first years of life, which provides space for the erupting deciduous teeth, and in many children there is also a surplus of space resulting in small gaps between the deciduous teeth. After the eruption of all deciduous teeth, the most marked change is that of progressive toothwear that can be substantial in many children. Weak-to-moderate correlations have been shown between wear facets on anterior primary teeth at 5 years of age and those of their permanent successors at age 14 and 18 (Nyström et al. 1990). It has also been reported that subjects with erosive lesions in their primary dentition have a significantly increased risk for toothwear in the permanent dentition (Ganss et al. 2001). A follow-up study of children and adolescents over 20 years of age found that toothwear at 15 years of age predicted increased anterior toothwear at age 35 (Carlsson et al. 2003). Furthermore, clinical observations indicate that occlusal erosion and toothwear in the deciduous dentition can influence the developing dentition and adversely affect OVD and craniofacial development (Fig. 10.7; see also Chapter 1, Fig. 1.14).

The mixed dentition starts when the permanent first molars erupt and the deciduous mandibular incisors are exfoliated, on average at 6 years of age. There is some variation in the order of eruption of the permanent teeth, but in general, the first molars and the incisors in both jaws will have erupted by 8.5 years of age. From age 10 the canines and premolars start erupting, with some differences in their sequence be-

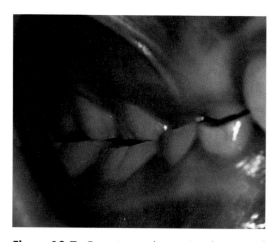

Figure 10.7 Extensive toothwear (combination of attrition, probably bruxism and erosion, caused by gastroesophageal reflux) of the deciduous dentition in a 12-year-old girl, which has created unfavourable alveolar compensatory growth of the posterior segment, thus affecting the occlusal vertical dimension. (With permission from Johansson & Carlsson 2006.)

tween the jaws. At age 12 the second molars erupt, after which there is a pause up to around age 20 when the eruption of the third molars, the wisdom teeth, usually occurs.

In young adults, the normal occlusal plane is established by the permanent incisors and the first molars. Enamel wear facets that may develop do not affect the overbite, overjet or the OVD substantially (Fig. 10.8).

However, as stated above, there is a correlation between the severity of wear on the deciduous teeth/mixed dentition with that found on the permanent teeth later in life in untreated patients. So, it comes as no surprise that many patients in their early teens may, in addition to exaggerated wear facets on their permanent teeth, also have developed toothwear of the incisal edges and erosion on marginal ridges of the upper central incisors and cuspal-'cupped' lesions on their lower first permanent molars. If this proceeds unchecked, the entire palatal surfaces of the incisors are degraded and the entire occlusal surfaces of the lower molars become eroded (Fig. 10.9). This may lead to a change in the OVD, needing therapeutic considerations (see below).

A further disruption of the anterior occlusal plane is found where the lower incisors show only minor attrition and overerupt. Upper molars which are generally less worn than their lower counterparts also overerupt. This may have treatment implications, which are discussed below.

The development of intermaxillary relations is governed by many factors, including different patterns of growth of the jaws, the order of exfoliation of the deciduous teeth and premature tooth loss. Throughout the stages of development there is much variability, which eventually results in wide interindividual variation in occlusal relationships. Many textbooks have described an ideal occlusion as a predetermined standard of perfect, harmonious tooth relationships to be striven for in both the natural and therapeutic (restored) dentitions. It is evident, however, that such an ideal occlusal

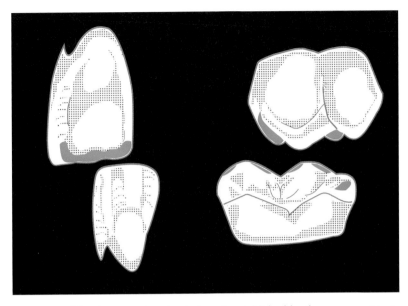

Figure 10.8 In young adults, the normal occlusal plane is established by the permanent incisors and the first molars. Enamel wear facets that may develop do not affect the overbite, overjet or OVD substantially.

template is highly theoretical and seldom found in the population. High prevalences of sagittal, vertical and transverse occlusal anomalies have been recorded in both adolescents and adults.

Instead of ideal occlusion, a concept of 'physiological occlusion' has been advocated, which is an occlusion that deviates in one or more ways from the theoretically ideal, yet is well adapted,

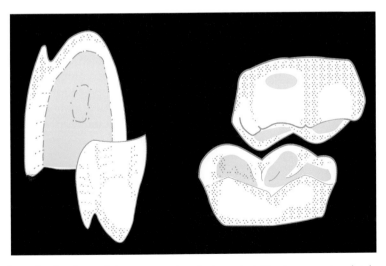

Figure 10.9 The palatal surface of the upper incisor is degraded. The large mesiopalatal cusp of the upper first molar and the five cusps with the entire occlusal basin of the lower molar are eroded. This extensive erosion alters the OVD substantially. Also note that the shallow, non-carious lesion over the palatal cervical margin may later fuse with the occlusal lesion degrading the entire mesiopalatal cusp.

is aesthetically satisfactory and has no pathological manifestations or dysfunctional problems (Mohl et al. 1988).

Occlusal parameters

In the description of occlusal relationships
a large number of terms are used. The maxillomandibular position at which maximal
intercuspation of the teeth occurs is usually
called the *intercuspal position* (ICP; in the current Glossary of Prosthodontic Terms 2005, it
is called maximal intercuspal position [MIP]).
Much attention has been devoted to studies and
discussion of the most retruded position of the
jaws, called centric relation (CR), or when teeth
are in contact, the retruded contact position
(RCP). The relationship between the maxillary
and mandibular teeth is of special interest.
The horizontal overlap is termed *overjet* and
the vertical overlap *overbite*. The *incisal guidance*
means the movement (e.g. protrusion) of the
mandibular incisors on the palatal surfaces
of the maxillary incisors. The corresponding
movements of the canines and posterior teeth in
lateral excursion are termed *canine guidance* and
posterior guidance (group function), amongst
others.

It is well established that the great majority
(≥90%) of dentate individuals have a distance
of up to 1 mm between RCP and MIP/ICP.
Some authors have believed that with advanced toothwear this distance would increase.
In Beyron's sample of Australian aborigines
with progressive toothwear with age (see Fig.
10.5), there was, however, little difference
between age groups for the RCP and MIP/ICP
distance. On the other hand, increased distance
between RCP and MIP/ICP is often found in
edentulous subjects with old complete dentures as well as in patients with TMJ diseases,
such as rheumatoid arthritis and osteoarth-
ritis.

Newly erupted teeth have a distinct morphology, which changes with time in response
to a wide range of factors, toothwear being the
most important. Toothwear is influenced by a
number of factors, such as function and parafunction, type of diet and occlusal forces used.
These are described elsewhere throughout. The
structural components of the dentition such as
number of teeth, jaw relations and occlusal contacts also have an influence on the toothwear
experienced.

In regard to functional contact relationships,
Beyron (1954) was able to demonstrate, in
his serial investigation of the occlusal changes
in the dentitions of 44 adult subjects, that
extensive dental attrition and abrasion with
time resulted in group function. In modern
populations, the development from a normal
canine/anterior-protected occlusion to group
function may be attributed not only to attrition
and abrasion, but also to erosion. Similarly, the
observation that young Western adults possess
canine guidance more frequently than group
function, and that such a population experiences only mild occlusal wear, need not necessarily imply a dependence of minimal wear
on the presence of canine guidance; an absence
of other factors considered to be aetiologic in
toothwear may alternatively be responsible for
the minimal wear experienced by such a population (Johansson et al. 2008).

With respect to the importance of various
types of occlusion and malocclusion, the results are often contradictory (Paesani 2010).
Deep bite and postnormal occlusion have been
associated with a high degree of incisor wear.
Studies also found correlations between toothwear and other anterior spatial relationships
(Van't Spijker et al. 2007). In a longitudinal
study of children and adolescents over 20 years
of age, toothwear was minimal in most subjects
and statistically significant only for incisors
and canines (Magnusson et al. 2005). Three
variables at the first examination predicted
toothwear on incisors and canines measured at
the 20-year follow-up, namely postnormal occlusion, wear on anterior teeth and premolars,
and postnormal occlusion (OR 7.3; $P = 0.001$). A
negative predictor for anterior toothwear was

non-working-side interferences (OR 0.26; $P = 0.03$), indicating that those with such interferences had a four times reduced risk of exhibiting severe anterior toothwear.

Canine and anterior guidances dictate contacts in horizontal movements solely on canines or in combination with incisors, respectively. As the canines wear, group function develops, which leads to contact on several teeth in lateral excursive and protrusive mandibular movements; the resultant occlusal wear is regarded as physiological and desirable.

In his studies on Australian aborigines, Beyron (1964) noted a remarkably regular pattern in chewing, alternating between the two sides of the mouth. This was consistent with previous findings that the preferred side for chewing was on the side with the greatest number of teeth in contact during lateral gliding. The toothwear was consistently symmetrical on the left and right sides in this sample. Besides being more regular, the masticatory cycle showed in general a wider range of contact gliding than reported in European studies.

Theoretically, anterior and canine guidance will disclude the posterior teeth during jaw movements, resulting in less occlusal wear on premolars and molars than in dentitions with posterior guidance. This theory has not been convincingly supported in scientific studies (Johansson 1992), and therefore it is not surprising that there is no sound evidence for recommending a certain occlusion-based treatment protocol above another in the management of attrition (Van't Spijker et al. 2007).

The ideal occlusion is defined as one that has a large number of occlusal contacts distributed across the entire dental arches, often two or three contacts on each premolar and molar. It is suggested that this classical contact relationship helps to maintain occlusal stability and that flattening of the cusps with wear might disturb the stability. However, there is no strong evidence that this occurs in the natural dentition as clinical studies have demonstrated that the number of contacts varies considerably and is on average less than one per occluding tooth pair, and also depends on biting force in healthy subjects (Riise & Ericsson 1983).

An important occlusal parameter is the number of teeth present. It has been shown that toothwear increases with a reduced number of teeth (Ekfeldt et al. 1990; Johansson 1992). A simple explanation might be that the functional stress on a reduced dentition leads to more wear on the remaining teeth. Surprisingly, a systematic review found no studies, suggesting that absent posterior support necessarily leads to increased toothwear, but acknowledged the above finding of a relationship between number of teeth and toothwear (Van't Spijker et al. 2007; Figs. 10.10a & b).

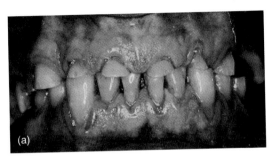 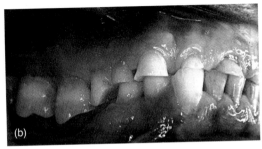

Figure 10.10 (a & b) A 60-year-old man with absent posterior support, which most likely has contributed to the severe toothwear on the remaining anterior teeth due to increased occlusal load producing attritional wear.

PATTERNS OF TOOTHWEAR ON ANTERIOR PALATAL AND POSTERIOR OCCLUSAL SURFACES AND ANGLE'S CLASSIFICATION

In contrast to findings in historical skull materials that posterior teeth had the most extensive toothwear, studies of contemporary samples have reported more wear on anterior teeth (Carlsson et al. 1985; Johansson 1992; Paesani 2010). Erosive wear also affects anterior teeth, especially maxillary incisors, often more so than they do other teeth (Johansson 1996; Khan et al. 1998).

Occlusal vertical dimension

Changes in the morphology of teeth – both the posterior occlusal surfaces and the anterior palatal surfaces – in response to severe toothwear are, in the main, accompanied by dentoalveolar compensation. The extent of this compensatory mechanism is varied and can give rise to different outcomes in terms of changes to the OVD, and the implications this might have for prosthodontic treatment, should this be necessary. Extensive wear may be accompanied by little compensation, and thus possibly an increased interocclusal space. However, it has been shown that dentoalveolar compensation may cause the OVD to remain relatively constant, or even increased, despite toothwear. This would mean that any increase in OVD as part of a reconstruction would be unnecessary. If, on the other hand, restoration is necessary, and the interarch restorative space required for restoration in intercuspal position (ICP) is inadequate for technical reasons, such as retention and resistance form, or should there be an aesthetic consideration, such as shortened anterior teeth that need to have a proper height re-established, then an increase in OVD may be indicated (refer Chapters 11 and 12).

In cases of generalised toothwear that need prosthodontic treatment, it is generally recommended that OVD, even if reduced, be so maintained. If possible, the patient's adapted, 'worn-in occlusion', in the absence of any functional problems, should be conformed to. Re-establishing OVD to some predetermined 'standard of normality' is not essential. However, in those cases where interocclusal space problems or aesthetic considerations are especially critical, there need be no doubts about increasing the OVD. There are seldom any adaptive problems. However, while there are hardly any difficulties involved in increasing the OVD in healthy individuals, a cautious approach is advocated with such procedures in patients exhibiting signs or symptoms of temporomandibular disorders (TMD). Such patients should first be treated with reversible methods to reduce the signs and symptoms of TMD and normalise function before any prosthodontic therapy is started (Johansson et al. 2008). As stated earlier, even if extensive toothwear is present, the OVD could well be unaffected due to compensatory eruption, which is an additional reason to leave it unchanged if possible.

Dahl concepts applied

The problem of restoring worn anterior teeth when little available interocclusal space exists had long challenged prosthodontists. The Dahl appliance has been designed to intrude the lower incisors and allow lower molars to erupt passively. This creates space for restorations on the palatal surfaces of the upper incisors. This is a less radical alternative to complete occlusal reconstruction, which had been the only interventional option until the Dahl method was presented (Dahl & Krogstad 1985). The appliance and the method are described in Chapter 12. Several variations of the Dahl method have been reported in the literature. Instead of the metal splint, composite palatal onlay build-ups or temporary crowns can be used with the

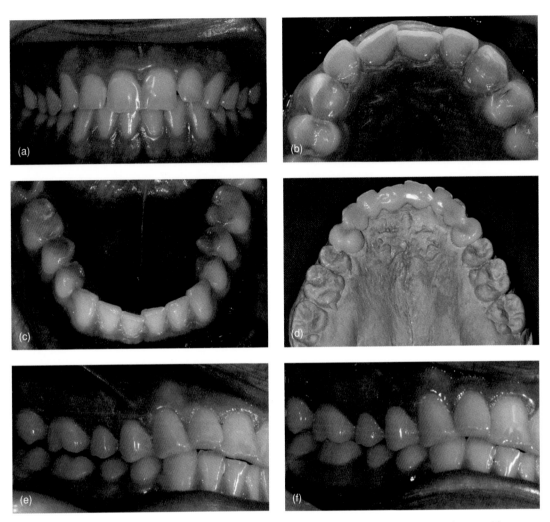

Figure 10.11 A 19-year-old man with extensive toothwear affecting maxillary anterior teeth caused by excessive soft drink intake with retaining drinking technique (a–c). Note especially the pronounced wear on palatal and buccal surfaces with shoulder formations (b). The patient is provided with palatal acrylic onlays ad modum Dahl (cemented with resin cement) producing posterior disclusion (d & e). After 4 months the posterior occlusal relationship has normalized (f), (*continued*)

same purpose. An example of the latter technique is presented in Figs. 10.11a–j and also in chapter 11.

Bruxism and toothwear

Some patients develop opposing, matched wear facets that are believed to be associated with intense tooth grinding (Fig. 10.12). However, such faceting may not be 'typical' of bruxism alone and is more likely the result of a combination of different factors (Khan et al. 1998). Toothwear is a cumulative record of both functional and parafunctional wear, and neither it proves ongoing bruxism activity, nor can it indicate if the subject has static tooth clenching.

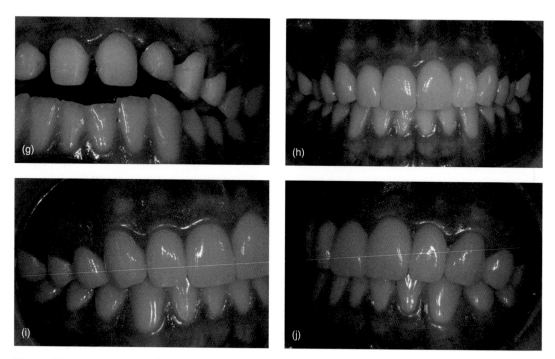

Figure 10.11   (*Cont.*) and after preparation, there is enough space for the restorations (g). Full-ceramic Empress crowns cemented on teeth 14–24 (h–j). (By courtesy to Dr. Fredrik Blomqvist, Postgraduate Dental Education Center, Örebro, Sweden.)

In addition, a diagnosis of bruxism is generally based on the dentist's opinion and seldom verified by an accurate diagnostic test (e.g. somnography or video/audio recordings). Even given a reliable diagnosis of bruxism, its frequency and intensity over time in that patient are seldom known (Koyano et al. 2008).

It is also the case that severe toothwear often shows clinical signs of erosive damage, while 'attrition-like', bruxing-induced wear as the sole feature is rare. The commonly expressed opinion among the dental profession that toothwear is mainly the result of bruxing activity may border more on the anecdotal than scientific and is not supported by the literature (Lavigne et al. 2008). Most of the studies reporting such an association are population studies based on self-reported bruxism, which is unreliable.

That bruxism is not the major cause of toothwear has considerable documented support. In a group of subjects with extensive toothwear, many factors apart from bruxism were found to have contributed to the wear (Carlsson et al. 1985), while elsewhere a variety of types of wear were found in a consecutive series of referred patients (Al-Omiri et al. 2006). Awareness of bruxism was not associated with wear scores and should not be used to define bruxist groups (Seligman et al. 1988). Similar findings have been reported by others (Johansson 1992; Nyström et al. 1990). In a large epidemiological study, it was concluded that the contribution of bruxism to the overall experience of toothwear was only 3% (Ekfeldt et al. 1990). Among 30-year-old Japanese subjects, toothwear status was not predictive of ongoing bruxing activity as measured by an intrasplint

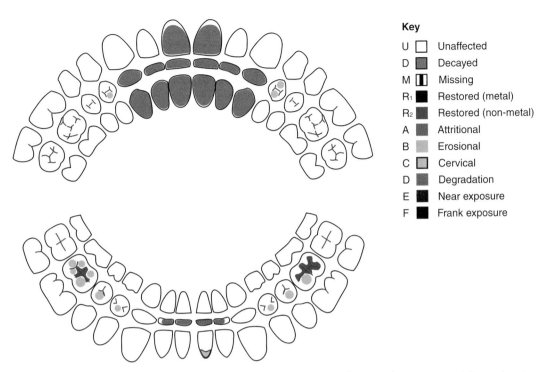

Key

U	☐	Unaffected
D	▨	Decayed
M	▯▯	Missing
R₁	■	Restored (metal)
R₂	▨	Restored (non-metal)
A	▨	Attritional
B	▨	Erosional
C	☐	Cervical
D	▨	Degradation
E	■	Near exposure
F	■	Frank exposure

Figure 10.12 Well-matching opposing facets that are considered to be typical in patients with heavy bruxism. (With permission from Johansson & Carlsson 2006.)

bruxing detection system (Baba et al. 2004). In another well-designed study it was concluded that dental erosion, and not attrition, was the more likely cause of the loss of tooth tissue in patients with bruxism (Khan et al. 1998). In sleep laboratory studies, confirmed moderate-to-severe tooth grinders did not exhibit noteworthy toothwear, while some patients with little tooth grinding activity during sleep presented more toothwear (Lavigne et al. 2008).

In cases of suspected bruxism, it is often suggested that a full-coverage occlusal splint could be constructed to protect teeth and restorations. In spite of its frequent use in such a manner, there is no evidence about the effectiveness of occlusal splints to prevent either bruxism or its effects (Macedo et al. 2007). To our knowledge, neither is there compelling evidence that occlusal splints can prevent toothwear or techni-

cal restorative failures. If dental erosion is the main perceived cause of the wear, an occlusal splint may not be protective and could even worsen the situation by retaining acidic substances in the splint during sleep.

CONCLUSION

It is reasonable to state that toothwear has an effect on the occlusion. This manifests directly as alterations in the way that opposing tooth contacts meet. Indirectly, toothwear contributes to dentoalveolar compensatory mechanisms, as well as craniofacial morphological changes, and this is more so as the severity of the process increases. At the same time, occlusion has the potential to influence the outcome and progression of toothwear through, for example, the jaw relationship, number of occluding teeth and occlusal contacts in jaw function and parafunction.

The interdependence between occlusion and toothwear is therefore clear, but it is also complex. This may have implications for outcomes in terms of functional comfort and aesthetic satisfaction, as well as the process and longevity of rehabilitation.

References

Al-Omiri, M.K., Lamey, P.J., Clifford, T. (2006) Impact of tooth wear on daily living. *International Journal of Prosthodontics*, **19**, 601–605.

Baba, K., Haketa, T., Clark, G.T., et al. (2004) Does tooth wear status predict ongoing sleep bruxism in 30-year-old Japanese subjects? *International Journal of Prosthodontics*, **17**, 39–44.

Bartlett, D.W. (2005) The role of erosion in tooth wear: aetiology, prevention and management. *International Dental Journal*, **55**(Suppl 1), 277–284.

Begg, P.R., Kesling, P.C. (1977) Correct occlusion, the basis of orthodontics. In: *Orthodontic Theory and Practice* (eds P. R. Begg & P.C. Kesling), 3rd edn. pp. 7–50. W.B. Saunders Co., London.

Beyron, H. (1954) Occlusal changes in adult dentition. *Journal of the American Dental Association*, **48**, 674–686.

Beyron, H. (1964) Occlusal relations and mastication in Australian aborigines. *Acta Odontologica Scandinavica*, **22**, 597–678.

Carlsson, G.E., Egermark, I., Magnusson, T. (2003) Predictors of bruxism, other oral parafunctions, and tooth wear in subjects over a 20-year follow-up. *Journal of Orofacial Pain*, **17**, 50–57.

Carlsson, G.E., Johansson, A., Lundqvist, S. (1985) Occlusal wear. A follow-up study of 18 subjects with extremely worn dentitions. *Acta Odontologica Scandinavica*, **22**, 83–90.

Creanor, S.L., Noble, H.W. (1994) Comparative functional anatomy. In: *Temporomandibu-lar Joint and Masticatory Muscle Disorders* (eds G.A. Zarb, G.E. Carlsson, B.J. Sessle, et al.), 2nd edn. pp. 17–47. Munksgaard, Copenhagen.

Dahl, B.L., Krogstad, O. (1985) Long-term observations of an increased occlusal face height obtained by a combined orthodontic/prosthetic approach. *Journal of Oral Rehabilitation*, **12**, 173–176.

Ekfeldt, A., Hugoson, A., Bergendal, T., et al. (1990) An individual tooth wear index and an analysis of factors correlated to incisal and occlusal wear in an adult Swedish population. *Acta Odontologica Scandinavica*, **48**, 343–349.

Ganss, C., Klimek, J., Giese, K. (2001) Dental erosion in children and adolescents – a cross-sectional and longitudinal investigation using study models. *Community Dentistry and Oral Epidemiology*, **29**, 264–271.

Hylander, W.L. (1977) Morphological changes in human teeth and jaws in a high-attrition environment. In: *Orofacial Growth and Development* (eds A.A. Dahlberg & T.M. Graber), pp. 301–330. Mouton Publishers, Paris.

Ingervall, B. (1988) Development of the occlusion. In: *A Textbook of Occlusion* (eds N.D. Mohl, G.A. Zarb, G.E. Carlsson, et al.), pp. 43–56. Quintessence, Chicago.

Johansson, A. (1992) A cross-cultural study of occlusal tooth wear. *Swedish Dental Journal*, (Suppl 86), 1–59.

Johansson, A., Johansson, A.-K., Omar, R., et al. (2008) Rehabilitation of the worn dentition. *Journal of Oral Rehabilitation*, **35**, 548–566.

Johansson, A.K. (2002) On dental erosion and associated factors. *Swedish Dental Journal*, (Suppl 156), 1–77.

Johansson, A.-K., Carlsson, G.E. (2006) *Dental erosion-bakgrund och kliniska aspekter.* Forlagshuset Gothia, Stockholm.

Johansson, A.K., Johansson, A., Birkhed, D., et al. (1996) Dental erosion, soft-drink intake, and oral health in young Saudi men, and the development of a system for assessing erosive anterior tooth wear. *Acta Odontol Scand*, **54**, 369–378.

Khan, F., Young, W.G., Daley, T.J. (1998) Dental erosion and bruxism. A tooth wear analysis from south east Queensland. *Australian Dental Journal*, **43**, 117–127.

Kiliaridis, S., Johansson, A., Haraldson, T., et al. (1995) Craniofacial morphology, occlusal traits, and bite force in persons with advanced occlusal tooth wear. *American Journal of Orthodontics and Dentofacial Orthopedics*, **107**, 286–292.

Kollias, I., Krogstad, O. (1999) Adult craniocervical and pharyngeal changes – a longitudinal cephalometric study between 22 and 42 years of age. Part I: Morphological craniocervical and hyoid bone changes. *European Journal of Orthodontics*, **21**, 333–344.

Koyano, K., Tsukiyama, Y., Ichiki, R., et al. (2008) Assessment of bruxism in the clinic. *Journal of Oral Rehabilitation*, **35**, 495–508.

Lavigne, G.J., Khoury, S., Abe, S., et al. (2008) Bruxism physiology and pathology: an overview for clinicians. *Journal of Oral Rehabilitation*, **35**, 476–494.

Macedo, C.R., Silva, A.B., Machado, M.A., et al. (2007) Occlusal splints for treating sleep bruxism (tooth grinding). *Cochrane Database System Reviews* (4), CD005514.

Magnusson, T., Egermark, I., Carlsson, G.E. (2005) A prospective investigation over two decades on signs and symptoms of temporomandibular disorders and associated variables. A final summary. *Acta Odontologica Scandinavica*, **63**, 99–109.

Mohl, N.D., Zarb, G.A., Carlsson, G.E., et al. (eds) (1988) *A Textbook of Occlusion*. Quintessence, Chicago.

Nyström, M., Könonen, M., Alaluusua, S., et al. (1990) Development of horizontal tooth wear in maxillary anterior teeth from five to 18 years of age. *Journal of Dental Research*, **69**, 1765–1770.

Paesani, D.A. (2010) Tooth wear. In: *Bruxism. Theory and Practice* (ed D.A. Paesani), pp. 123–148. Quintessence, London.

Riise, C., Ericsson, S.G. (1983) A clinical study of the distribution of occlusal tooth contacts in the intercuspal position at light and hard pressures in adults. *Journal of Oral Rehabilitation*, **10**, 473–480.

Seligman, D.A., Pullinger, A.G., Solberg, W.K. (1988) The prevalence of dental attrition and its association with factors of age, gender, occlusion, and TMJ symptomatology. *Journal of Dental Research*, **67**, 1323–1333.

Thilander, B. (2009) Dentoalveolar development in subjects with normal occlusion. A longitudinal study between the ages of 5 and 31 years. *European Journal of Orthodontics*, **31**, 109–120.

Van't Spijker, A., Kreulen, C.M., Creugers, N.H.J. (2007) Attrition, occlusion, (dys)function, and intervention: a systematic review. *Clinical Oral Implants Research*, **18**(Suppl 3), 117–126.

Wedel, A., Borrman, H., Carlsson, G.E. (1998) Tooth wear and temporomandibular joint morphology in a skull material from the 17th century. *Swedish Dental Journal*, **22**, 85–95.

Restoration of the worn dentition

Ian Meyers and Farid Khan

The restorative management of patients with toothwear can range from simple restorations through to complex full-mouth rehabilitations and is dependent on the severity and progression of the tooth surface loss. Pertinent to the topic are the restorative challenges the worn dentition presents, the techniques available, the stability of the oral environment, the consideration of case selection, the patient's demands and aspirations, the stages of wear and how they affect restorative choices.

TO RESTORE OR NOT TO RESTORE IS A CENTRAL QUESTION

Clinically, the decision to restore dental caries is made through assessment of the extent of cavitation, the caries susceptibility of the individual, the patient's ability to regularly maintain the region relatively free of plaque and the risk of progression. The previously considered di-agnostic modalities utilised for dental caries include radiographs, transillumination and laser diagnostics (chapter 7). However, for regions of toothwear, the decision is more difficult, given no such diagnostic modalities are applicable. In regions of toothwear, no cavitation exists. Affected surfaces have no 'infected zone' of bacteria or carious surfaces that need to be removed and instead surfaces have been eroded by extrinsic or intrinsic acids, with or without the influence of attrition and abrasive processes.

As considered in Chapter 8, a patient who is of good health, through normal intake of food and beverages, over a lifetime, will experience a certain amount of wear that would be classified as acceptable and non-pathological. Physiological wear is another term for non-pathological wear. It is when an individual experiences extreme deviation from the norm that accelerated rates of tooth structure loss could lead to 'pathological' wear. Smith and Knight (1984) considered whether a tooth surviving the rate of wear could form the basis of distinguishing acceptable and pathological wear

Toothwear: The ABC of the Worn Dentition, First Edition. Edited by Farid Khan and William George Young.
© 2011 John Wiley & Sons, Ltd. Published 2011 by John Wiley & Sons, Ltd.

at any given age. Hence, it follows that at any given age, a certain amount of toothwear is non-pathological, physiological and normal for that age. Whilst theoretically providing an arbitrary and conceptual approach upon which to base the decision to restore a tooth or not, unless toothwear is extreme or the patient insists on pursuing intervention, it is often difficult to determine this clinically. If a patient is managed optimally with preventive advice, lifestyle and dietary advice, and remineralisation products, could the toothwear be stabilised, and if so, why then restore? The state of balance of the oral environment is one important determinant. In deciding to restore or not to restore, consideration must be given to the benefits and risks of restorative intervention, any restorative challenges, the stage of wear, the patient's demands and aspirations, as well as the clinician's skills and preferences and case selection, all of which are further considered.

PRE-RESTORATIVE TREATMENT – PREPARATION AND PLANNING

Prior to the commencement of any restorative treatment to replace lost tooth structure from toothwear, it is essential to ensure that the oral environment is stable and toothwear and disease have been controlled and particular indicators should be looked for (Fig. 11.1).

When restoring toothwear, it should always be aimed to do so within a balanced oral environment. In cases where the balance cannot be created and, at the extreme, remains heavily unbalanced, a compromised result is envisaged from the start. Cases where the underlying loss of salivary protection cannot be corrected, such as due to medication-induced reduction from a medication that cannot be altered, or patients with chronic reflux conditions, where

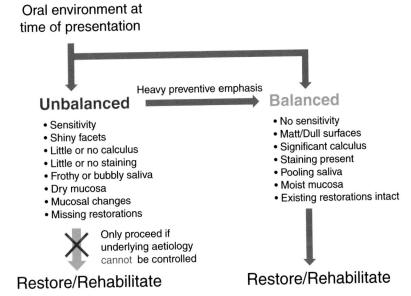

Figure 11.1 Consideration of the oral environment is given at the time of assessment to assist the decision-making process in deciding to commence restoration or rehabilitation of the worn dentition. (From Khan et al., 2010, with permission from Copyright Publishing Pty Ltd.)

despite medical intervention and medications, no further improvement can be achieved, will challenge restorative materials. If underlying factors cannot be altered through preventive efforts and adjuncts, limited improvement in the balance of the oral environment will be achieved. Restorative options should be thoroughly discussed with such patients. The restorative result is likely to offer some protection, but its longevity will be significantly reduced.

Raising the patient's awareness of the causative factors of the toothwear and minimising further damage are essential in this pre-restorative phase of treatment. Changing the balance from demineralisation to remineralisation not only prevents further tooth structure loss but may reduce sensitivity caused by an active erosion process (Prati et al. 2003). This remineralisation is also critical in establishing a stable substrate for adhesive restorations. In the absence of a remineralisation potential, mineral from tooth structure is lost and the resultant demineralised surface is weak, unsupported and prone to breakdown. This surface is also unsuitable for restorative adhesion as the interface between restorative material and tooth substrate will be compromised, and it has been shown that bond strengths to hypomineralised enamel are significantly lower than those to unaffected enamel (William et al. 2006). This hypomineralised surface not only leads to adhesive failures with the restorative material, but it is also possible to obtain cohesive failures within the tooth surface related to weakness in the demineralised surface. To minimise the risk of failure, it is therefore necessary, prior to any restorative treatment, for the tooth surface to be remineralised and strengthened to optimise interface adhesion. Preventive advice, modalities and adjunctive products available are further discussed in Chapter 7. The important role the oral environment and influence of intrinsic and extrinsic acids play in determining restorative success should not be underestimated as restorative clinicians are most often preoccu-

pied in restoring areas of imbalance, namely the sites of low salivary protection and high exposure to acids.

RESTORATIVE CHALLENGES

At the patient level, maintaining a balance in the oral environment and patient compliance to continue with preventive modalities are the primary challenges to restorative success. Health, lifestyle, dietary, work- and sports-related factors will hence have an impact.

At the dentition level, as toothwear progresses, changes in the vertical dimension of occlusion quickly ensue. Whilst in cases of rampant dental caries and coronal breakdown, some changes may be noted, toothwear processes pose a far greater threat to the vertical dimension. In a moderately or severely worn dentition, the sheer numbers of occluding surfaces present a challenge. Treatment more often than not requires multiple teeth to be restored.

The surface area of toothwear lesions is greater. At the tooth level, more dentine is exposed and less enamel is available to bond to. Enamel is often the first surface to be lost, and more often than not, dentine forms the predominant surface to be restored. Whilst the bond strengths of dentine adhesives are improving, these have not reached the bond strengths achievable between composite resin and enamel.

RESTORING THE STAGES OF WEAR

Depending on severity, restoration of a worn dentition varies greatly from placement of a few selective restorations to protect certain areas of wear from progressing to elaborate staged rehabilitation. This process may involve a few or many visits over a considerable time frame of months to years or even an interdisciplinary approach. Clinically, the restorative management of lesions of dental caries differs greatly. Variations in the site specificity and lesion morphology of toothwear have been considered in Chapter 4 and are quite different from those of dental caries. Hence, approaches for restoring dental caries are not applicable for management of toothwear lesions.

Due to differences in exposure and clearance levels of intrinsic and extrinsic acids, attritional and abrasive influences, and salivary protection, it is rare to find lesions of only one stage of wear within a dentition. The more severe the stage of wear affecting a tooth is, the more complex the restorative requirements are likely to be. The importance of offering pulpal protection increases as well. Therefore, consideration is next given to restorative aspects applicable for differing types of toothwear.

Restoring stage A – attrition

Attrition facets are by definition from tooth-to-tooth interaction, hence offering restricted or nill restorative space without changing the occlusion. When found affecting only the enamel, facets do not require restoration. Mandibular anterior teeth are often found to have attritional facets incisally, but are less of an aesthetic concern compared to those on maxillary incisor teeth, which may be affected in severe cases where forward posturing of the mandible has created an edge-to-edge bite, or this was pre-existing. In normal class I occlusion, patients with severe attrition may require restoration of palatal surfaces of the maxillary anterior teeth to offer pulpal protection. Those facets involving dentine exposures on the posterior teeth pose a significant clinical challenge. Over time the direction of the shearing force across the facet affects the margin on the leading edge and the body of the restoration. The same applies, but with lesser forces, to the restorations of the incisal edges of the anterior teeth. In cases of dentine exposure, lack of interarch space restricts use of the glass ionomer and composite resin sandwich technique. Composite resin remains the material of choice.

Restoring stage B – erosion

The chipped and worn incisal edges of the anterior teeth are commonly observed in patients with erosion and often restored given the aesthetic changes. Thinning of enamel and exposure of underlying dentine may, with further lesion progression, result in a deep scooping effect similar to the cupping seen in the premolar and molar teeth. Whilst only the incisal edges are affected, sufficient enamel remains on facial surfaces to allow bevelled extensions of resin restorations to be placed for improved retention, resistance and aesthetics. Cup lesions are characteristically seen on the cuspal inclines or apices of the molar and premolar teeth. These lesions are undercut free. Whilst in time gone by amalgam may have been used to restore these area, placement of undercuts on these surfaces contravenes conservation of tooth structure principles. Placement of a glass ionomer liner for improved dentine bonding and a covering layer of composite, as per the sandwich technique, is the ideal management for lesions extending into dentine, particularly in the mandibular molar teeth, which compared with the maxillary molar teeth are far more commonly and extensively affected by these lesions (Khan et al. 2001). Glass ionomers, may dissolve with time in a highly acidic oral environment or under conditions of low saliva flow. Their wear resistance when placed on occlusal surfaces, unless resin reinforced, is inadequate.

Restoring stage C – cervical lesions

Indications for restorations include the provision of pulpal protection in deeper cervical regions, particularly where underlying lifestyle, dietary and health factors cannot be controlled. Complicating factors in terms of restoration placement mirror those of caries lesions on class V surfaces in that the close proximity to the gingival margins, gingival crevicular fluid and bonding surfaces available all affect restoration longevity, plaque retention, periodontal changes and recurrent caries.

Placing a restoration in order to 'treat' sensitivity is conceptually difficult to justify. Deep cervical lesions encroaching upon pulpal regions should be restored to offer protection, providing justification for restorative intervention. Cervical grooved restorations on the facial surfaces of maxillary incisor teeth are well restored with composite veneers or traditional veneers to improve aesthetics of the affected areas. However, the need for restorative intervention for shallow cervical lesions remains uncertain. In a review of the literature on non-carious cervical lesions, Wood et al. (2008) concluded that the value in restoring non-carious cervical lesions is unclear and occlusal adjustments to prevent lesion progression or improve retention of restorations cannot be supported. It follows that tooth flexure and abfraction are not sustainable answers to explain why certain cervical restorations in non-carious regions fail prematurely. Sakool-namarka et al. (2002) and Tyas and Burrow (2007a, b) considered bond strengths of various dentine-bonding agents and restoration of non-carious cervical lesions, as well as possible reasons for restorative failure of bonded restorations attributable to the differences compared to regions of normal dentine. They concluded that significant doubt exists as to the importance of the involvement of abfraction in restorative failure and instead considered non-carious cervical lesion surfaces to:

1. have a lower phosphate-to-silicon ratio compared with normal dentine;
2. have dentine surfaces that were more highly mineralised with greater proportions of obliterated dentinal tubules;
3. lack a smear layer, such that etching exposed far more collagen fibres compared with normal dentine;
4. create a thinner hybrid layer when bonded to.

If the decision is made to restore non-carious cervical lesions, principles of conservation of tooth structure dictate that ideally no further cavity preparation occurs other than a fine bevel along the coronal enamel margin. Mild pumicing and mild etching are beneficial. However etch times should be reduced.

Restoring stage D – degradation

Degradation describes lesions resulting from the fusion of occlusal and cervical or incisal and cervical regions, involving considerable loss of tooth structure and significant dentine exposure, often with minimal enamel remaining. Posteriorly, few molar teeth reach stage D as cervical lesions are less common. It is the maxillary and mandibular premolar teeth and maxillary incisor teeth that are most commonly affected and require restoration. The direct restorative materials selected are those with stronger dentine-bonding abilities. At the expense of further tooth preparation, the utilisation of onlays, veneers and crowns may offer a longer term option.

Restoring stages E and F – near-exposure and frank exposure

Near-exposures require pulp capping to protect vital structure, and the maxillary anterior and premolar teeth are most commonly affected. Restoring such areas changes the occlusion given the often tight interarch spacing that exists. Enamel available is restricted to gingival margin areas only. The bite opening created requires neighbouring teeth to also be restored, as discussed later. Deep cervical lesions with near-exposures pose a different challenge, namely, at the gingival margin. Moisture control and marginal accuracy are imperative for long-term restorative success. Plaque retention around margins may create potential for periodontal or caries-related changes. Frank exposures involve irreversible pulpitis and involve root canal treatment. The health of the remaining dentition is assessed when deciding the strategic value of the affected tooth, and alternative treatment options include extraction with or without replacement. When a patient presents with a frank exposure, often multiple neighbouring teeth will have near-exposures, warranting restoration to protect vital structures.

PATIENT DEMANDS, ASPIRATIONS, AESTHETICS AND CASE SELECTION

The demands and expectations a patient presents with range from relief of acute symptoms to full-mouth occlusal rehabilitation and requests for smile makeovers. A patient may be concerned about a particular tooth or their entire dentition. Immense variation between patients exists as to what longevity they expect from the result. This needs to be carefully discussed and potential pitfalls identified given the challenges the worn dentition may present. Treatment costs, the number of appointments required and the need for ongoing maintenance are important discussion points. Informed consent is required.

Trends within society are changing. A set of flat and heavily worn teeth is a deviation from the perceived smile curve that resembles 'good health'. In most parts of the developed world it is rare to encounter people with missing anterior teeth in public. Most would seek immediate replacement of an anterior tooth. Previously, worn incisal edges were more commonly identified as age related, whilst these days patients are more likely to request restoration regardless of their age. Restorative considerations relevant to toothwear are detailed in Table 11.1. Before and after photographs of any such treatment are important and should be documented for more elaborate cases.

Of the more elaborate and challenging cases, the clinician should choose to restore clinical cases in which a confident diagnosis was reached and thereafter appropriately managed with preventive modalities which have stabilised the oral environment. Furthermore, the patient and clinician both should agree on the further interventions and be satisfied with the treatment processes and risks involved to achieve the outcome. The patient should demonstrate a high level of compliance to assist the dental team in achieving the desired result and maintaining this. Patient

Table 11.1 Aesthetic considerations.

Treatment parameters for aesthetic restorations:

Does the clinical crown need restoration to an aesthetically pleasing height?

Can the incisal edge be restored aesthetically and be able to resist biting stresses?

Has reduction of clinical crown height permitted passive eruption of the opposing teeth?

What adjustments need to be made to the occlusal vertical dimension to allow sufficient material thickness to resist the forces of the occlusion?

Does intact proximal enamel need to be removed for indirect restorations?

Will the restoration thickness be sufficient for the selected dental materials to mask out underlying dentine shades/colour to achieve the aesthetic outcome desired?

Will the cervical margin be compatible with gingival health?

What materials(s) are needed to cover the lingual or buccal degraded dentine surface to obtain retention and protect the pulp?

compliance may vary significantly over time, and whilst many patients are keen early on, their interest may reduce with time or where multiple restorative failures are encountered or their lifestyle and work-related interests restrict their dental attendance levels. Where the patient continues to exhibit an imbalanced oral environment despite the preventive modalities implemented, the clinician should not feel pressured to proceed with elaborate restorative treatment and instead should be careful to discuss and document their concerns and any effects this imbalance is likely to have on restorative prognosis. Indirect crown and bridge approaches in such patients should be avoided and instead focus should remain on conservative restorative options.

CONSERVATIVE RESTORATIVE OPTIONS FOR PARTIAL OR FULL-MOUTH OCCLUSAL RECONSTRUCTION

Often it is not until toothwear is well advanced that patients seek treatment, at which time the aesthetics are notably affected and/or teeth are hypersensitive (Lussi et al. 2006). It has previously been considered that the definitive restorative treatment for moderate and severe toothwear encompasses multiple crowns and bridges to restore form and function (Thongthammachat-Thavornthanasarn 2007). These indirect restorative treatments tend to be complex, highly invasive and costly, and many patients are not in the position to commence treatment immediately and prefer to delay it until they perceive it becomes essential. Consequently, the extent of toothwear may become even more severe before any definitive treatment is provided, which may further compromise the success of the treatment. Christensen (2005) reported that there has been a tendency in modern dental practice to place more full crowns than may be necessary, and

contrary to popular belief among dentists, conservative restorations can demonstrate good service longevity. Newer materials and techniques are available which enable cost-effective and conservative alternatives for the restorative management of patients with toothwear, and these make restorative options easier, more accessible and more attractive for dentists and patients, such that restorative interventions can commence at an earlier stage.

There are multiple options that now exist for the use of direct adhesive restorative materials to address the immediate functional and aesthetic concerns of the patient and thereby minimise further damage (Hemmings et al. 2000; Mahonen & Virtanen 1991; Poyser et al. 2007; Strassler & Serio 2004). In a well-stabilised oral environment these treatments can provide an intermediate restorative option aiming towards the long-term occlusal rehabilitation of the worn dentition. Careful case selection and preparation involving diagnostic records, diagnostic wax-ups and an understanding of the limitations of the direct restorative materials can provide an alternative solution for these complex cases. The use of preformed templates and keys for the reconstruction of lost tooth structure has been well established (Doan & Goldstein 2007; Vargas 2006), and these techniques can be extended to the use of transparent polyvinyl siloxane templates constructed from the diagnostic wax-up to rapidly reproduce the anatomical structure with direct restorative materials in the mouth (Liebenberg 1996; Meyers 2008). In some cases, a combination of direct and indirect restorative procedures may be utilised to achieve the desired outcome.

Complex rehabilitation and indirect restorations are detailed in the next chapter. Restoratively, however, a number of approaches have been reported to replace lost tooth structure with direct restorative techniques (Mizrahi 2004; Reis et al. 2009; Robinson et al 2008; Soares et al. 2005; Strassler & Serio 2004). These techniques involve the use of wax-ups, silicone putty keys and crown forms and focus primarily on the anterior teeth. Utilising laboratory-formed polyvinyl siloxane templates facilitates *en masse* composite restoration of multiple teeth is achievable in one or more appointments, reducing chairside time involved in individual and direct restoration of heavily worn teeth. The techniques detailed in the following two cases are applicable to most cases of moderate and severe toothwear.

Template technique for direct anterior composite resin restorations

The first case is that of a 52-year-old male patient who presented complaining that his teeth were wearing down, had sharp edges and were occasionally sensitive to cold. He reported that previous restorations did not last and his teeth continued to fracture. Due to the ongoing cost of treatment, the patient had not returned for any further crowns. He admitted that his diet was poor and drank three to four cans of soft drink (either lemon squash, lemonade or black cola drink) at work daily, as he tended to get hot and perspire in the work environment. He drank water only occasionally and usually had one or two glasses of white wine with his evening meal. The clinical examination revealed a heavily restored and eroded dentition (Fig. 11.2). Plaque control was good with healthy gingival condition, and no pocketing or bleeding on probing was observed. Numerous areas of fractured enamel were present, and arrested caries, staining and marginal breakdown of restorations were evident (Fig. 11.2). A salivary evaluation indicated slightly frothy saliva with reduced volume, and the patient reported that he occasionally felt he had a dry mouth, mainly whilst at work.

The patient was instructed to follow the WATCH strategy. The major concern was the dehydration at work followed by rehydration with acidic soft drinks. The further concerns of the possible side effect of dry mouth from the antihypertensive medication and the

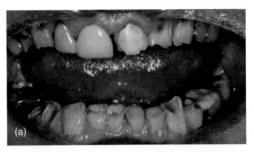

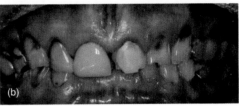

Figure 11.2 The heavily worn dentition of a 52-year-old male patient, who reported sharp, worn-down teeth that were occasionally sensitive to cold (a). The patient reported to have been taking antihypertensive medications for the past 7 years and admitted his diet was poor, drinking three to four cans of soft drink daily, working in warm and dehydrating conditions constructing fibreglass mouldings for motor vehicle accessories. Multiple restorations were reported to have fractured over time and previous restorative attempts had limited life spans. The maxillary right central incisor was reported to have had root canal treatment and a post and core crown placed 3 years prior to presentation. Upon closing, the debilitated state of the occlusion is evident (b), with multiple regions showing breakdown of restorations, staining around margins and arrested dental caries in previously restored areas. The gingivae were healthy and the level of plaque control good.

acidic nature of the white wine were advised. The patient was informed that restorative treatment would be successful only once the oral environment was stabilised and remineralisation strategies commenced to improve the remaining dental structures. Water consumption was encouraged and various preventive adjuncts, including fluoride, chewing gum and caseine phosphopeptide-amorphous calcium phosphate formulation, recommended.

At the first review appointment, the saliva was rechecked and a marked improvement in quantity was noted. The patient also commented that sensitivity to cold had been less noticeable. The options for treatment were discussed with the patient and the agreed decision was made to rebuild the teeth with direct adhesive composite resins. Treatment was to be provided over two appointments, the first to rebuild the anterior teeth and the second, one month later, to restore the posterior teeth.

Diagnostic wax-ups (Fig. 11.3) were completed to establish the required tooth shape, size, and the overbite and overjet relationships. The amount of vertical opening was determined by evaluating the space required to enable restoration, yet being mindful of the functional interocclusal space. This wax-up was used to discuss the anticipated outcomes for the patient and explain the required increase in occlusal opening to accommodate the new

restorations. Once an understanding, agreement and consent were obtained from the patient, the diagnostic wax-up was then used for the construction of transparent polyvinyl siloxane templates to act as guides for the re-establishment of anatomical contour. Due to the presence of the porcelain fused to metal crown on the upper right central, the decision was made to leave this tooth as is and restore all other incisor and canine teeth.

The decision to restore the anterior teeth as the first stage of treatment was based on obtaining an acceptable aesthetic result and ensuring the patient could adapt to the new increased vertical dimension. While numerous other restorative techniques using silicone putty templates or individual celluloid crown forms could have been used to rebuild each individual tooth, the construction of a clear silicone template allows multiple teeth to be restored while conforming to the anatomy of the diagnostic wax-up, reducing chairside time involved in placement and polishing. The translucent template was constructed by taking an impression of the diagnostic wax-up with a transparent polyvinyl siloxane occlusal registration paste (Regofix Transparent, Dreve) with interproximal celluloid-separating strips placed between the individual teeth (Fig. 11.4).

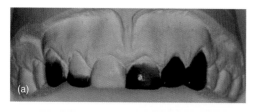

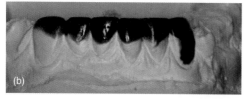

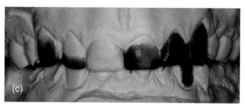

Figure 11.3 Diagnostic wax-ups of the anterior teeth on plaster and stone models of the dentition of the patient shown in Fig. 11.12 were completed in the laboratory on the maxillary (a) and mandibular (b) incisor and canine teeth with anticipated aesthetic incisal heights. Upon occluding the maxillary and mandibular arches, the extent of posterior open bite created is evident (c).

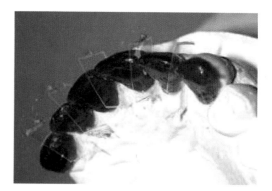

Figure 11.4 Interproximal celluloid strips were utilised to separate the wax-up on the plaster models, facilitating template formation and reducing chairside time required for separating and polishing restorations.

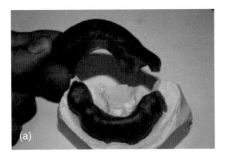

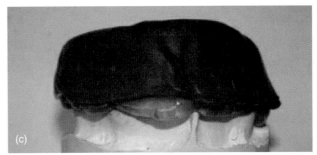

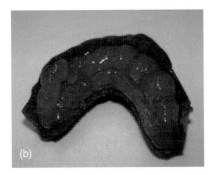

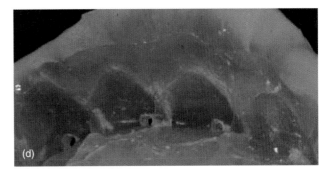

Figure 11.5 A wax spacer and tray is formed on the plaster or stone model (a) for the transparent polyvinyl siloxane material (b) template to be constructed (c). Small vent holes are drilled into the template in the incisal regions of each anterior tooth to facilitate flow of excess composite resin out of overfilled regions prior to polymerisation (d). Note the presence of thin, clear separating strips within the template.

This enables the template to act like individual crown forms for each tooth, which are incorporated into the one template that can be seated in one application. During the diagnostic wax-up procedure, it is important to prepare the dental model with adequate separation to accommodate the separating strips prior to taking the replica impression. Accurate placement of the separating strips will ensure the anterior teeth are not bonded to each other during the resin placement phase. Prior to template construction, the laboratory technician should use a heated lacron carver to melt the ends of the separating strips to enhance their retention within the template. This is particularly important upon removal from the working plaster or stone model.

To ensure an even thickness of silicone over the teeth, a spacer consisting of two sheets of modelling wax is adapted over the wax-up, followed by a sheet of modelling wax moulded over this spacer to act as an impression tray for the silicone (Fig. 11.5). The modelling wax can easily be removed from the set silicone impression. The silicone material is accurate enough to adapt precisely to the wax-up and rigid enough to displace the composite resin when seating back in the mouth. On removal of the silicone, the celluloid interproximal strips remain embedded in the silicone and a vent hole can be drilled in the incisal edge of each tooth to enable release of excess material and any entrapped air (Fig. 11.5).

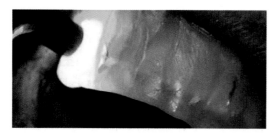

Figure 11.6 Photopolymerisation of the composite resin through the clear template. Upon removal of the template, further light curing of restorations is required to ensure adequate polymerisation.

The preparation of the teeth prior to restoration requires that all old restorative material and weakened tooth structure is removed. Any remaining enamel is kept and utilised for adhesive bonding to the resin. Etching, adhesive bonding, linings and initial increments of resin can then be made to the teeth in preparation for the outer layer of composite resin to be formed using the template. A minimal amount of interproximal separation of the teeth is required prior to placement of the template to enable the template to be seated without distorting or bending the interproximal strips. Composite resin is then placed in the template and the template seated fully over the teeth. Excess material is removed and the resin photopolymerised through the transparent silicone (Fig. 11.6).

The selection of composite resin material used for this restorative procedure must be based on the ability of the material to adapt to the tooth surface while having sufficient physical properties to withstand occlusal load and wear. A low-viscosity composite should not be used as the physical properties are not sufficient for long-term stability of the restorations. Likewise a very high viscosity composite should not be used as it will not adapt to the teeth and distort as the template will be deformed or displaced on placement. It is possible to use most hybrid composite resin materials as the silicone template material is quite firm when set. The transparent silicone

bite registration material should have enough rigidity and resistance to allow placement of the composite without distortion. It must, however generally be no greater than 2–3 mm in thickness to retain this rigidity, as a template that is too thin will distort. In addition, when placing the template it is important to slowly seat the template to allow the composite material to adapt to the teeth and flow onto the surface. A gentle agitation of the template when seating allows this to occur, and as the composite warms up slightly to mouth temperature, this seating process becomes even easier. Sufficient time should be taken to seat the template and ensure it is fully adapted, and excess resin is removed from the vent holes. It is also important not to excessively overfill the template as this makes seating difficult, but the template must not be underfilled as voids will otherwise occur. While dual-cure composite resin materials may be used, in most cases a light-cured composite resin is preferred as it allows time to seat the template. As the thickness of the template reduces the light intensity reaching the composite, it is essential that large bulk placements of resin are avoided. To overcome this, very worn or badly broken-down teeth which require large additions are built up with glass ionomer cement restorative or composite resin prior to template placement. This enables the last increment of composite resin in the template to be kept to a minimum thickness of 2–3 mm. This also allows easier seating of the template without distortion as there is less resistance in this thinner layer. It is essential that not only the composite is cured through the silicone template from labial, incisal and lingual surfaces, but a second curing stage is performed once the template is removed to fully polymerise the resin. Recent literature has suggested that adequate polymerisation can be achieved well beyond 2 mm (Ceballos et al. 2009; Krämer et al. 2008; Rahiotis et al. 2010); however, it is still advisable that the composite thickness in the template, as the final increment for restoration, should only be a maximum of

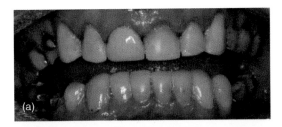

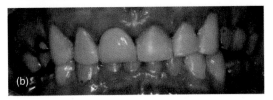

Figure 11.7 Immediate result upon removal of templates with reproduced anatomical result (a) and reproduction of new vertical height with notable disclusion of the posterior teeth (b).

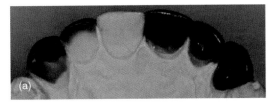

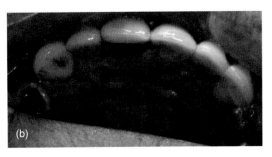

Figure 11.8 Attention to detail at the time of waxing up the plaster or stone model (a) improves the success rates in achieving an appropriate reproduction clinically (b).

2–3 mm. Final shaping and polishing of the restorations is then required to remove any gingival excess and make adjustments on the occlusion to ensure even contact across the anterior teeth (Fig. 11.7).

The duplication of anatomical contour and detail of the wax-up can be seen in the final restorations (Fig. 11.8). Due to the increase in thickness of the maxillary anterior teeth and the increase in length of the mandibular anterior teeth, contact is limited to the anterior teeth from the canine forward with the posterior teeth separated. The patient, having been previously advised that there would be only occlusal contact on the anterior, is left for between 2 and 4 weeks to adapt to this new vertical dimension prior to restoration of the posterior teeth. In most instances, patients adapt to this anterior occlusion within a week and have adequate function until the posterior teeth are restored. In this patient case, the posterior teeth were badly broken down, and after 1 month, direct composite resin restorations were placed on the posterior teeth to recreate posterior contact using conventional posterior restorative techniques. The use of the

translucent silicone template technique is not recommended for direct placement of composites in posterior teeth as it is impossible to achieve correct interproximal contact anatomy with sufficient contact tightness to prevent food trapping. Posterior restoration requires a different technique using alternative direct or indirect restorative techniques.

In cases of localised anterior wear, there is often loss of occlusal height anteriorly, with little or no tooth height loss in the posterior segments. In these cases, the patients can be left to function on the anterior teeth alone until posterior overeruption occurs following the Dahl principle (Briggs et al. 1997; Dahl et al. 1975; Dahl & Krogstadt 1983; Mizrahi 2006; Poyser et al. 2005; Yip et al. 2003). This orthodontic re-establishment of the occlusion may take up to 3 months, but provides a fully functional occlusion without the need to restore the posterior teeth. The Dahl technique is further discussed in Chapter 12.

In the current case, the patient was required to continue with the WATCH strategy and preventive adjuncts on an ongoing basis, and at the 6-month recall, all restorations were performing well and quantity and quality of saliva had remained high (Fig. 11.9).

The ongoing success of this case is dependent on good patient compliance and achieving stabilisation and remineralisation prior to restoration. Eighteen month and three-year appearance of the restorations is shown in Figs. 11.9c and d respectively. The overall longevity of restorations from this technique is very much dependent on the individual and the care and maintenance provided. Large composite restorations should be considered as a medium-term conservative management strategy, and act as medium- to long-term provisional restorations for those who cannot afford complex crown work. Patients report good levels of satisfaction with the composite resin restorations and evidence would suggest that an estimate of the serviceable lifetime for these restorations would be in the 5–10 year range (Schmidlin 2009). This allows patients to consider the following:

1. Leaving and maintaining these restorations, replacing any failed restorations as required over time
2. In rare cases of not tolerating a change in the vertical dimension well or being dissatisfied with the result, having the restorations adjusted, ground back or removed
3. Replacement with longer term indirect crowns on a staged, year-by-year basis to spread the one off-cost of having all crowns done at once
4. Or alternatively after a period of monitoring the composite rebuild, having all heavily restored teeth crowned at once or by arch. Rehabilitation options are detailed in the next chapter.

Prior to use of indirect restorative techniques, a composite rebuild also allows time to ensure any underlying tooth erosion or oral environment imbalance has been stabilised.

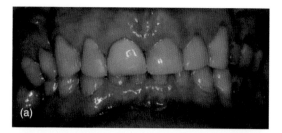

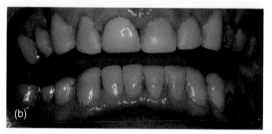

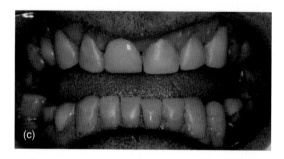

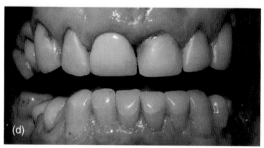

Figure 11.9 Full-occlusal contact was achieved by the 6-month recall (a) with some overeruption of posterior and mild intrusion of the anterior teeth. Comparison of the restorative result at 6 months (b), 18 months (c) and 3 years (d) highlights the balance achievable with direct restorative materials utilising templates. Plaque control and gingival health have remained good throughout this time.

The patient's understanding of the condition and the successful control of the pathological process make it possible over time to undertake replacement restorations with more definitive fixed prosthodontic option when required.

Full-occlusal reconstruction using direct anterior and indirect posterior composite resin restorations

This case involves utilising translucent silicone templates for direct anterior and indirect posterior composite resin restorations. The 27-year-old male patient shown in Fig. 11.10 presented with severe toothwear on all teeth. His occupation as a building supervisor and concurrent high soft drink consumption, particularly at times of dehydration, predisposed this patient to developing severe toothwear, despite his otherwise good oral hygiene practices. The patient was keen to have some definitive treatment on his teeth as he realised the tooth structure was reducing and the sensitivity was increasing. The cost of complex indirect crown work had prevented him from undertaking this treatment; however, he was most interested in

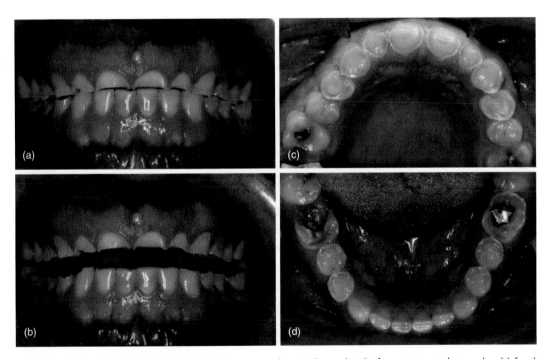

Figure 11.10 This 27-year-old male patient reported a moderate level of sensitivity to hot and cold foods and beverages and presented with severe toothwear on all teeth. The patient reported that he was currently a site supervisor for a building company, and had previously worked as a carpenter in the construction industry, consuming 1.5–2.0 L of cola drinks on a daily basis with little or no water consumption. An edge-to-edge incisal relationship was evident (a) with significant loss of coronal tooth structure across the dentition (b). Near-exposures (stage E) were noted on all maxillary anterior teeth; however, all these teeth responded positively to pulp sensibility testing (c) and cervical lesions affected all premolar teeth buccally. Previous restorative treatment included some small amalgam restorations in the posterior molar teeth, and endodontic therapy on the broken-down lower right first molar tooth (d). The soft tissue lesion seen on the labial gingival adjacent to the frenum (a & b) was an asymptomatic benign soft tissue growth unrelated to the teeth.

improving the appearance of his smile. The patient was advised of the nature and causes of his tooth surface loss and stabilisation and remineralisation strategies implemented as previously discussed. Impressions were taken of the teeth for a diagnostic wax-up and an orthopantomogram (OPG) reviewed to assess root structure and bone support and to ensure there was no other underlying pathology. An important diagnostic feature of many toothwear cases, as evident in this case, is the presence of a small band of enamel at the gingival margin (Fig. 11.10). This enamel remains less affected by the ongoing acid erosion and there is additional erosion protection provided by gingival crevice fluid flow. It is critical that this small band of residual enamel is retained as it provides a peripheral bond and seal for the composite resin, which will be used to restore the teeth. This marginal enamel not only enhances the adhesion of the resins to the remaining tooth surface, but also minimises marginal leakage and reduces the potential for caries to develop under the restoration.

To assist the laboratory technician with the diagnostic wax-up, a photograph illustrating the original shape and size of the teeth prior to the toothwear was provided by the patient. This also assisted in determining the amount of vertical opening by evaluating the space required to rebuild the tooth anatomy to the required dimensions. In this case where there was excessive anterior tooth loss, the laboratory technician was able to adapt and incorporate acrylic denture teeth into the diagnostic wax-up (Fig. 11.11).

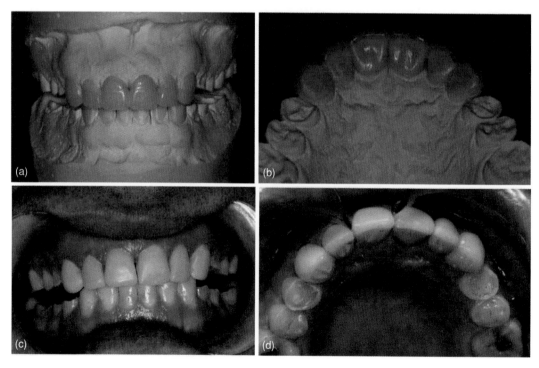

Figure 11.11 The initial diagnostic wax-up of the anterior teeth was achieved using prefabricated acrylic denture teeth adapted to the study cast (a), which enabled construction of the translucent silicone template for restoration of the anterior teeth (b) with an accurate reproduction of the anatomical contour of the wax-up translated to the clinical restorations (c & d).

The first restorative phase for this involved the restoration of the maxillary and mandibular anterior teeth using translucent silicone templates, as described in the previous case. This allowed duplication of the diagnostic wax-up and allowed the patient to evaluate the aesthetics and the new vertical dimension (Fig. 11.11). In preparation for the second restorative phase, the posterior occlusal amalgams were removed and replaced with composite resin and a provisional glass ionomer restoration placed in the fractured lower right molar. All occlusal undercuts were restored with composite resin, and putty and wash silicone impressions were taken to provide die-stone diagnostic models of

the restored anterior teeth and worn posterior teeth. An occlusal registration record was also taken to verify the occlusal relationship prior to the final stages of the diagnostic wax-up. The remaining stage of the diagnostic wax-up was then completed with the posterior occlusion restored (Fig. 11.12).

A replica cast was constructed from the wax-up to provide a model for construction of composite resin onlays. A further impression of this model was taken with the translucent silicone material to provide a template for construction of these resin inlays (Fig. 11.13).

The construction of the posterior composite resin inlays could then be undertaken by

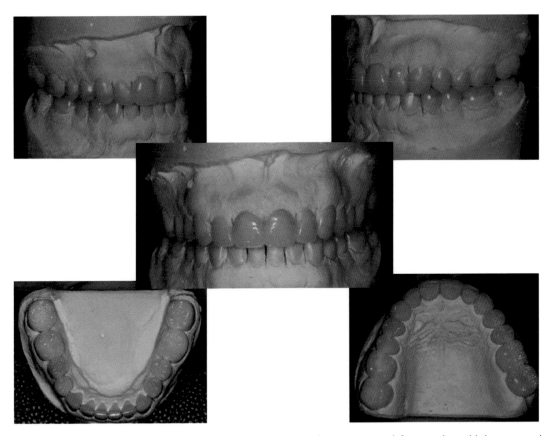

Figure 11.12 The complete occlusal wax-up aims to reproduce anatomical form and establishes a good functional occlusion. Attention to detail in the wax-up and the interocclusal relationship of the teeth ensures the final clinical restorations based on the wax-up require minimal adjustment.

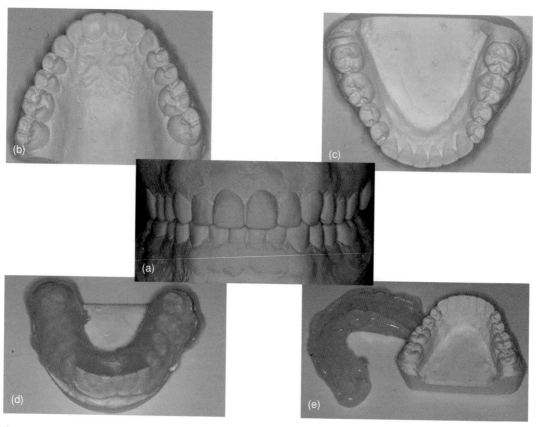

Figure 11.13   Replica stone models from the wax-up (a–c) are used to construct the silicone template (d & e) for the posterior inlays.

utilising this translucent silicone template and placing this on the diagnostic die-stone models of the restored anterior teeth and worn posterior teeth (Fig. 11.14). Removal of the anterior labial section of the silicone allows visualisation of the adaptation of the template to the model to ensure it is correctly seated, and the resultant void above the posterior teeth can be clearly seen (Fig. 11.14).

Composite resin restorative material can then be placed into the posterior sections of the template and carefully seated onto the die-stone model to allow adaptation of the resin to the occlusal surface of the worn teeth while maintaining the occlusal anatomy created by the diagnostic wax-up. The composite resin can

then be polymerised through the template to provide an initial cure. Final polymerisation is achieved once the silicone template is removed (Fig. 11.15).

To ensure the composite resin does not adhere to the die-stone model, two layers of die-separating solution are painted over the die-stone model and allowed to completely dry before adapting the composite resin to the surface. Once fully polymerised, the posterior composite resin inlays can be removed from the die-stone model and carefully separated and sandblasted to remove any surface contaminants (Fig. 1.16).

Each individual onlay can then be identified for cementation onto the tooth at the second

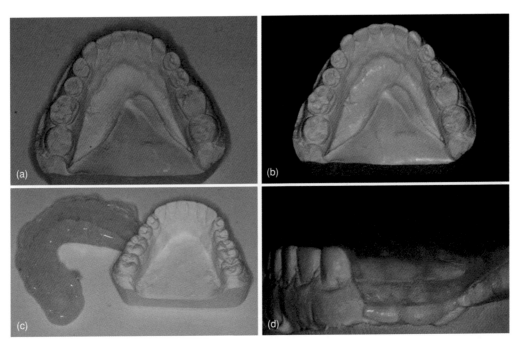

Figure 11.14 To ensure the composite resin does not adhere to the die-stone model (a), several layers of separating medium are painted onto the teeth and surrounding tissue (b). The anterior segment is cut away from the silicone template (c) and the template placed on the die-stone model to demonstrate the amount of lost tooth structure in the posterior teeth (d).

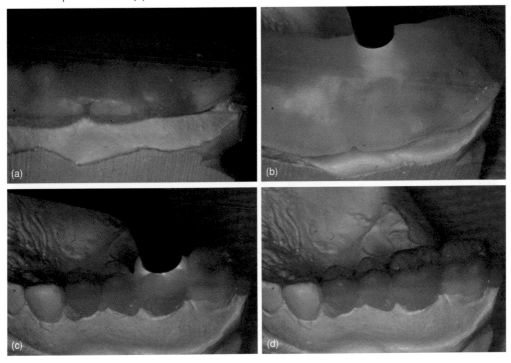

Figure 11.15 Composite resin is placed into the silicone template and seated onto the die-stone model (a) and initial polymerisation of the resin undertaken (b). Upon removal of the template, the composite resin must have a final cure to ensure full polymerisation (c) such that the final onlays can then be checked for any voids or discrepancies (d).

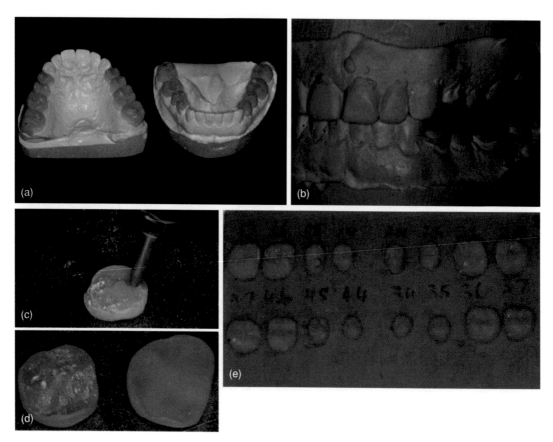

Figure 11.16 The completed onlays (a) are checked to ensure occlusal contact has been maintained (b) and the inlays carefully removed from the die-stone model, separated and the fitting surface cleaned and sandblasted (c & d). The prepared restorations are then individually identified ready for cementation (e).

restorative visit. As minimal preparation was undertaken in the mouth and all undercuts previously restored, it is possible to seat each onlay onto the tooth without any additional tooth preparation other than etching and conditioning as required for cementation. The use of an all-resin cement to bond the inlays to the worn tooth surface is recommended as it can flow freely onto the surface and is able to fill any small voids that may be present under the onlay or at the onlay margins (Fig. 11.17).

Final occlusal adjustments can then be made to ensure there are no occlusal interferences of high spots. The final restorative outcome for this patient was very successful and the new vertical dimension well tolerated (Fig. 11.18).

The two restorative phases provided both the patient and the clinician an opportunity to assess the aesthetics and occlusal height increases while allowing scope for easy adjustment or replacement of restorations should the need arise. In some instances, particularly with the bruxing patient, it may be necessary to construct an occlusal splint to provide some protection against wear and fracture of the restorations. Longer term management can then be considered and planning for future replacement of the composite resins with ceramic or gold crowns.

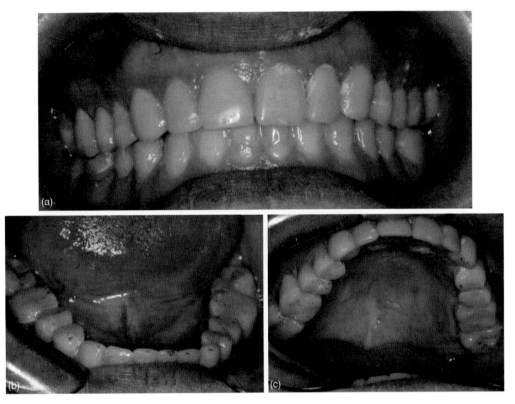

Figure 11.17 The final restorations are cemented onto the mandibular (a) and maxillary (b) teeth using an all-resin cement and the final occlusion checked and adjusted (c).

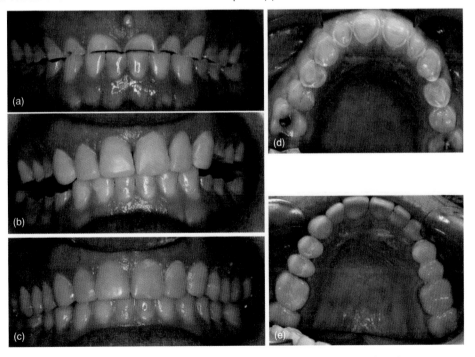

Figure 11.18 The two-stage approach to restore a severely worn dentition (a) with a direct anterior template as the first stage (b) and indirect posterior cemented onlays (c) allows for rapid replacement of lost tooth structure and reconstruction of a debilitated occlusion (d & e).

SUMMARY

The preceding cases highlight the need for prevention from a young age. Preventive efforts should begin through discussion of dietary and lifestyle advice with parents and their children. Ideals, whilst always aimed for, may not be achieved and hence in many patients, a need to restore or rehabilitate a worn dentition already exists at the time of presentation. Whilst challenging conventional restorative materials and operator skill in such cases, success rates also rely heavily upon the compliance of the patient to make lifestyle changes and follow the advice of their practitioner in protecting the result.

The restorative management of patients presenting with toothwear is rarely confined to restorative interventions alone. Long-term successful management requires recognition of the problem, stabilisation of the oral environment, remineralisation of the tooth structure and when appropriate, restoration. Adoption of a patient management strategy which involves both the patient and the oral health team and addresses all the underlying aspects of the toothwear condition will ensure improved outcomes for all patients.

Patients who present with evidence of limited toothwear may not require any restoration. Those with moderate toothwear can usually be treated simply and with traditional restorative approaches. In cases of more severe toothwear, the techniques for repair and reconstruction tend to be more complex and time consuming. In all cases, preventive management strategies are paramount.

The option to restore or not is one of clinical judgement, which should be based on clear principles, considering the risks and benefits of doing so. The patient's demands and aspirations increasingly direct the course of dental treatments. Considering functional and aesthetic parameters and the stages of wear identified across the patient's dentition, decisions can be made to instigate restorative treatment. The key rules in restoring the worn dentition are to bond, fill and polish more so than drill and fill. Strict adherence to guidelines of conservation of tooth structure is indicated. In patients, where the oral environment has been balanced using preventive modalities and restorations are required, most teeth with stage A, B and C wear can be treated with adhesive, non-invasive dentistry, whilst more complex restorations and pulpal protection are often required in stages D, E and F. Conservative restorative options using glass ionomer and composite resin materials, with or without laboratory formed templates, offer an alternative to indirect restorations. This mode of restoration will likely be increasingly utilised as further improvement in adhesive tooth-coloured restorative materials is achieved.

References

Briggs, P.F., Bishop, K., Djemal, S. (1997) The clinical evolution of the 'Dahl Principle'. *British Dental Journal*, **183**, 171–176.

Ceballos, L., Fuentes, M.V., Tafalla, H., et al. (2009) Curing effectiveness of resin composites at different exposure times using LED and halogen units. *Medicina Oral, Patologia Oraly Cirugia Bucal*, **14**(1), E51–E56.

Christensen, G.J. (2005) What has happened to conservative tooth restorations? *Journal of the American Dental Association*, **136**(10), 1435–1437.

Dahl, B.L., Krogstad, O. (1983) The effect of a partial bite-raising splint on the inclination of upper and lower front teeth. *Acta Odontologica Scandinavica*, **41**, 311–314.

Dahl, B.L., Krogstad, O., Karlsen, K. (1975) An alternative treatment in cases with advanced localized attrition. *Journal of Oral Rehabilitation*, **2**, 209–214.

Doan, P.D., Goldstein, G.R. (2007) The use of a diagnostic matrix in the management of the severely worn dentition. *Journal of Prosthodontics*, **16**, 277–281.

Hemmings, K.W., Darbar, U.R., Vaughan, S. (2000) Toothwear treated with direct composite restorations at an increased vertical dimension: results at 30 months. *Journal of Prosthetic Dentistry*, **83**, 287–293.

Khan, F., Young, W.G., Law, V., et al. (2001) Cupped lesions of early onset dental erosion in young Southeast Queensland adults. *Australian Dental Journal*, **46**, 100–107.

Khan, F., Young, W.G., Taji, S.S. (2010) *Toothwear: A Guide for Oral Health Practitioners*. Copyright Publishing Pty Ltd. Brisbane, Australia.

Krämer, N., Lohbauer, U., García-Godoy, F., et al. (2008) Light curing of resin-based composites in the LED era. *American Journal of Dentistry*, **21**(3), 135–142.

Liebenberg, W.H. (1996) Occlusal index-assisted restitution of esthetic and functional anatomy in direct tooth-colored restorations. *Quintessence International*, **27**, 81–88.

Lussi, A., Hellwig, E., Zero, D., et al. (2006) Erosive tooth wear: diagnosis, risk factors and prevention. *American Journal of Dentistry*, **19**, 319–325.

Mahonen, K.T., Virtanen, K.K. (1991) An alternative treatment for excessive toothwear. A clinical report. *Journal of Prosthetic Dentistry*, **65**, 463–465.

Meyers, I.A. (2008) Diagnosis and management of the worn dentition: conservative restorative options. *Annuals of the Royal Australasian College of Dental Surgeons*, **19**, 31–34.

Mizrahi, B. (2004) A technique for simple and aesthetic treatment of anterior toothwear. *Dental Update*, **31**(2), 109–114.

Mizrahi, B. (2006) The Dahl principle: creating space and improving the biomechanical prognosis of anterior crowns. *Quintessence International*, **37**, 245–251.

Poyser, N.J., Briggs, P.F.A., Chana H.S., et al. (2007) The evaluation of direct composite restorations for the worn mandibular anterior dentition – clinical performance and patient satisfaction. *Journal of Oral Rehabilitation*, **34**, 361–376.

Poyser, N.J., Porter, R.W., Briggs, P.F., et al. (2005) The Dahl Concept: past, present and future. *British Dental Journal*, **198**, 669–676.

Prati, C., Montebugnoli, L., Suppa P., et al. (2003) Permeability and morphology of dentin after erosion induced by acidic drinks. *Journal of Periodontology*, **74**, 428–436.

Rahiotis, C., Patsouri, K., Silikas N., et al. (2010) Curing efficiency of high-intensity light-emitting diode (LED) devices. *Journal of Oral Science*, **52**(2), 187–195.

Reis, A., Higashi, C., Loguercio, A.D. (2009) Re-anatomization of anterior eroded teeth by stratification with direct composite resin. *Journal of Esthetic Restorative Dentistry*, **21**(5), 304–316.

Robinson, S., Nixon, P.J., Gahan, M.J., et al. (2008) Techniques for restoring worn anterior teeth with direct composite resin. *Dental Update*, **35**(8), 551–552, 555–558.

Sakoolnamarka, R., Burrow, M.F., Tyas, M.J. (2002) Micromorphological study of resin-dentin interface of non-carious cervical lesions. *Operative Dentistry*, **27**, 493–499.

Schmidlin, P.R., Filli, T., Imfeld, C., et al. (2009) Three-year evaluation of posterior vertical bite reconstruction using direct resin composite – a case series. *Operative Dentistry*, **34**(1), 102–108.

Smith, B.G., Knight, J.K. (1984) An index for measuring the wear of teeth. *British Dental Journal*, **156**, 435–438.

Soares, C.J., Pizi, E.C., Fonseca, R.B., et al. (2005) Direct restoration of worn maxillary anterior teeth with a combination of composite resin materials: a case report. *Journal of Esthetic Restorative Dentistry*, **17**(2), 85–91.

Strassler, H.E., Serio, C.L. (2004) Conservative treatment of the worn dentition with adhesive composite resin. *Dentistry Today*, **23**(8), 79–80, 82–83.

Thongthammachat-Thavornthanasarn, S. (2007) Treatment of a patient with severely worn dentition: a clinical report. *Journal of Prosthodontics*, **16**, 219–225.

Tyas, M.J., Burrow, M.F. (2007a) Five-year clinical evaluation of One-Up Bond F in non-carious cervical lesions. *American Journal of Dentistry*, **20**(6), 361–364.

Tyas, M.J., Burrow, M.F. (2007b) Clinical evaluation of three adhesive systems for the restoration of non-carious cervical lesions. *Operative Dentistry*, **32**(1), 11–15.

Vargas, M. (2006) Conservative aesthetic enhancement of the anterior dentition using a predictable direct resin protocol. *Practical Procedural Aesthetic Dentistry*, **18**, 501–507.

William, V., Burrow, M.F., Palamara, J.E., et al. (2006) Microshear bond strength of resin composite to teeth affected by molar hypomineralization using 2 adhesive systems. *Pediatric Dentistry*, **28**, 233–241.

Wood, I., Jawad, Z., Paisley C., et al. (2008) Non-carious cervical tooth surface loss: a literature review. *Journal of Dentistry*, **35**, 759–766.

Yip, K.H., Smales, R.J., Kaidonis, J.A. (2003) Dahl appliances used for the restorative management of localized anterior tooth erosion. *General Dentistry*, **51**, 54–57.

Rehabilitation of the worn dentition

Ridwaan Omar and Ann-Katrin Johansson

In general, there are few objective criteria for evaluating the need for prosthodontic treatment, but toothwear-based criteria may be the exception. For most people, toothwear is a natural part of ageing, and replacement of lost tooth substance is only infrequently a necessity. Even patients with extensively worn dentitions do not automatically require oral rehabilitation if their functional adaptation is good. But if the toothwear is considered to be so severe or its rate of progression threatens, for example, endodontic integrity, that rehabilitation is indicated, there are several possibilities for treatment.

This chapter reviews the evolution of rehabilitative concepts and techniques from the traditional approach to ones that are increasingly favoured today. Wherever possible, the account given is based on an appraisal of the available literature (Johansson et al. 2008). Realistically, however, the literature on toothwear provides very little scientific evidence that can be said to support unambiguous recommendations about its management. The question of what the best approach to rehabilitation of given toothwear scenarios is, is therefore often based on evidence of lower scientific strength than randomised controlled trials (RCTs).

Within the general scheme of a book on toothwear, the title of this chapter would, to most readers, suggest an account of the rehabilitation of the *severely* worn dentition. It would likely also imply the severe loss of predominantly *posterior occlusal*, but also *anterior palatal*, tooth substance, with the host of clinical challenges related to the management of such conditions. The approach to rehabilitation has traditionally been an 'all-or-none' one, which – once the need for treatment has been decided – uses invasive, irreversible and, in most cases, clinically and technically demanding full-mouth reconstruction. The net result of this has been a complex decision-making process with a tendency to defer treatment until the toothwear is well advanced.

The fact that erosive toothwear is increasingly seen in younger individuals has, in more recent times, seen the emergence of another

Toothwear: The ABC of the Worn Dentition, First Edition. Edited by Farid Khan and William George Young.
© 2011 John Wiley & Sons, Ltd. Published 2011 by John Wiley & Sons, Ltd.

treatment approach. The method focuses on meeting greater aesthetic demands while also being conservative of further tooth substance reduction and showing favourable longevity in early reports. The most severe lesions that affect the occlusion occur on the occlusal surfaces of the first permanent molars and the palatal surfaces of the upper central incisors, as discussed in Chapter 10. It follows that there are vertical as well as horizontal dimensions to the resultant toothwear (Johansson 2002). A better understanding of this characteristic localisation of toothwear and how its subsequent effect on the occlusion complicates rehabilitation has prompted the development of specific treatment methods that aim to address the problem through more conservative, and frequently site-specific, solutions. Increasingly, these techniques are applied to older patients who would otherwise have been treated with conventional prosthodontic methods. Besides the rehabilitative challenges posed by occlusal and palatal toothwear, erosion is suggested to be the primary aetiological factor for non-carious cervical lesions (NCCLs). The term 'degradation' has been used to describe the presence of such lesions together with occlusal wear (Khan et al. 1999), and presents another dimension to the rehabilitative challenge.

There is now recognition that early diagnosis of toothwear is possible and a proper investigation of its aetiology a necessity. Frequently, although not invariably, this will result in preventing, or at least slowing, further damage. However, even as our understanding of the aetiology and pathogenesis of toothwear gradually increases, it remains some way off the level of knowledge that exists about other comparable dental conditions, such as dental caries. Such limitations add to the management complexities, especially with regards to rehabilitation. Fortunately, there are a number of promising, and some would say alluring, developments towards more conservative treatment approaches afforded by, albeit still

limited, research as well as rapid developments in dental materials science.

PRINCIPLES AND STRATEGIES FOR REHABILITATING WORN DENTITIONS

The clinical challenge

Toothwear is generally slowly progressive, and its early signs do not inevitably lead to further deterioration. Any symptoms or patient dissatisfaction is similarly slow to present. The unpredictability of the rate and the likely periodicity of progression will, on an individual basis, have therapeutic implications. Its irreversible nature and multifactorial aetiology make toothwear one of the most difficult clinical problems to deal with. An especially vexing aspect of toothwear is that because most dentists examine patients for the first time at an unknown point in its progression, a dilemma arises regarding the decision to intervene restoratively and/or prosthodontically, or not. Precisely what an acceptable severity and rate of wear is, is not easy to decide, but such a judgement should always be individually evaluated. Consideration should be given to the age and life expectancy of the individual, as well as aetiological factors and host defence mechanisms that may be operating (see Chapter 7). At the same time, one has to consider the risk of 'supervised neglect' of the patient's condition (Bartlett 2010). Early diagnosis and awareness on the part of the patient of an unacceptable level of wear would appear to be key to prevention and management.

Management strategies

The definitive *treatment* of toothwear can be performed in a number of different ways. However, its broader *management* is an inclusive process, comprising a thoroughly methodical clinical examination and assessment of possible causative factors, including a systematic history, diagnoses, prevention, monitoring and, in some cases, definitive rehabilitation. In an article that sought to present some clinical guidelines, its authors cautioned, 'There are no hard and fast rules and the need for treatment should be established after considering: the degree of wear relative to the age of the patient; the aetiology; the symptoms; the patient's wishes' (Davies et al. 2002). On the basis of current knowledge, there is little reason to contest this statement from almost 10 years ago.

On the basis of the history, clinical examination and diagnosis, management should be directed towards first eliminating the aetiological factors and strengthening any modifying factors. Since toothwear is usually a relatively slow process, urgent restoration will, in many patients, not be necessary. Proceeding with caution is important especially for younger individuals since the longevity of restorations is finite and frequently quite limited. However, for a patient suffering from demonstrably progressive wear or severe sensitivity or pain, it becomes important to hasten the investigatory phase in order to retard or prevent further deterioration or symptoms.

Rehabilitative considerations

The question of rehabilitation arises when the patient's needs, severity of the wear and potential for unacceptable progression are of concern. There is no evidence that the presence of toothwear will inevitably lead to severe wear, with fluctuations in its rate of progression making it difficult to estimate future deterioration. Costly conventional prosthodontics was, and still is, the mainstay of rehabilitation of the severely worn dentition when treatment is indicated. Such treatment is also complex and generally highly invasive. As has already been mentioned, the tendency has, therefore, been to defer it if at all possible, with the result that wear was usually well advanced by the time definitive restorative treatment was commenced. On the other hand, there are those who

advocate early diagnosis and timely treatment 'to prevent the tooth from wear beyond a point of acceptable restoration' (Dawson 2007).

Besides the traditional 'subtractive' approach to rehabilitation of the worn dentition, a gradual shift towards greater conservatism by an 'additive' approach seems to be under way in the form of direct and indirect resin composite restorations (see Chapter 11), bonded cast metal restorations, implant-supported removable partial dentures (RPDs), orthodontic treatment and protective splints, amongst others. While this trend may be more apparent in some parts of the world than in others, the rationale for it and the developments in dental materials science and more reliable accompanying clinical techniques are both relevant and promising. More about these developments is discussed later in the chapter.

As regards the efficacy of any one of the aforementioned treatment options or comparisons among them, a recent search of the literature on rehabilitation of toothwear (covering the period up to November 2007) was unable to identify a single paper with an RCT design (Johansson et al. 2008). In preparing for this chapter, a further literature search was performed using the same parameters as in our previous report, and this again failed to identify any paper on the topic as at May 2010. A systematic review similarly failed to find any support for the efficacy of any one occlusion-based treatment modality over another (van't Spijker et al. 2007), and it can be concluded that there are no sufficiently robust, documented outcomes regarding different approaches to the rehabilitation of the worn dentition.

However, even though the RCT is considered the most reliable design for evaluating the effectiveness of treatment, just as in most other areas of dentistry, RCTs are rarely found in prosthodontics. It has been reported that RCTs made up only 1.7% of all articles in the three leading prosthodontic journals between 1990 and 1998 (Dumbrigue et al. 1999), and even then many are judged to be of poor methodological quality (Jokstad et al. 2002). More recently, it was reported that most RCTs on implant dentistry had inadequate randomisation procedures (Dumbrigue et al. 2006). Even systematic reviews on the prosthodontic treatment options for single-tooth replacement have concluded that a lack of comparable comparative studies limits any clear recommendations from being made (Salinas & Eckert 2007; Torabinejad et al. 2007). Bearing such constraints in mind, the discussion and recommendations that follow are necessarily based on studies whose designs are considered to be of less scientific rigour than RCTs, on the opinions of respected authorities and on our own clinical experience.

Dentoalveolar compensation

Severe occlusal toothwear may result in changes to the occlusal vertical dimension (OVD), with a possible increase in interocclusal space. This potentially has significant implications for rehabilitation. It has been shown that dentoalveolar compensation may cause the OVD to remain relatively constant, or even increase, despite toothwear. This would mean that any re-establishment of OVD (for the purpose of restoring facial height, for example) would not ordinarily be a *de facto* part of rehabilitation.

Instead, the important question, if rehabilitation is necessary, will be whether sufficient interarch restorative space required for restorations that also meet aesthetic requirements is available in the maximum intercuspal position (MIP) and whether retention and resistance, particularly so for conventionally cemented restorations, will be adequate. If such 'restorative space' exists, restoration in MIP is probably going to be relatively straightforward using a conformative approach (Wise 1977). If, on the other hand, there is not sufficient space, the next question will be whether the wear is largely localised or generalised (Fig. 12.1a). For localised wear, vertical space can be gained by reversing

the effects of dentoalveolar compensation using the 'Dahl technique' (Dahl et al. 1975; Chapter 10). In this regard, it will be recalled that the most severe lesions that affect the occlusion occur on the occlusal surfaces on the first permanent molars and the palatal surfaces of the upper central incisors. Passive eruption of upper molars and lower incisors then introduces both vertical and horizontal changes to alter the occlusal plane. Although this complicates rehabilitation, the 'Dahl technique' is capable of addressing it in a relatively simple way. By this means, treatment is confined to the worn teeth and avoids it being disproportionately broadened to more teeth (which may well be unaffected by wear) than necessary (Fig. 12.1b). Several modifications of the technique have been described following the original report, including placement of single or multiple bonded restorations at increased OVD in anticipation of rapid re-establishment of full intercuspation being attained by the non-occluding teeth (Poyser et al. 2005). Orthodontic treatment is increasingly common in adults, and several types of tooth movements, including selective intrusion or extrusion, may be provided for the purpose of increasing interocclusal 'restorative space' in the anterior region, but increasingly also in localised posterior sites.

Generalised wear, on the other hand, will in most cases require a reorganised approach (Wise 1977), with or without an increase in OVD, and this is discussed later (Fig. 12.1b).

Biomechanical factors

When conventional fixed prosthodontic rehabilitation is necessary, extensive tooth preparation is invariably going to be needed. This raises a paradox whereby more tooth substance removal is needed in the therapeutic pursuit of making good the damage caused by a process of tooth substance loss itself. The difficulty of achieving adequate mechanical retention and resistance forms for conventionally cemented restorations, and the potentially greater load on

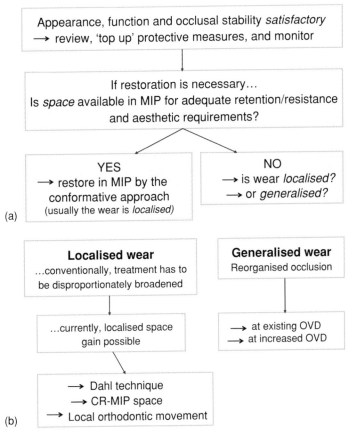

Figure 12.1 Interocclusal restorative space considerations once treatment has been decided upon: (a) Implications of space adequacy or inadequacy; (b) approaches that can be used when space is not adequate for restorative purposes.

restorations if there is bruxism, heavy chewing forces or unfavourable loading directions between teeth means that caution is needed in the design of restorations.

Single crowns should be provided whenever possible and fixed dental prostheses (FDPs) should be of minimal extension. Nevertheless, many restorations fail as a result of stress concentration from differential wear and poorly planned occlusal contacts, a risk that is greater if there is heavy loading, perhaps 'directly' through bruxism or 'indirectly' if there are few remaining occluding units. Inadequate retention and resistance of crowns on short

abutments can be improved in several ways (Box 12.1).

Box 12.1 Methods of improving retention and resistance for conventionally cemented restorations.

- Extending the finish line apically
- Preparing vertical grooves or boxes with parallel sides
- Including parallel pins in the preparation
- Preparing occlusal pits with parallel walls
- Crown-lengthening surgery
- Use of resin-based cements

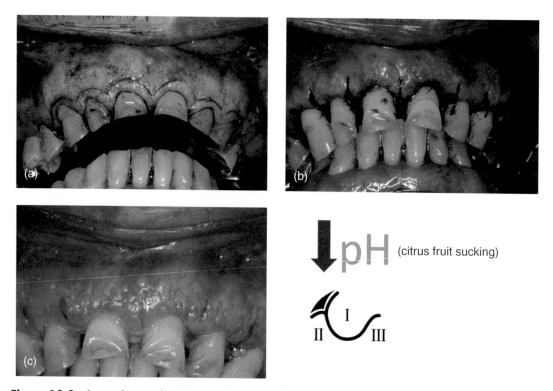

(citrus fruit sucking)

Figure 12.2   Surgical crown lengthening of worn maxillary anterior teeth prior to provision of metal–ceramic crowns: (a) inverse bevel incision prior to raising mucoperiosteal flap; (b) sutured mucoperiosteal flap after osseous recontouring; (c) one-week postsurgical condition shows adequate clinical crown length to allow appropriate abutment preparation and restoration. (Courtesy of Dr. Fadel Kamber, Kuwait University, Kuwait.)

Increasing the length of a short clinical crown and extending the finish line apically can be achieved by crown-lengthening surgery, which implies removal of parts of the periodontal tissues, with or without osseous recontouring (Fig. 12.2). Elective devitalisation of a tooth in order to place a post and core should be considered only when there is no other way to increase retention and resistance form as vital teeth (perhaps even short ones) generally survive longer as abutments than ones that are endodontically treated (de Backer et al. 2007). Fortunately, the techniques of surgical crown lengthening and devitalisation that were once popular seem to be abating as non-preparation, adhesive-bonding techniques, as well as techniques that regain vertical space by reversing the effects of dentoalveolar compensation are developed.

Splinting should be avoided whenever possible, and is not recommended in cases of confirmed bruxism. Similarly, splinting additional abutments in order to compensate for a short, poorly retentive primary abutment is contraindicated: the risks of cementation failure followed by secondary caries or mechanical problems, such as fracture of porcelain or connectors, rather than being reduced, will probably be as great at the short abutment, irrespective of the inclusion of secondary abutments. Thus, physiological tooth mobility will be unrestrained, torquing forces minimised, and in case of cementation failure, the condition easily detected and more easily correctable.

It is often suggested that occlusal splint therapy should be provided in the form of a full-coverage appliance overlaying the restored teeth. In spite of its frequent use in such a manner and strong recommendation by some authorities (Dawson 2007), there is no evidence about the effectiveness of occlusal splints to prevent future restorative failure.

Conventional rehabilitative techniques

For clarification, this section refers to prosthodontic methods that were considered standard before the era of adhesives. That being said, it is reasonable to assert that traditionally, restorative techniques developed in response to the need to restore teeth damaged by dental caries. The greater the carious damage, the greater was the complexity of the restoration called for, and when direct restorative techniques were no longer capable of fulfilling restorative objectives, full-coverage indirect restorations could both restore and protect the weakened tooth. Strict adherence to the principles of tooth preparation and technical precision were considered essential for the success of such restorations.

Although the severity of caries may, after its excavation, sometimes result in a tooth that resembles a severely worn tooth (in terms of quantity of substance loss), the morphological features are generally quite different: one of the most striking differences is short clinical crowns in severely worn teeth. Yet the very same fixed prosthodontic methods, in the absence of any obvious alternative, have been almost identically applied to rehabilitating the severely worn dentition. Although the strategies needed to rehabilitate a severely worn dentition would seem to be different from those needed for teeth that are relatively unworn, the ingenuity of salvage techniques that have been used over the years has been impressive, adding to the quality of life of many patients. However, the methods are largely anecdotal and lack rigorous scientific scrutiny of their outcomes.

Conventional fixed restorations

Despite the lack of information on outcomes of conventionally cemented restorations to restore teeth damaged by toothwear, they are widely used, specifically full-coverage metal–ceramic restorations. They offer some flexibility as regards appearance, design of restoration and thus degree of tooth reduction required, as well as the possibility of replacing missing teeth.

In many cases, localised toothwear affects only the anterior segments. These are also the most commonly affected teeth, particularly so due to an erosive factor, and rarely would the complete dentition be equally affected. The problem of restoring worn anterior teeth when little available interocclusal space exists is apparent. In this regard, a less radical alternative to complete arch occlusal rehabilitation was first described by Dahl and coworkers (1975), as a two-stage process. To achieve this, a bite-raising removable anterior cobalt–chromium splint was originally utilised as the first stage. By this means, a combination of forced intrusion of anterior teeth and supraeruption of posterior teeth takes places, resulting in the re-establishment of initially opened posterior tooth contacts. Such an approach can greatly simplify and curtail treatment to only the affected anterior teeth (the second stage of the process), obviating the need for full-coverage restorations of frequently sound (albeit sometimes mildly worn) posterior teeth. The sequence of treatment is illustrated in Fig. 12.3, in a patient who has severe erosive toothwear affecting the anterior teeth. Treatment is required, but is complicated by insufficient restorative space. In the first stage, a cast removable anterior splint provides canine-to-canine occlusion only, and creation of adequate restorative space after 2 months' continuous use; in the second stage, metal–ceramic crowns are provided without need for tooth preparation of palatal

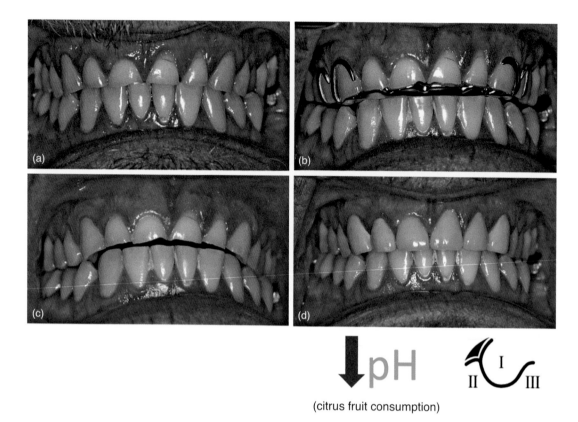

↓pH

(citrus fruit consumption)

Figure 12.3 A 36-year-old Swedish sailor with a long history of frequent citrus fruit consumption: (a) His anterior maxillary teeth are extremely worn, with reduced buccolingual dimension and little available space for full-coverage restorations. (b) Cobalt–chromium splint providing anterior tooth separation of 2 mm and incorporating retentive clasps. (c) After 2 months' continuous use of the splint, adequate space had been created to provide anterior crowns (without undue tooth tissue sacrifice), and definitive reconstruction needs to be performed without delay. (d) Final metal–ceramic crowns on 13–23 after cementation. Although full posterior intercuspation posteriorly is not yet evident, there are posterior contacts. Note that the first premolar that had previously been clasped has achieved occlusion in the short period following discontinuation of the splint. (Reprinted with permission from Johansson et al. 2008.)

(except for margin definition) or incisal aspects, which would otherwise have jeopardised remaining tooth integrity.

Relapse of the anterior interocclusal space so gained has been shown to be negligible in long-term follow-ups (Dahl & Krogstad 1985), but even if this were not the case, simplification of treatment would have been facilitated by the method. Such a relatively conservative treatment modality is generally appropriate when severe wear affects the anterior segments only, and particularly so in the younger patient. The

method has successfully withstood long-term scrutiny. Further, even if adequate interocclusal space exists for restoring the anterior teeth, the 'Dahl technique' can be used to increase the OVD so as to allow for more aesthetically optimal anterior restorations to be provided.

In contrast to the procedural rigidity of most conventional treatment methods used for rehabilitating toothwear, variations on the original 'Dahl technique' are regularly reported in the literature (Johansson et al. 2008). Coupled with adhesive techniques, the method has been steadily developed so that the use of removable metal splints is almost a thing of the past. Resin-bonded cast metal, or resin composite, palatal onlays or temporary crowns can be used with the same purpose. The use of acrylic resin temporary crowns cemented temporarily as a 'Dahl appliance', following initial tooth preparation, is illustrated in Fig. 12.4. After posterior occlusion was re-established, the second stage was performed in the form of bonded all-ceramic crowns.

Notably, because the concept is a dynamic process and it is difficult to preoperatively predict the final occlusal contacts, a one-stage, instead of a two-stage, process has evolved in recent years (Fig. 12.5).

Several case reports have been published following the Dahl concept, but with definitively placed restorations (even if sometimes temporarily cemented for a 'trial' period) from the outset. Figure 12.6 illustrates the one-stage approach using a 6-unit cobalt–chromium splinted onlay cemented to the eroded palatal surfaces of the maxillary anterior teeth with Panavia®. The case represents one of the early attempts at modifying the 'Dahl technique' and explains the caution that was exercised in opting for splinting the onlays. As mentioned earlier, however, single units are generally preferable, and when cemented with a high-bond-strength luting agent such as the one that was used in this case, would probably serve

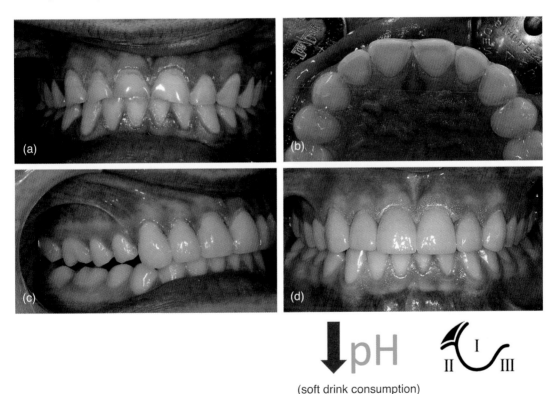

(soft drink consumption)

Figure 12.4 (a & b) A 20-year-old man with severe toothwear affecting the whole dentition, caused by frequent soft drink consumption during his teens. (c) Anterior bite-raising temporary fixed dental prosthesis was cemented with a temporary cement for a period of 5 months to create space anteriorly and allow for increasing the crown height of the planned permanent restorations. (d) IPS Empress® crowns were bonded to 14–23. (*Note:* The patient had stopped drinking soft drinks, uses home-based fluoride prophylaxis and attends regular check-ups). (Reprinted with permission from Johansson et al. 2008.)

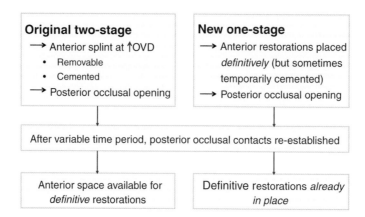

Figure 12.5   The 'Dahl technique' illustrating the original two-stage and newer one-stage approaches for achieving intrusion of anterior teeth and supraeruption of posterior teeth.

as well as splinted units. Further, if there is a plan to remove the onlays at some future date, a glass ionomer luting cement would be preferred.

The one-stage modification would seem to be particularly well suited to younger patients with anterior toothwear, as shown in this 15-year-old who presented with cola drinking–induced palatal erosion of the maxillary incisors and a dry mouth (Fig. 12.7). Posterior occlusion was re-established within only 6 weeks of placement of palatal resin composite restorations. How these methods are categorised in terms of 'temporary', 'semipermanent' or 'long-term' is not a straightforward matter. However, if it is recognised that the choice of treatment opted for is dependent on a wide range of patient and technical considerations, the point about terminology is probably a secondary one.

In addition to the 'Dahl technique', space may also be gained, in certain cases, if occlusal analysis reveals a large horizontal discrepancy between centric relation (CR) and maximum intercuspal position (MIP), but with little vertical discrepancy. Occlusal adjustment of the 'centric interferences' causing the CR–MIP discrepancy will produce a significantly more distal MIP, and thus adequate palatal space so that full-coverage anterior restorations can

be constructed. In cases of extensive anterior wear, such an approach can maintain the original OVD, although in cases that are *planned* for an increased OVD, the use of CR as the new reference maxillomandibular position is in any case implicit. The net space gained in such a reorganised approach to occlusal reconstruction would then have been achieved by a combination of the corrected CR–MIP slide and the increase in OVD. Many patients with severe toothwear will be older adults who will frequently have additional dental problems such as defective large restorations, caries and missing teeth. The 68-year-old man shown in Figure 12.8 is fairly representative of such patients.

He was unhappy with the shape of his lower front teeth, but mostly concerned about losing any more of his teeth. After detailed examination and discussions with the patient, it was agreed that his dentition be rehabilitated by conventional fixed prostheses. The sequence of procedures used to treat this patient would be considered standard by many prosthodontists, and a review of these procedures is presented in Box 12.2.

Orthodontic methods may also be applied for the creation of anterior space, such as intruding lower incisors or proclining upper incisors, for example.

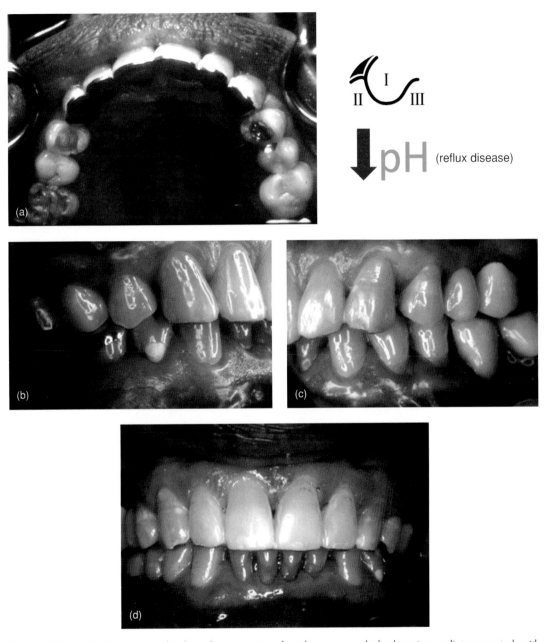

(reflux disease)

Figure 12.6 (a) Extensive palatal toothwear restored with a cast cobalt–chromium splint cemented with Panavia® according to the one-stage 'Dahl technique'. (b & c) Posterior space at the time of cementation. (d) Posterior space closure 8 weeks after cementation. (*Note:* The splint produced no untoward aesthetic effect and continues to serve satisfactorily without further need for treatment 15 years after placement.) (Courtesy of Dr. Raj Raja Rayan, London, England; laboratory work by Mr. Nadim Kurban.)

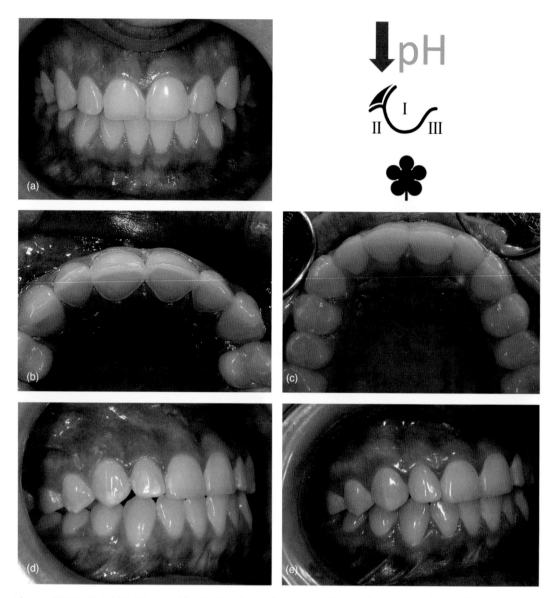

Figure 12.7 (a & b) A 15-year-old girl with cola drinking–induced palatal erosion on the maxillary central and lateral incisors. (c & d) Palatal resin composite restorations initially produce a bilateral posterior open bite. (e) Six weeks later the occlusion has returned to normal through compensatory eruption of posterior teeth. (Reprinted with permission from Johansson et al. 2008.)

In some cases, severe toothwear will affect the entire dentition. A reduction of the OVD may well be associated with the wear, in which case it is generally recommended that it is so maintained. If possible, the patient's adapted, 'worn-in occlusion', in the absence of any functional problems, should be conformed to; increasing the OVD according to some predetermined 'standard of normality' for the sake of gaining better occlusal stability is not

(Normal salivary flow)

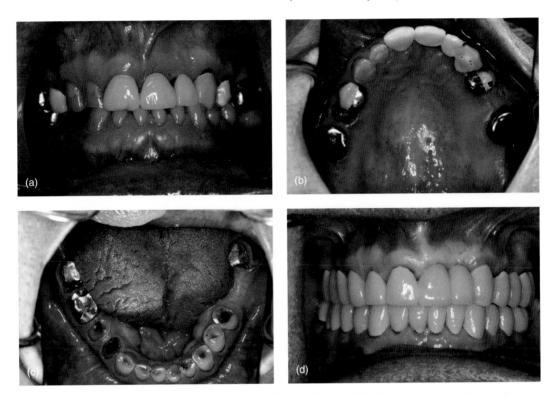

Figure 12.8 (a–c) A 68-year-old man with generalised toothwear, failed previous restorations and missing teeth. (d) Treatment included increasing the OVD by 2 mm anteriorly, establishment of the new maxillomandibular relationship at a more distal mandibular position in CR, selective crown-lengthening procedures, endodontic treatments, two further extractions, and full-arch, full-coverage metal–ceramic restorations. (Courtesy of Dr. Yacoub Al-Tarakemah, Kuwait University, Kuwait.)

essential. However, increasing the OVD becomes necessary in those cases where interocclusal space problems or aesthetic considerations are especially critical. In such instances, there need not be undue hesitation in increasing the OVD. Conventional methods of determining the new OVD should be used, and there are seldom any adaptive problems (see Fig. 12.8). Techniques for doing so include trial periods with bite-raising occlusal appliances; also, the

addition of interim resin composite to selected posterior teeth whilst the anterior segments are restored with temporary crowns to the new OVD has also been described. Although these more conventional methods have been applied by clinicians for a long time, many innovative methods facilitated by adhesives have rapidly, albeit empirically, sprung up.

While there are hardly any difficulties involved in increasing the OVD in healthy

Box 12.2 Considerations in rehabilitating advanced toothwear by conventional fixed prosthodontic methods.*

Phase I: Elimination of pathology and preliminary procedures
- Oral hygiene instruction and periodontal therapy as needed
- Caries removal
- Endodontic therapy as needed
- Extractions as needed

Phase II: Diagnostic procedures and stabilisation
- Occlusal examination
  - 0.5 mm anterior 'slide in centric' from CR to MIP
  - Non-working side interferences in right and left excursions
  - Lack of anterior guidance
  - Reduced OVD with about 5-mm interocclusal space at rest (which was considered excessive)
  - Severely compromised occlusal plane
- Diagnostic casts
  - Mounted in CR in a semiadjustable articulator
  - Occlusal adjustment was carried out on the casts and then in the mouth
  - New diagnostic casts were then mounted in CR
- Preliminary diagnostic wax-up carried out according to prosthodontic, aesthetic and anatomical guidelines
  - Accordingly, an increase in OVD was considered to be necessary and the incisal pin was raised by 2.5 mm
- Heat-processed occlusal device modelled to diagnostic wax-up was fabricated
  - Evaluated over 8 weeks for comfort and function
  - Casts remounted to new CR record at new OVD
- Final diagnostic wax-up performed at new, tested OVD
- Provisional restorations fabricated according to diagnostic wax-up template
- Tooth preparations and foundation build-ups in standard fashion
- Provisional restorations cemented and monitored according to functional aesthetic and biomechanical parameters

Phase III: Definitive phase
- Up to this point, the design and development of the new occlusion would have followed the *reorganised approach* to occlusal reconstruction
- Once functional criteria were met, a *conformative approach* was followed in copying the newly established occlusion into the definitive restorations

Phase IV: Maintenance phase
- Custom recall programme to monitor periodontal and prosthodontic conditions
- Continuation of daily fluoride application

*Using the case in Fig. 12.8 as illustration.

individuals, a cautious approach is advocated with such procedures in patients exhibiting signs or symptoms of temporomandibular disorders (TMD). Such patients should first be treated with reversible methods (e.g. splints or muscle exercises, depending on the TMD diagnosis) to reduce the signs and symptoms of TMD and normalise function before any prosthodontic therapy is started (De Boever et al. 2000). As stated earlier, even if extensive toothwear is present, the OVD could well be unaffected due to compensatory eruption, which is an additional reason to leave it unchanged if possible.

Removable prostheses

Fixed prostheses are expensive and not affordable for many patients who require rehabilitation of worn dentitions. In many countries where removable prostheses are common due to reasons of tradition or economics, total extraction followed by complete dentures is the commonly suggested therapy for managing such patients' rehabilitative needs. Such treatment results in gradual resorption of the residual alveolar ridges, leading to a deteriorating situation as regards denture instability and poor retention. The possibility for future implant treatment also worsens. If single teeth or roots can be retained as overdenture abutments, the risk of progressive resorption of the alveolar ridge is decreased. If the patient can maintain good oral hygiene and the abutment teeth receive intensive fluoride prophylaxis regularly, a conventional overdenture is a relatively inexpensive option with a good prognosis. Such a case is illustrated in Fig. 12.9. Few heavily worn mandibular teeth remained as well as a significantly reduced OVD (with excessive interocclusal rest space). A complete overdenture at an increased OVD was the treatment of choice due to economic constraints. As mentioned, with proper preventive measures the remaining teeth will continue to serve well.

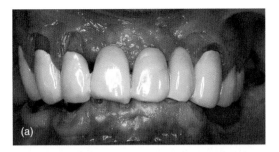

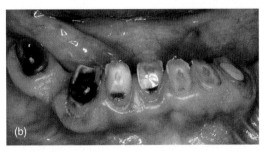

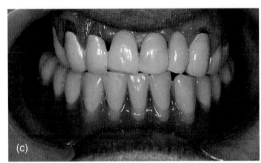

Figure 12.9 (a & b) A 66-year-old woman who has been on antidepressant medication for many years. She has pronounced xerostomia with documented hyposalivation and is a heavy bruxer. The maxillary porcelain restorations are likely to have contributed to the severe wear seen on the remaining mandibular teeth. The risks in prescribing fixed prostheses are high, which the patient can neither afford. (c) She was provided with an overdenture supported by remaining roots which have been restored with resin composite. (*Note:* A preventive regimen with fluoride gel inside the prosthesis was prescribed; follow-up after 1 year showed that the prosthesis had functioned well and there were no further dental problems.) (Reprinted with permission from Johansson et al. 2008.)

The use of gold copings on the abutment teeth supporting overdentures may produce surprisingly good long-term results.

RPDs with occlusal overlays can also be used to re-establish OVD in patients with non-compensated wear that would result in excessive interocclusal space and reduced anterior lower facial height. RPDs might also be the realistic or preferred option for patients with poorly distributed remaining teeth. In cases of severe anterior wear, appearance can be managed with complete facings with or without a flange, or a butt joint onto the standing teeth. The materials can be purpose-made acrylic facings, hollowed-out denture teeth or custom-made in the mouth with autopolymerising resin, composite or light-curing resin. The patient in Fig. 12.10 was aware of his worn teeth, but his chief complaint was chewing discomfort due to few remaining occluding teeth and their sharpness. Following examination and discussions with the patient, maxillary and mandibular overlay RPDs were felt to be the treatment of choice. Occlusal examination showed a reduced OVD with an interocclusal resting space of 6 mm and a severely compromised occlusal plane. Standard prosthodontic procedures included an altered cast impression technique for the bilateral distal extension lower jaw, facebow transfer of the upper cast to a semiadjustable articulator, mounting of the lower cast with the aid of a CR record at an increase in OVD by 4 mm and the use of purpose-made heat-cured shell acrylic facings, supported by the metal framework, for the worn anterior teeth. As for patients with tooth-supported overdentures, frequent fluoride gel application was advised, with which the patient complied. At recall visits, the patient reported good chewing function and satisfaction with his appearance. An overlay denture would be considered a high-maintenance prosthesis in order to maintain, in particular, the acrylic facings. In this case, the facing at 21 fractured (most likely due to its thinness) not long after the RPDs were delivered, and was repaired intraorally.

Implants

In some dentitions affected by severe wear, there may be missing teeth. Usually, rehabilitation by means of conventional fixed restorations will allow the replacement of such teeth. The possibilities offered by implants in restoring spaces, especially when unfavourably distributed in the arch, mean that the adjunctive use of implants as part of the rehabilitation of the worn dentition cannot be discounted. However, whereas bruxism is not a major aetiological factor in toothwear, it is considered by some clinicians to be a risk factor for technical complications in implant-supported restorations, albeit not for the implants themselves (Lobbezoo et al. 2006).

Information on the outcome of implants as part of rehabilitation of the worn dentition is, at best, circumstantial. In the absence of good evidence, clinical experience would urge caution in their prescription, and especially so if excessive loading is judged to be present.

Materials

The choice of material to be used for a restoration could be crucial if it is opposed, for example, by natural teeth or if the patient is a heavy bruxer. Studies on the wear process affecting restorative materials are almost always experimental, laboratory trials, and extrapolating these results to the extremely variable conditions that apply clinically is difficult. In cases of an opposing occlusion of tooth enamel, most clinicians and researchers agree that a metal occlusal surface, and preferably one of high noble content, is preferred in order to minimise wear of the natural dentition. Unpolished ceramics could be detrimental to opposing natural teeth (see Fig. 12.9). However, there is a lack of long-term clinical studies to support any strong conclusions regarding choice of material for the restoration of worn teeth.

In cases of heavy occlusal load, the situation becomes very complex as we need to consider

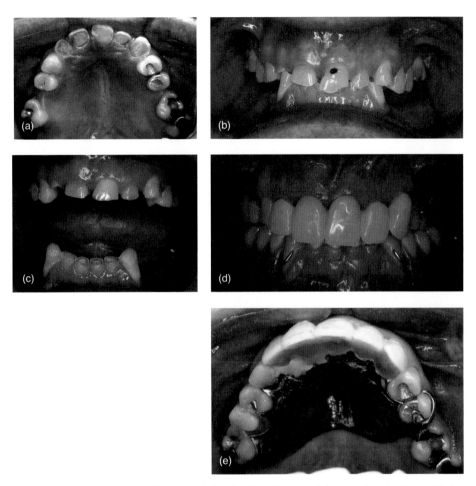

Figure 12.10 (a & b) A 58-year-old man with localised toothwear of the maxillary and mandibular anterior teeth, loss of posterior many teeth, loss of OVD and resultant increased interocclusal space. The patient was a pensioner with limited economic resources. (c) After provision of basic dental care in preparation for prosthodontic treatment. (d) Rehabilitation with cobalt–chromium overlay dentures at an increased OVD of 4 mm; the prostheses incorporated purpose-made acrylic facings for the upper anterior teeth and butt-joint coronal additions for the lower anterior teeth. (e) Palatal view of the upper prosthesis in the mouth showing the extent of coverage of the upper anterior teeth. (Courtesy of Prof. Peter Owen, University of the Witwatersrand, South Africa.) (f) Odontogram (on page 222) with charting of *The Stages of Wear*.

not only the risk of wear of the restorative material itself and the opposing natural dentition, but also the requirement that all the components of the superstructure are able to withstand the applied load. Besides the risk of mechanical failures under conditions of excessive load, biological failures are even more likely, for example, caries and endodontic problems following loss of retention and cement dissolution. Overall, metal or metal–ceramic restorations seem to be the safest choices in cases of high-load conditions, although under extreme conditions, there is no material that will last for very long. Because of the risk of chipping of ceramic veneers in metal–ceramic restorations many prosthodontists prefer gold–acrylic FDPs

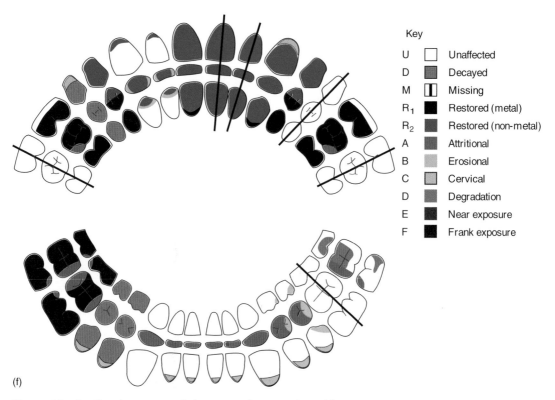

Key

U	☐	Unaffected
D	▨	Decayed
M	🔳	Missing
R₁	■	Restored (metal)
R₂	▨	Restored (non-metal)
A	▨	Attritional
B	▨	Erosional
C	☐	Cervical
D	▨	Degradation
E	■	Near exposure
F	■	Frank exposure

(f)

Figure 12.10   (f) Odontogram with the Stages of Wear indicated for the same 58 year old male patient (shown on page 221).

for heavy bruxers. The few clinical studies published on wear of materials indicate only small differences in wear resistance of gold and ceramic materials, whereas resin-based materials show three to four times more substance loss than gold or ceramics (Dahl & Øilo 1996).

It is also important to consider other factors which influence the wear resistance of remaining natural teeth, including, amongst others, erosive influences, hyposalivation and salivary lubricatory factors.

Adhesive rehabilitative techniques

Traditionally, full-mouth rehabilitation based on full-coverage fixed restorations has been the recommended treatment for patients with severe occlusal wear. The approach would also appear to have been a *sine qua non* for the rehabilitation of generalised occlusal wear, although not exclusively so, and many clinicians today would still consider even localised toothwear to require full-mouth rehabilitation due to the technical difficulties posed if interocclusal space is compromised.

For many clinicians, however, the indications for conventionally cemented crowns appear to be declining. Thanks to improved adhesive techniques, a more conservative approach to the problem has evolved and is increasingly proposed in many case reports, describing a range of clinical protocols. A number of factors have already been mentioned that appear to be driving this shift away from the more traditional, 'subtractive' methods of rehabilitation. These include the availability of viable, less invasive, 'additive' materials and techniques, the demands of an increasingly younger group of patients in need of treatment and the recognition that even meticulously performed traditional rehabilitation has significant limitations. A recent report described the full-mouth rehabilitation of a 14-year-old with conventional crowns, which raises questions about the number of times that replacement of crowns will be needed, prognosis of the teeth, and remaining vitality of the teeth, to name a few (Van Roekel 2003).

The use of resin composites has been described in Chapter 11 and its specific application to the rehabilitation of severe occlusal and/or palatal toothwear is now further dealt with. While clinical evidence for the efficacy of adhesive technologies in restoring dentitions *uncomplicated by toothwear* is appearing more and more, this is not the case for the worn dentition. However, resin composites placed at an increased OVD have been shown to result in similar tooth movements as do other restorations and/or devices placed for this purpose. Several case reports have described favourable clinical outcomes as well as patient satisfaction with directly placed resin composite for anterior wear in a one-stage 'Dahl technique' (see Fig. 12.7). Promising results, using templates obtained from diagnostic wax-ups to avoid freehand build-up techniques (as described in Chapter 11), have been reported (Schmidlin et al. 2009). Such findings, however, do not concur with the conclusions from another case series study of a strong trend towards lower survivals for directly placed resin composite restorations than conventional indirect restorations (Smales & Berekally 2007).

As regards the adhesive bonding of indirect restorations in the worn dentition, evidence is even sparser. A report of three case histories, each with one or more teeth with complete loss of the clinical crown, found one case to have survived for 10 years, one failing at 6 years and

one treated too recently to report upon (Bartlett & Sundaram 2006). While the suggestion that the method is a possible prosthodontic management strategy may be viewed as optimistic, it does illustrate the needs and demands of patients suffering from the effects of severe wear and the ongoing challenges that the rehabilitation that such dentitions will continue to pose for clinicians.

As regards perhaps less demanding partial-coverage indirect restorations, the use of bonded palatal porcelain veneers in combination with initial orthodontic space creation has been advocated, although clinical follow-ups on retention and effects on opposing tooth surfaces are limited. In routine situations, labial porcelain veneers are now established as a predictable long-term treatment option with a low failure rate, at least in controlled clinical settings. Similarly, resin-bonded type III gold veneers showed close to 90% survival at a mean of 5 years, irrespective of being cemented high or to correct OVD. In such cases, prognosis would most likely be poorer in the presence of an active erosive process or unfavourable loading.

Long-term follow-ups of bonded full-coverage ceramic FDPs are scant, but show a higher failure rate compared to conventional fixed restorations. It seems that under such circumstances of limited information in even the unworn state, the more demanding conditions of restoring the worn dentition by these methods suggests that much greater caution is needed.

Adhesively retained ceramic restorations are becoming almost routinely and exclusively practised by some clinicians, but the procedures involved are technique sensitive and the method is not yet suitable in the hands of all dentists. Nevertheless, innovative case reports continue to appear, including combining space obtained from a CR–MIP discrepancy and the 'Dahl technique', to apply adhesive restorations; also described is the use of more or less traditional protocols, but

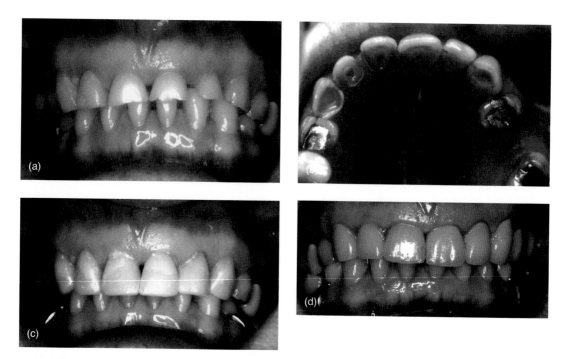

Figure 12.11 (a & b) Severe anterior toothwear in a 40-year-old woman with a past history of bulimia and parafunction. (c) Direct resin composite build-ups on upper anterior teeth using a template modelled on a diagnostic wax-up; a 'softer' compomer was used on the palatal aspects to allow her to 'wear in' her anterior guidance. (d) Metal–ceramic restorations designed to conform to the established anterior guidance were cemented with a temporary cement onto zinc phosphate–cemented cold copings. (*Note:* The rehabilitation serves satisfactorily 14 years later.) (Courtesy of Dr. Raj Raja Rayan, London, England; laboratory work by Mr. Nadim Kurban.)

utilising adhesives as opposed to conventional retention for restorations. Such processes, however, increasingly appear to be as exacting as for full-arch rehabilitation by conventional restorations, although there is the obvious benefit of conservation of tooth structure that adhesives permit. While cautiously welcoming these pioneering efforts, it needs to be kept in mind that an understanding of risks and an ability to more reliably predict prognosis through proper patient selection are the keys to good clinical outcomes. It is advisable to exercise some caution when it comes to restoring worn teeth with aesthetic alternatives that rely solely on adhesive bonding until more reports on its clinical longevity have appeared.

Conventional fixed prosthodontics, with its proven record of long service even if only in the context of the entirely lesser strategic demands of relatively unworn teeth (which these data relate to; de Backer et al. 2007), would seem in many instances still to be the treatment of choice for extensively worn teeth (see Fig. 12.8). However, nowadays even tried-and-trusted formulae cannot ignore the possibilities arising out of newer technologies. An example of how older prosthodontic procedures can be adapted to incorporate these advantages is the case shown in Fig. 12.11. The patient, who had a history of bulimia and parafunction, was treated conventionally with a metal–ceramic fixed reconstruction (cemented with a temporary cement on telescopic copings which were themselves cemented with zinc phosphate) in the upper jaw, and opposed by a combination of posterior crowns and a bounded RPD in the lower jaw. However, the interesting point in the prosthodontic management of the case was the use of adhesive methods to re-establish the lost anterior guidance. In this case, resin composite build-ups were performed with the aid of a template modelled on a diagnostic wax-up of the mounted casts (see Chapter 11); moreover, the palatal aspects were built in a 'softer' compomer, allowing the patient to 'wear in' her anterior guidance. This guidance was then reproduced in the definitive restorations in a conformative manner.

Concept of staged reconstruction

An alternative rehabilitative strategy was recently proposed based on the principle of reversibility (Creugers & van't Spijker 2007). Because the worn dentition usually produces slow occlusal breakdown, it permits most patients to *adapt* to the changing situation until a level of unacceptable function, biological risk or aesthetic dissatisfaction is reached. Contrasting with this, typical reconstructive methods represent a *sudden* change that precludes proper evaluation of the patient's ability to readapt to changed oral conditions. Just as the pathway to the worn status may vary, so too does the reconstructive process need to be guided, and this is suggested by the authors to be best achievable through staged reconstruction using adhesive techniques wherever possible. Even if the evidence for such a rationale is generally lacking, it seems possible that the all-too-frequent failures seen after traditional rehabilitative efforts may be more controllable through a staged, reversible reconstructive process that relies to a large extent on adhesive technology, including resin composite or similar materials. Conceptually, and given the

favourable reports, the 'Dahl technique' would seem to be in line with such an approach to reconstruction.

Maintenance phase

Because the original aetiological factors are often incompletely controlled and human nature is such that compliance is for a limited period, the aim should be to maintain stability in the oral environment.

Regular review of the rehabilitated dentition is necessary for several reasons. For example, a combination of short clinical crowns, differential wear and heavy loading increases the risks of cementation failure. Similarly, erosion-induced wear may continue even in the presence of teeth with full-coverage crowns and can progress cervical to the crowned tooth and on any remaining natural teeth if causal factors have not been eliminated (see Fig. 4.1). In addition, occlusal splint treatment in combined attrition (bruxism) and erosion cases may not be successful. Cases should be reviewed at least annually when new study casts and photographs should be taken for the purpose of serial monitoring.

A careful clinical and radiographic examination of abutments should be performed. For example, caries, failed retention, wear facets, porcelain integrity and, increasingly, adhesive bond integrity must be checked, recorded and treated as necessary. Individually designed preventive regimens should be prescribed and carried out with an interval determined on the basis of the supposed aetiology and future progression of the toothwear. These could comprise topical fluoride application, dietary advice and psychological motivation for lifestyle changes, amongst others. Unfortunately, one has to bear in mind that many such preventive measures may have a very small effect if patient compliance is poor. The lack of reliable information on the long-term results of rehabilitation of severe toothwear is a further reason for regular follow-ups.

CONCLUSION

Toothwear is a multifactorial process which can make it difficult to identify a single cause at the individual patient level. Its progress is usually slow, which characterises it as a physiological condition; when it threatens tooth survival or is of concern to the patient it may be regarded as pathological. Recognition of the early signs of wear, and especially erosion, could bring about timely prevention and improve the life span of teeth. The most obvious feature of wear is shortened clinical crowns, generally accompanied by dentoalveolar compensation. This may complicate definitive conventional rehabilitation, although research, newer technologies and materials offer broader possibilities for rationalising treatment modalities.

Rehabilitation of worn teeth will be needed in only some patients, and the measures with which need for treatment is assessed is one of the keys to a successful outcome. In broad terms, the decision to treat or not should be guided by the patient's stated and/or perceived need, severity of the wear as determined by morphological changes and potential for progression in the context of the patient's age. Thus, the same degree of toothwear does not necessarily mean the same treatment approach, and the decision will in most cases be tempered by the generally complex and expensive nature of rehabilitation of the worn dentition and the known risks of biomechanical failures. High costs can generate great resentment if failure occurs. Treatment methods that last well for severely worn, possibly previously restored teeth, in patients who are frequently of older age, are being learned the hard way; not all emerging technologies may be best suited to the task. Research that clarifies the particular needs and solutions for such dentitions is slow in appearing and still far from complete. This striking lack of evidence regarding long-term outcomes of reconstructive treatment of severe toothwear using different methods and materials calls for caution in decision making. The converse of this, namely disregarding the consequences of poor diagnosis, inappropriate management, overambitious intervention and uncertainty about prognosis, can only augur for very unfortunate outcomes. Nonetheless, rehabilitation of the worn dentition, whilst challenging, can be rewarding and satisfying to both the patient and the clinician if careful and thorough lead-up work has been completed in line with *The ABC of the Worn Dentition*.

References

Bartlett, D. (2010) A proposed system for screening tooth wear. *British Dental Journal*, **208**, 207–209.

Bartlett, D., Sundaram, G. (2006) An up to 3-year randomized clinical study comparing indirect and direct resin composites used to restore worn posterior teeth. *International Journal of Prosthodontics*, **19**, 613–617.

Creugers, N.H., van't Spijker, A. (2007) Tooth wear and occlusion: friends or foes? *International Journal of Prosthodontics*, **20**, 348–350.

Dahl, B., Øilo, G. (1996) Wear of teeth and restorative materials. In: *Prosthodontics. Principles and Management Strategies* (eds B. Öwall B, A.F. Käyser, G.E. Carlsson), pp. 187–200. Mosby-Wolfe, London.

Dahl, B.L., Krogstad, O. (1985) Long-term observations of an increased occlusal face height obtained by a combined orthodontic/prosthetic approach. *Journal of Oral Rehabilitation*, **12**, 173–176.

Dahl, B.L., Krogstad, O., Karlsen, K. (1975) An alternative treatment in cases with advanced localized attrition. *Journal of Oral Rehabilitation*, **2**, 209–214.

Davies, S.J., Gray, R.J., Qualtrough, A.J. (2002) Management of tooth surface loss. *British Dental Journal*, **192**, 11–23.

Dawson, P.E. (2007) *Functional Occlusion: From TMJ to Smile Design*. Mosby, St. Louis.

de Backer, H.G., Decock, V., van der Berghe, L. (2007) Long-term survival of complete crowns, fixed dental prostheses, and cantilever fixed dental prostheses with post and cores on root canal-treated teeth. *International Journal of Prosthodontics*, **20**, 229–234.

De Boever, J.A., Carlsson, G.E., Klineberg, I.J. (2000) Need for occlusal therapy and prosthodontic treatment in the management of temporomandibular disorders. Part II: Tooth loss and prosthodontic treatment. *Journal of Oral Rehabilitation*, **27**, 647–659.

Dumbrigue, H.B., Al-Bayat, M.I., Ng, C.C.H., et al. (2006) Assessment of bias in methodology for randomized controlled trials published on implant dentistry. *Journal of Prosthodontics*, **15**, 257–263.

Dumbrigue, H.B., Jones, J.S., Esquivel, J.F. (1999) Developing a register for randomized controlled trials in prosthodontics: results of a search from prosthodontic journals published in the United States. *Journal of Prothetic Dentistry*, **82**, 699–703.

Johansson, A., Johansson, A.-K., Omar, R., et al. (2008) Rehabilitation of the worn dentition. *Journal of Oral Rehabilitation*, **35**, 548–566.

Johansson, A.-K. (2002) On dental erosion and associated factors. *Swedish Dental Journal*, **156**(Suppl 156), 1–77.

Jokstad, A., Esposito, M., Coulthard, P., et al. (2002) The reporting of randomized controlled trials in prosthodontics. *International Journal of Prosthodontics*, **15**, 230–242.

Khan, F., Young, W.G., Shahabi, S., et al. (1999) Dental cervical erosions associated with occlusal erosion and attrition. *Australian Dental Journal*, **44**, 176–186.

Lobbezoo, F., van der Zaag, J., Naeije, M. (2006) Bruxism: its multiple causes and its effects on dental implasnts: an updated review. *Journal of Oral Rehabilitation*, **33**, 293–300.

Poyser, N.J., Porter, R.W., Briggs, P.F., et al. (2005) The Dahl concept: past, present and future. *British Dental Journal*, **198**, 669–676.

Salinas, T.J., Eckert, S.E. (2007) In patients requiring single-tooth replacement, what are the outcomes of implant – as compared to tooth-supported restorations? *International Journal of Oral and Maxillofacial Implants*, **22**(Suppl), 71–95.

Schmidlin, P., Filli, T., Imfeld, C., et al. (2009) Three-year evaluation of posterior vertical bite reconstruction using direct resin composite – a case series. *Operative Dentistry*, **34**, 102–108.

Smales, R.J., Berekally, T.L. (2007) Long-term survival of direct and indirect restorations placed for the treatment of advanced tooth wear. *European Journal of Prosthodontics and Restorative Dentistry*, **15**, 2–6.

Torabinejad, M., Anderson, P., Bader, J., et al. (2007) Outcomes of root canal treatment and restoration, implant-supported single crowns, fixed partial dentures, and extraction without replacement: a systematic review. *Journal of Prosthetic Dentistry*, **98**, 285–311.

Van Roekel, N.B. (2003) Gastroesophageal reflux disease, tooth erosion, and prosthodontic rehabilitation: a clinical report. *Journal of Prosthodontics*, **12**, 255–259.

van't Spijker, A., Kreulen, C.M., Creugers, N.H.J. (2007) Attrition, occlusion, (dys)function, and intervention: a systematic review. *Clinical Oral Implants Research*, **18**(Suppl 3), 117–126.

Wise, M.D. (1977) Occlusion and restorative dentistry. *British Dental Journal*, **143**, 45–52.

Index

Abfraction, 62–3, 186
Abrasion, 1–2, 62–6, 75, 91, 153–5
Acid wear, 1–3, 90
Acidic beverages, 4, 22, 35, 39–41, 94–5
Acids
    code numbers, 35–6
    extrinsic, 4, 22, 35, 39–41, 94–5, 115
    intrinsic, 4, 10, 23, 70, 94
Acquired enamel pellicle, 85–6
Adhesive techniques
    anterior toothwear, 30, 189–95
    posterior toothwear, 30–31, 195–201
    templates, 188, 191–2
Adjuncts, 28–9, 112, 117–26
Aesthetics, 34–5, 176, 186–8, 200
Aetiology
    abrasion, 1–2, 75, 153–5
    attrition, 1–2, 55–7, 75, 153–5
    erosion, 1–2, 41–2, 75, 153–5
    toothwear, 1–2, 16–17, 50, 70–71
Alcohol, 95, 118, 120
Alcoholism, 104–8, 115, 121
Amalgam, 35, 159, 165
Amelogenesis Imperfecta, 23–5, 28, 91
Anorexia nervosa, 7, 28, 95, 115

Anterior guidance, 174–5
Antidepressants, 121
Antihypertensive medications, 90, 92, 95, 121
Artificial saliva, 121
Asthma, 9, 20, 23, 37–9, 95, 121
Athletes, 4, 36, 94, 96–8, 115
Attrition, 1–2, 55–7, 90–91, 153–5

Bicarbonate, 79, 81–2, 84–5
Bicarbonate rinses, 120
Biomaterial wear, 155–61
Biomaterials, 153–67
Bite registration, 197
Bruxism, 8, 23, 28, 56, 90–91, 177–9, 209–10, 225
Buffering capacity, 84
Bulimia nervosa, 28, 94–5, 115, 120–21

Caffeine, 116, 118, 121
Calcium, 118, 120
Calcium phosphate, 77
Calcium phosphopeptide ACP, 29, 37, 86, 123–4
Calculus, 52
Canine guidance, 174–5
Cardiovascular disease, 39

Caries
    aetiology, 75–6
    differences to toothwear, 9–12, 19–20, 41–2,
        53, 86, 111–12, 182
    early childhood, 19–20
Centric relation, 174, 214
Cervical lesions
    grooved, 61, 185–6
    shallow, 58–61, 185–6
    wedge shaped, 61–4, 185–6
Cervical toothwear lesions, 58–64, 185–6
Charting toothwear lesions, 66–70
Chewing gum, 29, 86, 117–18, 120
Clenching, 91, 100
Clinical examination
    extraoral, 4–9, 52–3
    intraoral, 4–9, 52–3
Clinical history, 20–21, 52, 89–96
Clinical photography, 51–3
Compliance, 51, 187–8, 225
Composite resin, 28, 30, 158–9, 164–5, 192, 196,
        207, 214, 217, 220, 223–5
Computer models, 135
Congenital Rubella syndrome, 103–4
Conservation of tooth structure, 114
Contact stylus technique, 135
Conventional fixed restorations, 211–19
Conventional rehabilitative technique, 211
Corrosion, 1, 62, 153, 155
Counselling, 42–8, 113, 117–21
Crown & bridgework, 211–19
Crown lengthening surgery, 209
Cup & bowl shaped lesions, 17, 30, 53, 57–60,
        72, 141–5, 185–6

Dahl technique, 176–7, 193, 208, 211–14
Deciduous dentition, 9–10, 16–17, 27, 29, 171–2
Degradation, 64–6
Dehydration
    alcohol, 115
    sports, 4, 7, 36, 94, 96–8, 115
    work, 7, 94–5
Demineralisation, 122–3
Dental caries, 9–12, 19–20, 41–2, 75–6
Dental erosion
    adults, 57–8, 185
    aetiology, 1–2, 41–2, 153–5

children & adolescents, 9–10, 16–18, 35
    and dental caries, 41–2, 75–6
Dentinal hypersensitivity, 29, 64, 126–8, 188
Dentine bonding agents, 124
Dentinogenesis Imperfecta, 25, 28, 91
Dentoalveolar compensation, 176, 208, 210
Development of occlusion, 170–74
Developmental defects, 24–5
Diabetes mellitus, 39, 95
Diagnosis, 50–54, 71–2, 90–96
Diagnostic modalities, 50–54
Diagnostic models, 52–3, 139–41
Diagnostic wax-up, 188, 190, 197, 223
Diet, 35–7, 39–41
Diet analysis & advice, 27–8, 39–41, 117–20
Diet diary, 21, 44–6, 126
Dietary acids, 4, 22, 39–41, 43–7, 93–4, 118, 120,
        126–7
Dietary counselling, 42–8, 117–20
Dietary habits, 39–40
Down's syndrome, 91

Early childhood caries, 19–20
Eating disorders, 7, 28, 94–5, 115, 120–21
Enamel hypoplasia, 20, 24–5
Erosion
    adults, 57–8, 185
    aetiology, 1–2, 41–2, 153–5
    children & adolescents, 9–10, 16–18, 35
    and dental caries, 41–2, 86
Examination
    of dentition, 66–70
    of extraoral features, 4–9, 52–3
    of intraoral soft tissue, 4–9, 52–3
    odontogram, 6, 68–9
Exercise, 4, 36, 94, 96–8, 115
Extrinsic acids, 4, 22, 35, 39–41, 70, 93–4, 115

Fluoride, 86, 93, 123
Full mouth reconstruction, 205–27

Gastro-oesophageal reflux disease, 9, 20, 23, 27,
        75, 94, 115
Glass ionomer, 30, 159, 165
Greaves effect, 56–7
Group function, 174–5

Habits, 23, 28, 91, 115
Health, 114–5, 118, 121
Hereditary conditions
    dentine, 25
    enamel, 23–5, 28
Hybrid layer, 186
Hydroxyapatite, 77
Hypertension, 90, 95

Ideal occlusion, 172–3, 175
Implants, 220
Impressions, 139–41, 196–7
Interarch restorative space, 176, 208–9
Intercuspal position, 174
Intrinsic acids, 4, 20, 23, 70, 94, 115, 120

Lifestyle, 14, 34, 112, 114–16
Linea alba, 8, 91, 147

Management of toothwear
    adults, 111–31
    children, 25–31
Materials, 28, 30, 153–67
Maximal intercuspal position, 174, 208, 214
Measuring toothwear, 134–51
Medical history, 20, 95
Medications, 22–3, 28, 35, 95, 114–15, 121
Mixed dentition, 9, 27, 89, 171–3
Monitoring toothwear, 29, 129–30, 225
Multifactorial, 12–14, 70–71, 131

Non-parametric measurement, 134–5
Non-pathological wear, 182–3
Nutrition, 27, 35–7, 39, 42–6, 117–21

Obesity, 39, 95
Obtundent toothpastes, 124
Occlusal parameters, 174–5
Occlusal splints, 207, 211, 225
Occlusal stability, 175
Occlusal vertical dimension, 168, 172, 176, 184,
    208, 214, 216–17, 219
Occlusion, 8, 56, 168–81
Odontogram, 6, 68–9
Oral environment, 114, 162, 183–4
Oral habits, 23, 28, 91, 115

Oral hygiene, 93, 112
Orthodontic treatment, 207–8, 216, 223

Parafunction, 8, 23, 28, 177–9
Parametric measurement, 135–7
Patient
    aspirations, 187–8
    concerns, 34, 95–6
    compliance, 51, 187–8, 225
    demands, 187–8
    education, 25–8, 41–8
    habits, 23, 28
Physiological wear, 156, 182–3
Polishing, 154,
Posterior guidance, 174–5
Prader–Willi syndrome, 91, 99–103
Prevalence, 16, 34
Prevention of toothwear
    aimed at children, 25–28
    dietary advice, 27–8, 39–44
    for all ages, 111–31
    WATCH strategy, 117–21
Primary dentition, 9–10, 16–17, 27, 29, 171
Profilometry, 146–51
Protection hypothesis, 163–5
Pulp testing, 52
Pulpal exposure, 16, 22, 35, 66

Radiographs, 50–52
Recreational drugs, 51, 94
Rehabilitation, 205–27
Remineralisation, 86, 122–3
Removable prosthesis, 207, 219–20
Restoration, 30–31, 182–204
Restorative material
    amalgam, 35, 159, 165
    ceramics, 159, 178, 213
    composite resins, 28, 30, 158–9, 164–5, 192,
        196, 207, 214, 217, 220, 223–5
    glass ionomers, 30, 159, 165
    porcelain fused to metal, 211, 217, 221
    stainless steel crowns, 25, 30–31
Restorative treatment, 30–31, 182–204
Restoring sensitivity, 186
Retruded contact position, 174, 214
Review appointments, 29, 129–30, 225
Risk factors, 12–14, 21–5, 37–9, 90–96

Saliva
    buffering capacity, 84
    calcium, 4
    clearance, 61, 83
    components, 80–83
    flow rates, 79–80, 83
    pellicle, 76, 85–6
    Phosphate, 4, 77–8
    protection, 4, 17–18, 70, 84–6, 112
    sources, 78–80
Salivary gland aplasia, 80–81, 91
Salivary glands, 8, 79
Sandwich technique, 30, 185
Sclerotic dentine, 63, 66, 122, 124, 127
Semi-parametric measurement, 134–5
Sensitivity, 126–8
Sialadenosis, 9, 94–5
Site specificity of caries, 19–20, 53–4, 84
Sjögren's syndrome, 80, 95
Smear layer, 186
Splinting teeth, 210
Splints, 207, 211, 225
Stages of wear, 67
Stainless steel crowns, 25, 28, 30–31
Study models, 52–3, 139–41
Sugar-free chewing gum, 29, 86, 117–18, 120
Sugar-free lozenges, 120
Surface susceptibility, 19, 53–4, 71

Taste, 118–20
Templates for restoration, 188, 191–2
Temporomandibular disorders, 219
Temporomandibular joint, 7

Tongue indentations, 8, 91
Tooth mineral, 77
Toothbrushing, 92
Toothpastes
    abrasivity, 92
    Fluoride content, 25, 123
    obtundent, 124
    whitening, 92, 123
Toothwear
    charting, 66–70
    clinical history, 20–21, 52, 89–96
    clinical presentation, 16–20, 54–66
    and dental caries, 9–12, 19–20, 41–2, 53, 86,
        111–12, 182
    diagnosis, 50–53, 71–2
    management, 25–31
    measurement of, 134–51
Treatment planning, 128

Varnishes, 124
Veneers, 186, 221
Vertical dimension of occlusion, 168, 172, 176,
    184, 208, 214, 216–17, 219
Vitamin C, 93, 115

WATCH strategy, 117–21
Water, 27, 80, 118–20
Water fluoridation, 91, 121, 123
Wear couples, 157
Wedge-shaped lesions, 61–4
Wine tasters, 4, 115

Xerostomia, 80, 83–4